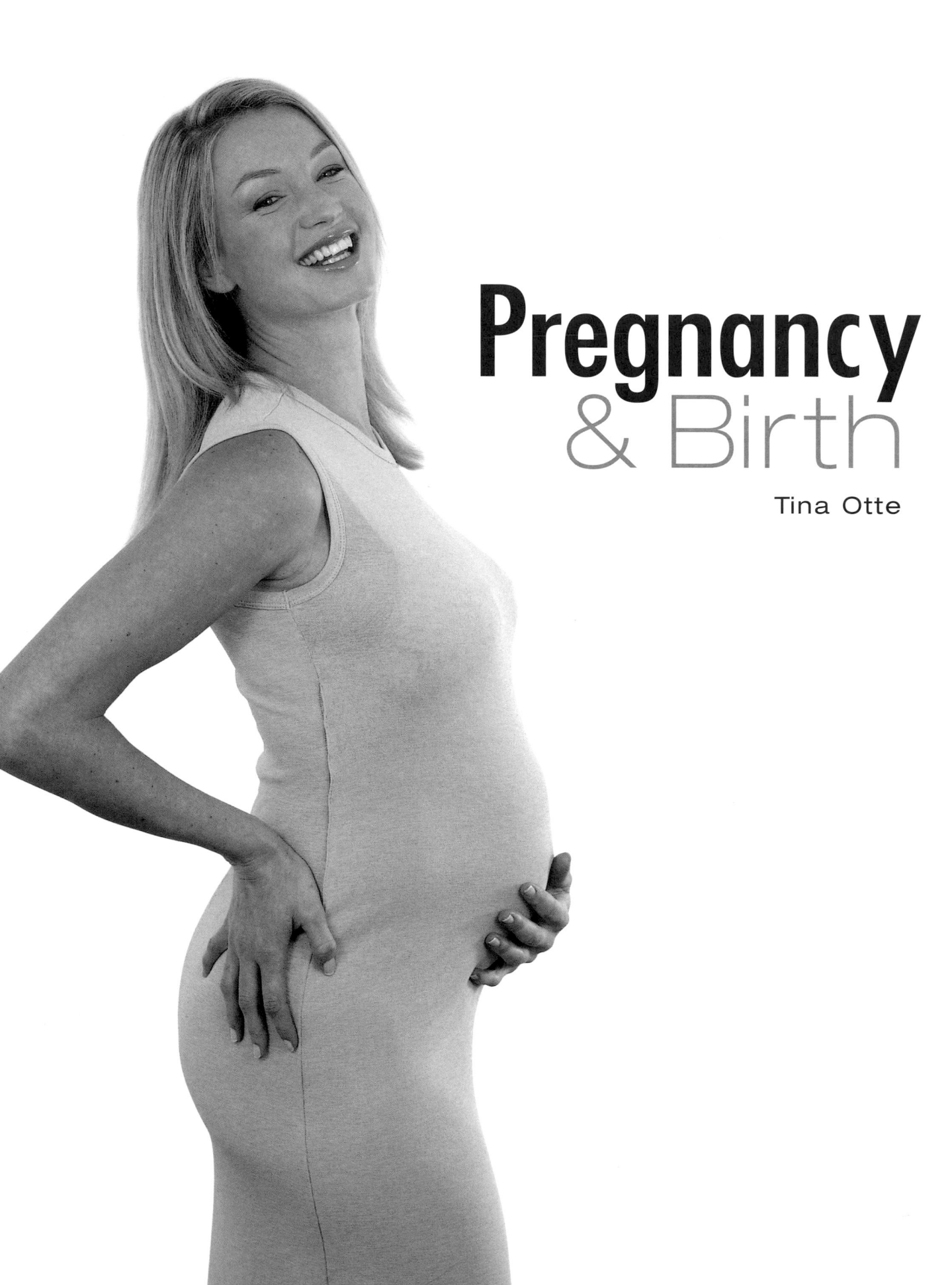

Pregnancy
& Birth

Tina Otte

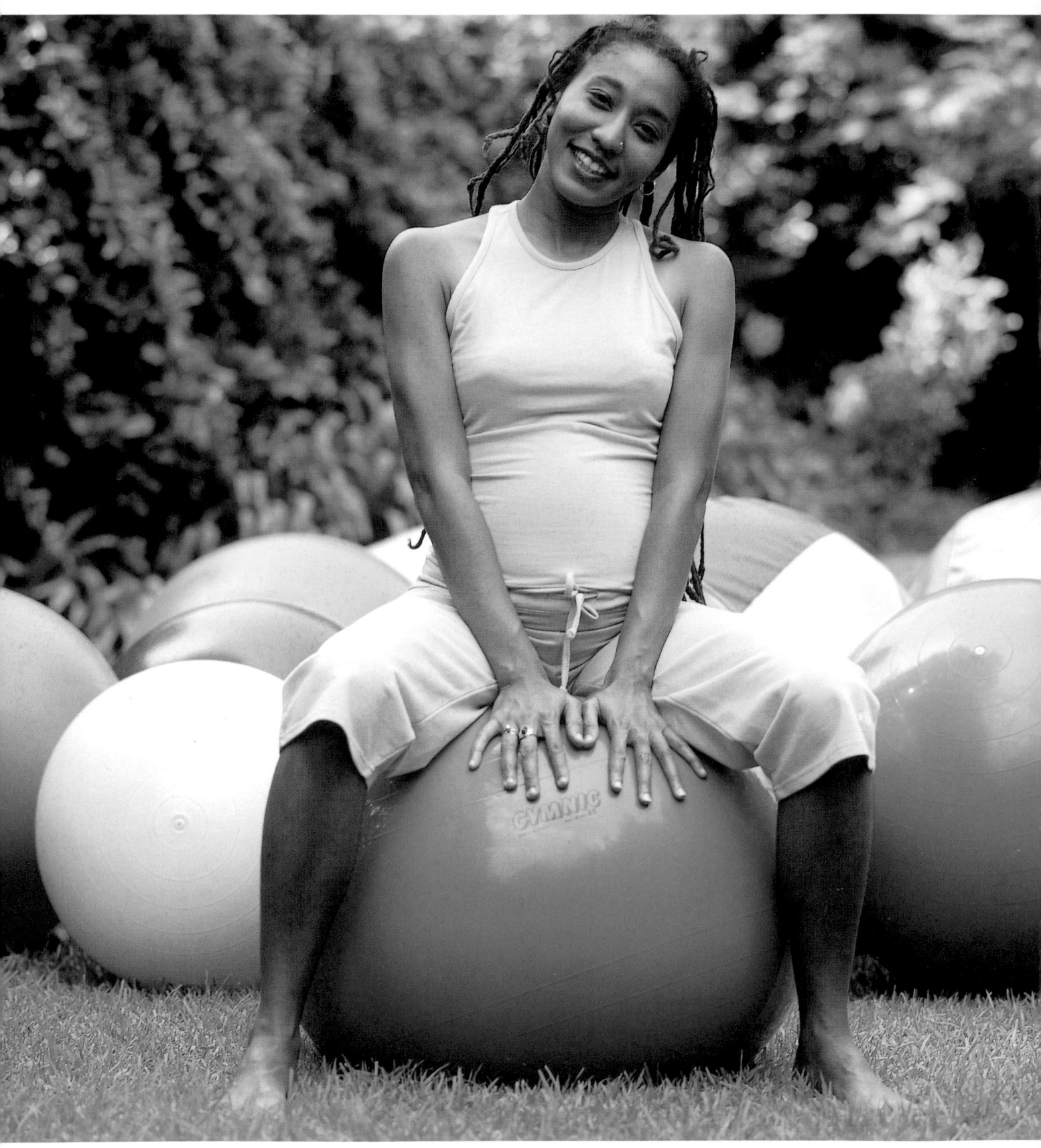

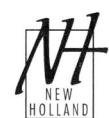

NEW HOLLAND

Pregnancy

& Birth

Tina Otte

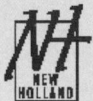

First published in 2005 by
New Holland Publishers
London • Cape Town • Sydney • Auckland
www.newhollandpublishers.com

86 Edgware Road
London W2 2EA
United Kingdom

80 McKenzie Street
Cape Town 8001
South Africa

14 Aquatic Drive
Frenchs Forest
NSW 2086
Australia

218 Lake Road
Northcote
Auckland
New Zealand

DISCLAIMER

The author and publishers have made every effort to ensure
that the information contained in this book was accurate at the
time of going to press, and accept no responsibility for any
injury or inconvenience sustained by any person using this book
or following the advice provided herein.

Publisher	Mariëlle Renssen
Publishing managers	Claudia dos Santos, Simon Pooley
Commissioning editor	Alfred LeMaitre
Editor	Leizel Brown
Designer	Christelle Marais
Illustrator	James Berrangé
Picture researchers	Karla Kik, Tamlyn McGeean
Production	Myrna Collins
Consultant	Dr Stephen Smith Consultant Obstetrician & Gynaecologist, Chesterfield and North Derbyshire District General Hospital NHS Trust
Proofreader	Anna Tanneberger

ISBN 1 84537 7028 7 (HB); 1 84537 029 5 (PB)

Reproduction by Resolution
Printed and bound in Singapore by Tien Wah Press (Pte) Ltd

10 9 8 7 6 5 4 3 2 1

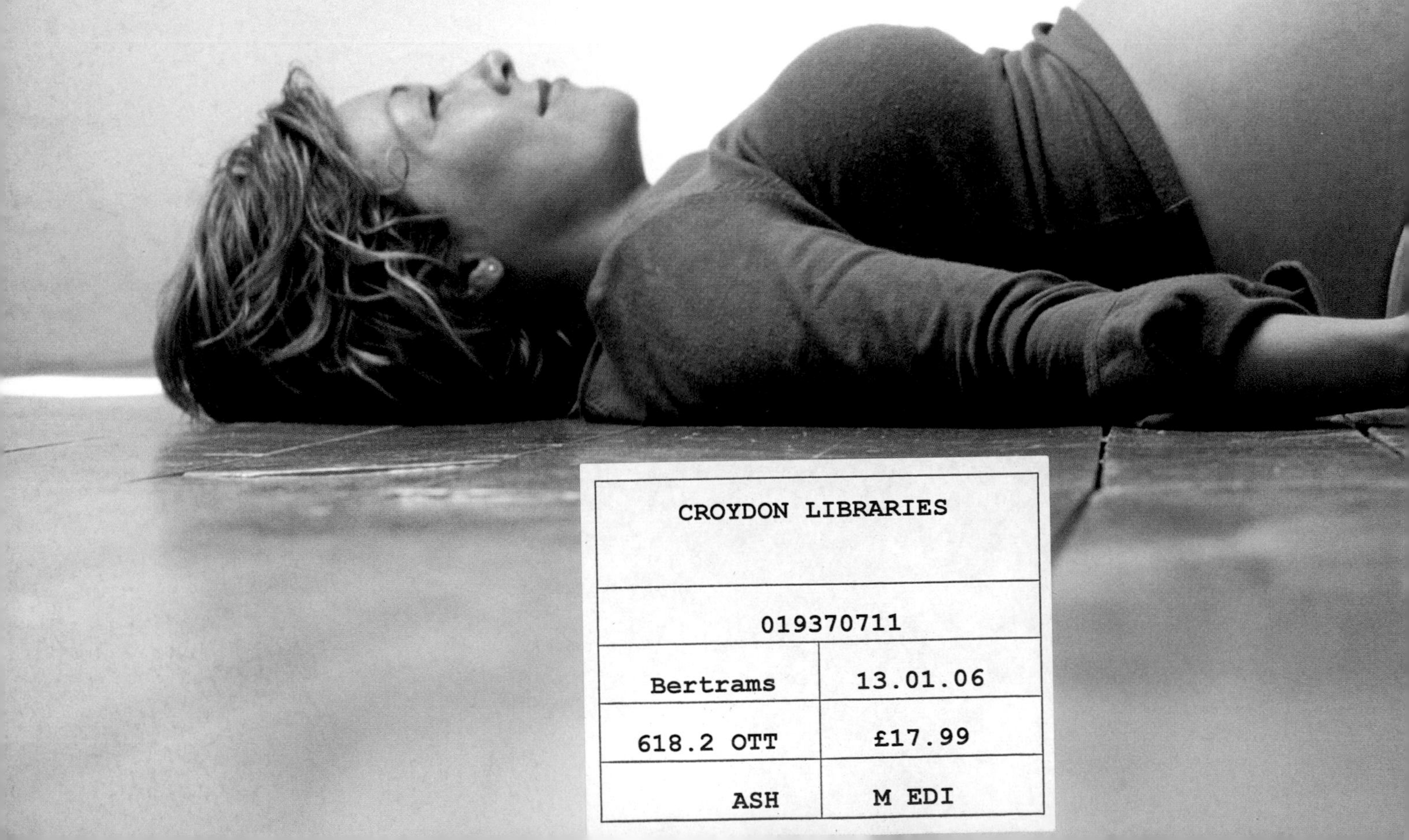

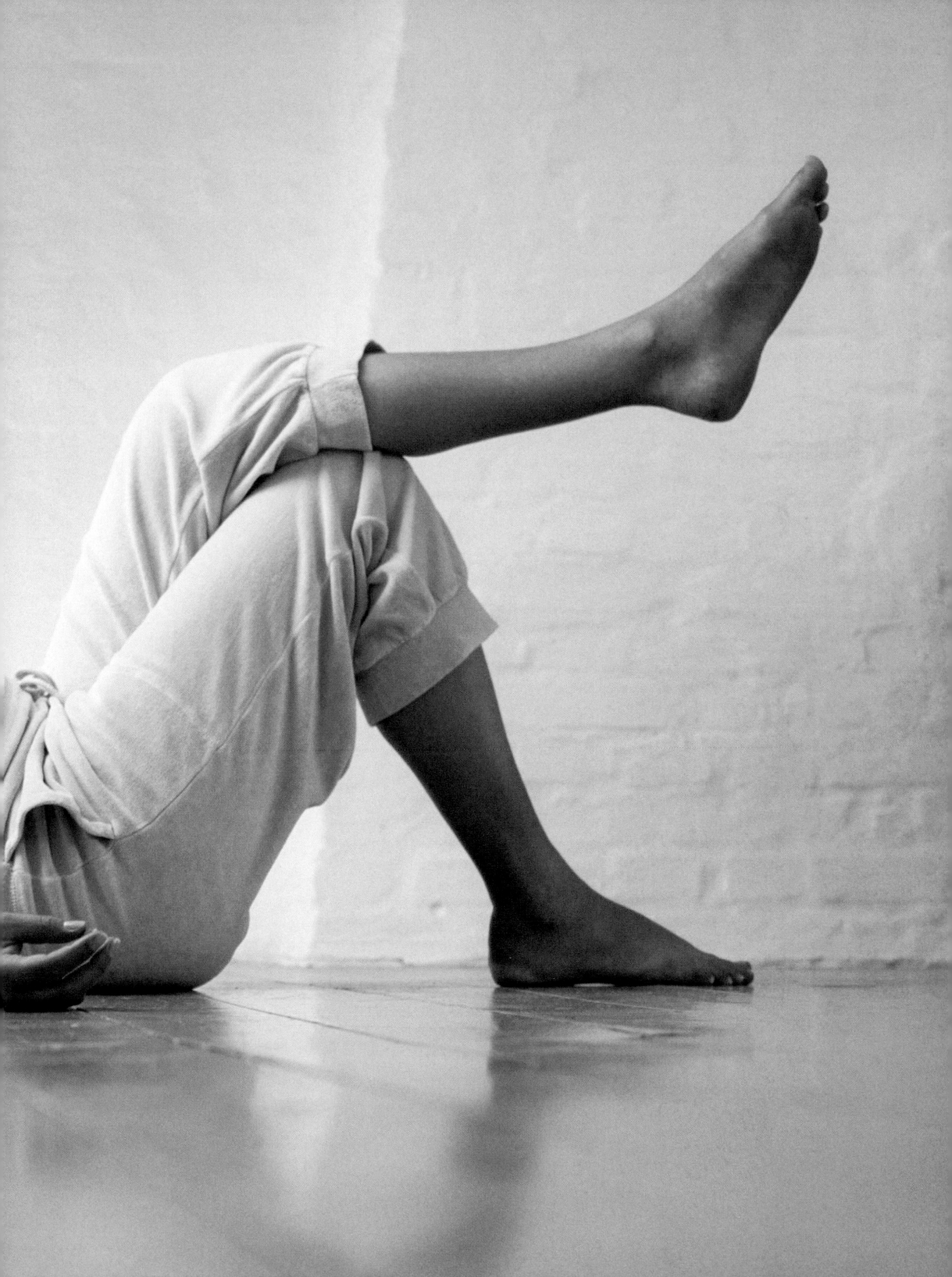

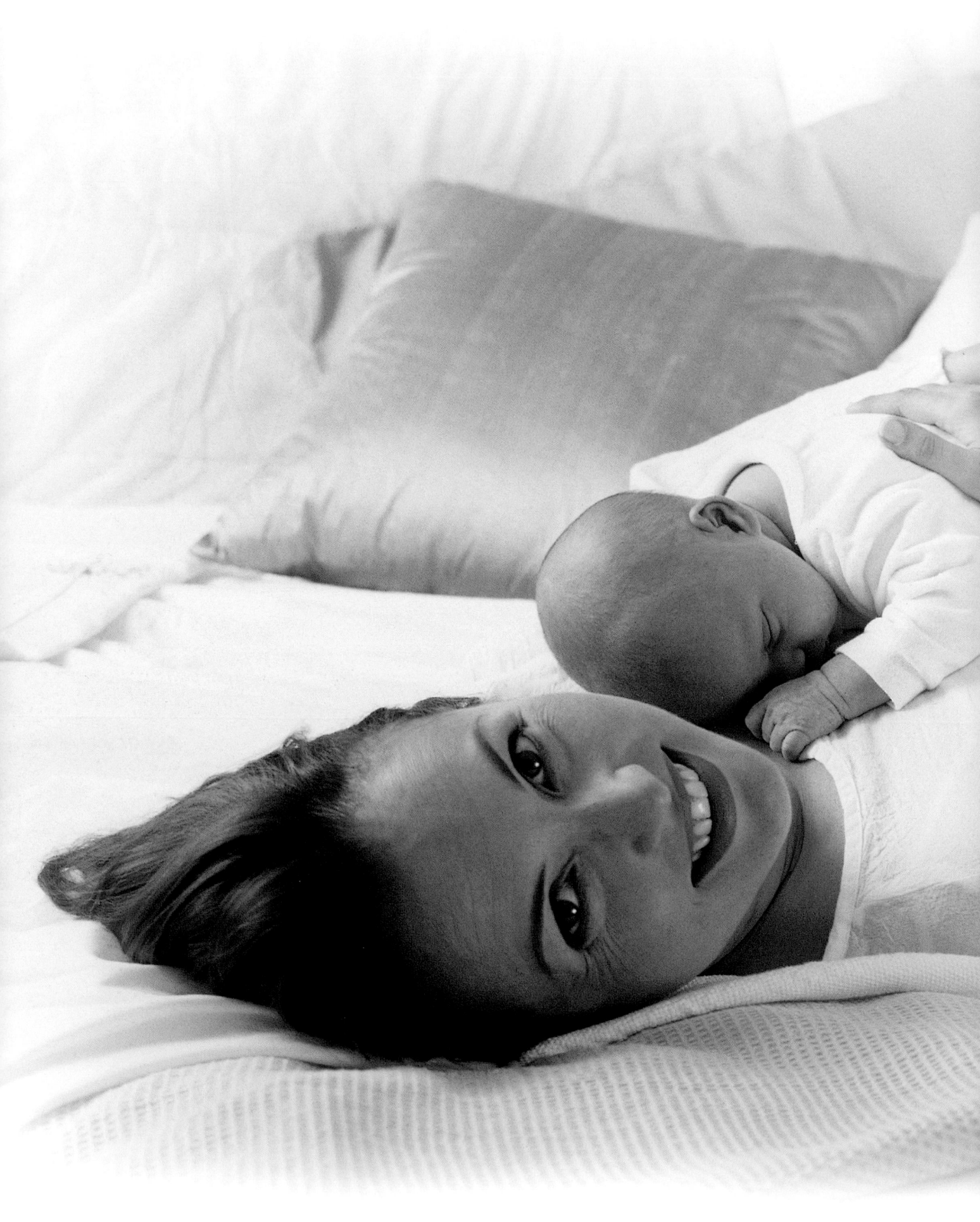

Contents

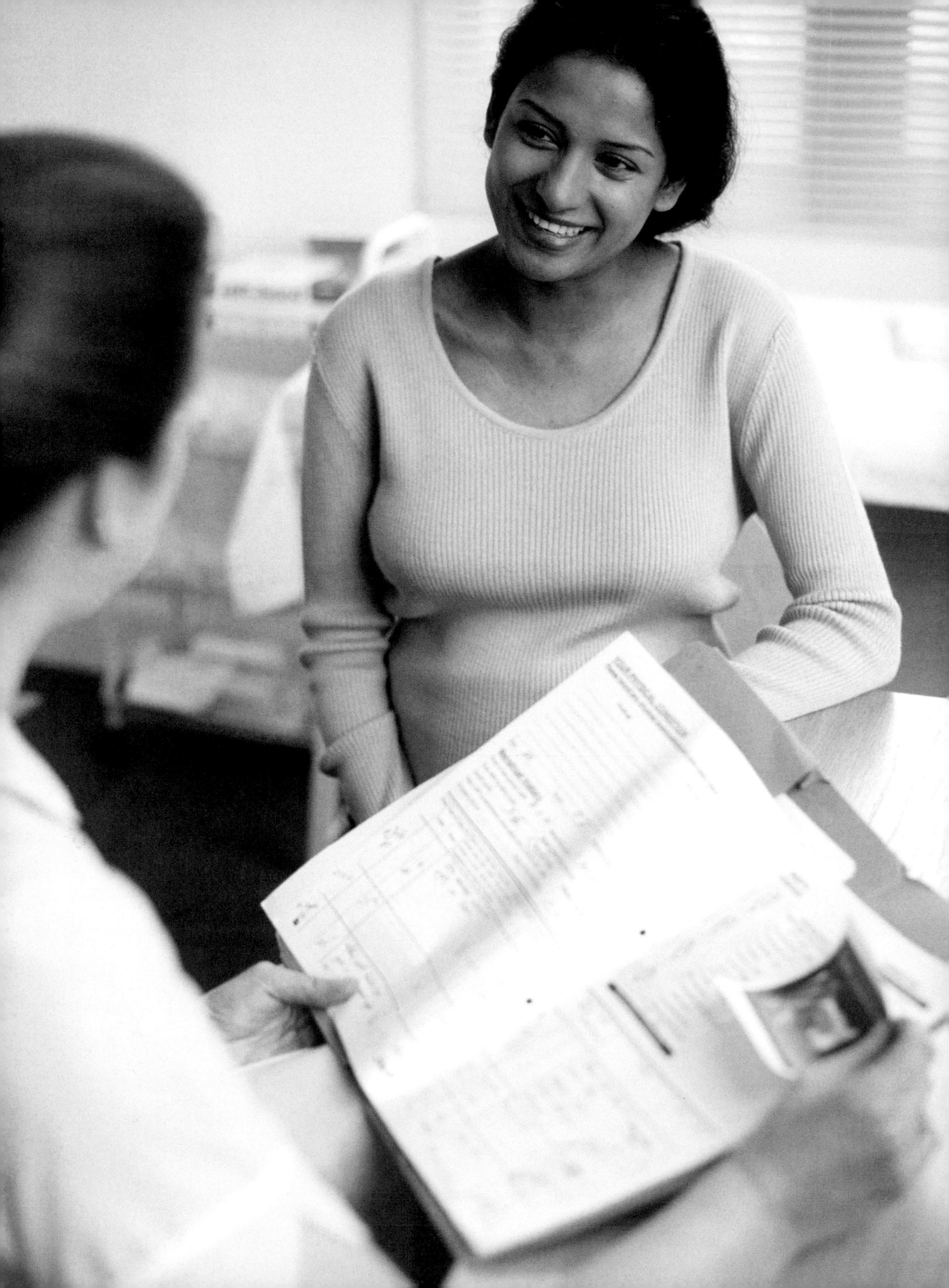

Part I
So you are going to have a baby

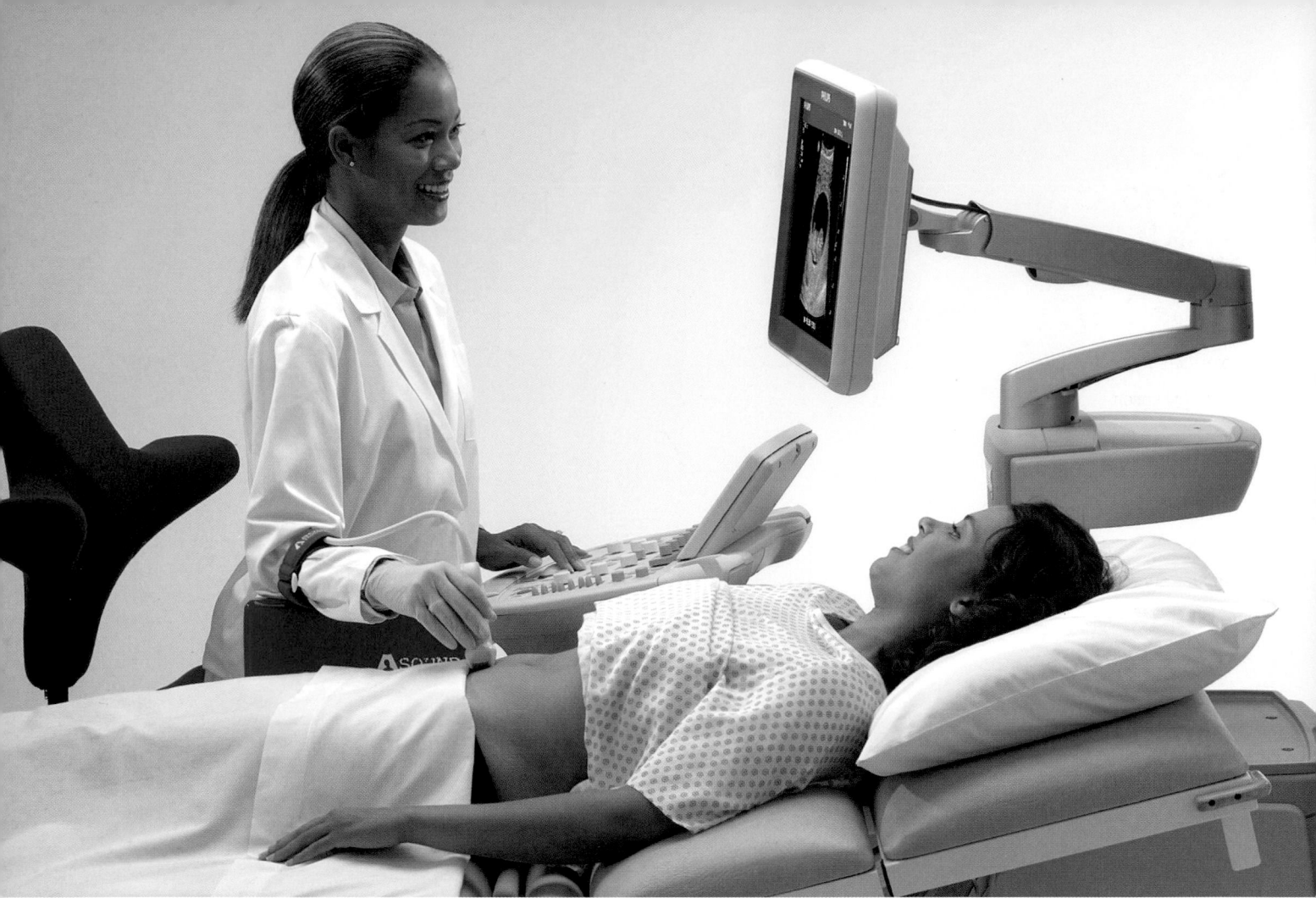

What to expect

There is no excuse to enter your pregnancy and birth experience in a fearful and ignorant manner. It is important to take responsibility for your body and your baby. You need to evaluate your options, and this can only be done if you are well informed of the changes that your body is going through. Having a baby will affect everything and everyone around you, and there is a lot you can do to make it a positive growth phase. While medical technology has come a long way, you need to retain your power in the birth arena – your future and the future of your offspring are at stake. Having a baby is a normal physiological event that your body knows how to do.

BE WELL INFORMED OF THE CHANGES YOUR BODY IS GOING THROUGH

Signs and confirmation of pregnancy

Some women can detect pregnancy soon after conception, especially those who have been pregnant before and experienced the hormonal changes that occur within days of conception. Other women do not experience any of the signs but know instinctively that they are pregnant. The earliest and most reliable sign of pregnancy for women who have a regular monthly cycle is a missed period.

Subtle signs

- **Breast changes** The breasts feel full and heavy, you may feel tenderness and tingling around the nipples and the areolae (circular area around the nipple) become darkened.
- **Frequent urination,** mainly at night.
- **Nausea,** and even vomiting, at any time during the day. This feeling may last for the first three months only or may persist for longer.
- **Increased vaginal discharge** without any redness, irritation or smell.
- **Sudden aversions** to things like tea, coffee, fatty food and tobacco smoke may develop.
- **Menstrual-like cramps** are normal provided they are mild and there is no bleeding – you may also feel full or bloated in the lower abdomen.
- **Tiredness** and drowsiness.

If you suspect that you are pregnant, the next step is to get a pregnancy test. Pregnancy tests check your urine or blood for human chorionic gonadotrophin (HCG), a hormone produced only during pregnancy.

Home urine tests are available from pharmacies. You can test a sample of urine from the first day of your missed period, which is from about two weeks after conception. The first urine passed in the morning is best to use because there is a build-up of HCG while you sleep. Ensure that the container you use to collect your sample is clean and free of soap.

A blood test, on the other hand, can be conducted within days of conception if pregnancy is suspected. Your caregiver will draw a sample of blood and the results are usually available within 24 hours. Whereas a positive result is almost always correct, a negative result is less reliable and you may have to try again after a week or so.

Once your pregnancy is confirmed, you may experience mixed emotions, especially if the pregnancy was unplanned. This is normal and you have to give yourself time to adjust to the idea. Try to attend antenatal classes from early on in your pregnancy; it will put you in touch with other pregnant women who are experiencing the same hormonal changes and similar emotions.

Deciding when to share the news with your family and friends is very personal and there is no right or wrong time to do it. In the past, many mothers-to-be were advised to keep the news of their pregnancy to themselves until they were past the critical, first three months. Many expectant mothers today choose to share the news shortly after the pregnancy is confirmed.

Below Once your pregnancy is confirmed, your caregiver will conduct a routine urine test.

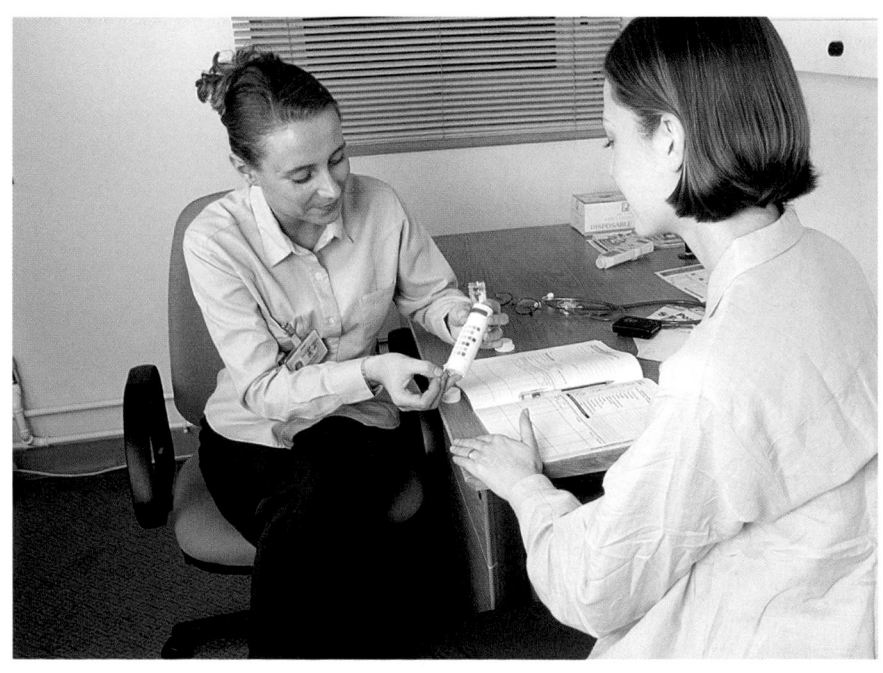

Calculating your due date

Although fertilization occurs about two weeks after your last menstrual period, pregnancy is calculated from the first day of that period and lasts an average of 280 days or 40 weeks. So, for example, when your doctor or midwife estimates your pregnancy at eight weeks, the foetus is, in actual fact, six weeks old. To calculate your expected date of delivery (EDD), your caregiver will subtract three months from the first day of your last menstrual period and add seven days. If your average cycle is longer or shorter than 28 days, the extra days are added to, or the shortfall subtracted from, the EDD. Sometimes counting ahead 266 days from the exact date of conception is more accurate, but not every woman knows when that was.

You may wish to use the table provided below to calculate your EDD. Look up the date of the first day of your last menstrual period in the months in bold print, and then look at the date immediately to the right to get an idea of your due date. (For example, if your last period started on 13 April, your EDD is 18 January.) Your EDD is an approximate date and, in fact, babies can be expected any time from three weeks before to two weeks after the EDD. Only five per cent of babies arrive on their due date and up to 70 per cent are born late.

Jan	Oct	Feb	Nov	Mar	Dec	Apr	Jan	May	Feb	Jun	Mar	Jul	Apr	Aug	May	Sep	Jun	Oct	Jul	Nov	Aug	Dec	Sep
1	8	1	8	1	6	1	6	1	5	1	8	1	7	1	8	1	8	1	8	1	8	1	7
2	9	2	9	2	7	2	7	2	6	2	9	2	8	2	9	2	9	2	9	2	9	2	8
3	10	3	10	3	8	3	8	3	7	3	10	3	9	3	10	3	10	3	10	3	10	3	9
4	11	4	11	4	9	4	9	4	8	4	11	4	10	4	11	4	11	4	11	4	11	4	10
5	12	5	12	5	10	5	10	5	9	5	12	5	11	5	12	5	12	5	12	5	12	5	11
6	13	6	13	6	11	6	11	6	10	6	13	6	12	6	13	6	13	6	13	6	13	6	12
7	14	7	14	7	12	7	12	7	11	7	14	7	13	7	14	7	14	7	14	7	14	7	13
8	15	8	15	8	13	8	13	8	12	8	15	8	14	8	15	8	15	8	15	8	15	8	14
9	16	9	16	9	14	9	14	9	13	9	16	9	15	9	16	9	16	9	16	9	16	9	15
10	17	10	17	10	15	10	15	10	14	10	17	10	16	10	17	10	17	10	17	10	17	10	16
11	18	11	18	11	16	11	16	11	15	11	18	11	17	11	18	11	18	11	18	11	18	11	17
12	19	12	19	12	17	12	17	12	16	12	19	12	18	12	19	12	19	12	19	12	19	12	18
13	20	13	20	13	18	13	18	13	17	13	20	13	19	13	20	13	20	13	20	13	20	13	19
14	21	14	21	14	19	14	19	14	18	14	21	14	20	14	21	14	21	14	21	14	21	14	20
15	22	15	22	15	20	15	20	15	19	15	22	15	21	15	22	15	22	15	22	15	22	15	21
16	23	16	23	16	21	16	21	16	20	16	23	16	22	16	23	16	23	16	23	16	23	16	22
17	24	17	24	17	22	17	22	17	21	17	24	17	23	17	24	17	24	17	24	17	24	17	23
18	25	18	25	18	23	18	23	18	22	18	25	18	24	18	25	18	25	18	25	18	25	18	24
19	26	19	26	19	24	19	24	19	23	19	26	19	25	19	26	19	26	19	26	19	26	19	25
20	27	20	27	20	25	20	25	20	24	20	27	20	26	20	27	20	27	20	27	20	27	20	26
21	28	21	28	21	26	21	26	21	25	21	28	21	27	21	28	21	28	21	28	21	28	21	27
22	29	22	29	22	27	22	27	22	26	22	29	22	28	22	29	22	29	22	29	22	29	22	28
23	30	23	30	23	28	23	28	23	27	23	30	23	29	23	30	23	30	23	30	23	30	23	29
24	31	24	1	24	29	24	29	24	28	24	31	24	30	24	31	24	1	24	31	24	31	24	30
25	1	25	2	25	30	25	30	25	1	25	1	25	1	25	1	25	2	25	1	25	1	25	31
26	2	26	3	26	31	26	31	26	2	26	2	26	2	26	2	26	3	26	2	26	2	26	1
27	3	27	4	27	1	27	1	27	3	27	3	27	3	27	3	27	4	27	3	27	3	27	2
28	4	28	5	28	2	28	2	28	4	28	4	28	4	28	4	28	5	28	4	28	4	28	3
29	5			29	3	29	3	29	5	29	5	29	5	29	5	29	6	29	5	29	5	29	4
30	6			30	4	30	4	30	6	30	6	30	6	30	6	30	7	30	6	30	6	30	5
31	7			31	5			31	7			31	7	31	7			31	7			31	6

Now that you are pregnant

Pregnancy is the ideal time to take stock and prioritize your life. This is the beginning of the many decisions and choices that parenthood will bring to you and your partner. Learn, and make the necessary changes in preparation for the arrival of your newborn.

Choosing a caregiver

The anticipation of birth brings to the surface a woman's deep feelings about many things – memories of her childhood, her sexuality, what she will be like during labour, her expectations of herself as a mother, and even her relationship with her partner. Your impressions from your labour and treatment will stay with you forever. It is therefore vital to find a caregiver who will guide you through your pregnancy by answering your questions and listening to your concerns. It will have to be someone whose expertise you trust, who will give you emotional support and encourage you to make certain decisions and plans regarding your baby's birth.

As long as pregnancy and birth remain normal, parents can, if they wish, play a big part in decision-making. If complications develop, the caregiver assumes a greater role in this process. When choosing a caregiver, it is also important to know at which hospital or clinic he or she will deliver your baby, so you can decide whether you are happy with this choice.

At first you may not know what questions to ask, so it is best to write down anything that may puzzle you or provoke questions.

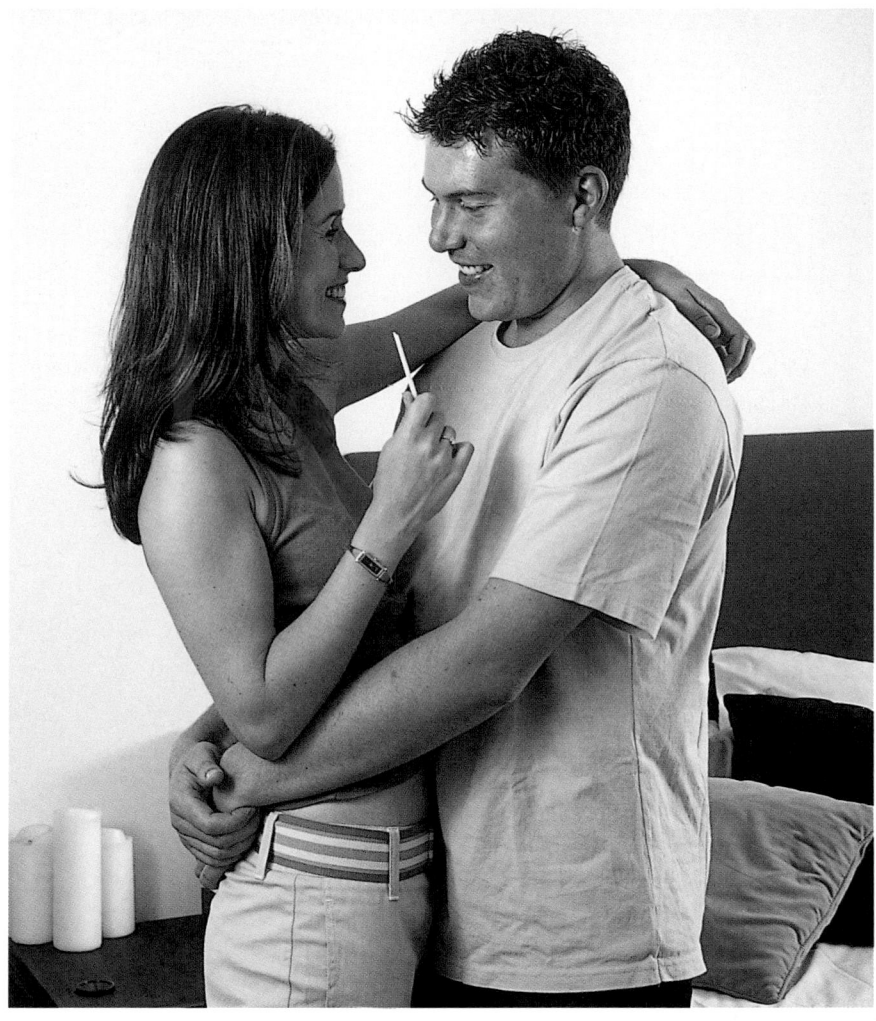

Do not feel intimidated or afraid to ask questions! You may find that once you have started childbirth classes, you have many more questions for your caregiver. You may want to draw up a 'wish list' (see p122).

Above *Sharing the news of your pregnancy with your partner is very exciting, especially if it was planned.*

What to ask
- What are your relevant qualifications and experience?
- Who will take calls when you are off duty or not on call?
- Do you have delivery privileges at more than one hospital?
- What are your fees?
- Will you be prepared to assist if I decide on home birth?

Gynaecologists/ obstetricians

A gynaecologist is a doctor who specializes in diseases of the female reproductive system. An obstetrician, however, specializes in managing both normal and complicated pregnancy and childbirth. A gynaecologist/ obstetrician almost always manages both disciplines and he or she is the only medical doctor who is qualified to perform Caesarean sections. In some hospitals, you may be seen by registrars (qualified doctors who are ranked below consultants).

Some gynaecologists run their own private practice, while others are employed by a hospital.

If you choose a private obstetrician, you will visit him in his rooms for the months before your baby's birth. These visits will start off monthly and will gradually increase until you will be seeing your obstetrician once a week.

Midwives

Midwives are practitioners in their own right and their speciality is delivering babies. They assist healthy women with a hospital, home or water birth. An experienced midwife will detect problems far in advance and get the mother to a specialist if need be. Midwives are usually qualified nurses who have trained for midwifery within their general course, which is usually completed within a four-year period. There are also advanced midwifery courses, which take one year to complete. The majority of midwives are female, and can be in private practice or employed by a hospital. Their approach focuses on the mother and her choices.

General practitioners

Although they are not specialists in obstetric care, general practitioners (GPs) often manage pregnancies, especially in smaller towns. In fact, in the UK the GP as caregiver is the norm (although midwives organize the births), and a gynaecologist/obstetrician is consulted only when a specialist is needed. Doctors study for six years with one year of housemanship. Their training also incorporates obstetrics. Some GPs take further training, such as a Diploma in Obstetrics. GPs may be in private practice or employed by a clinic. In terms of approach, they view pregnancy as natural, but are also trained to 'manage' childbirth.

Below Choose a caregiver with whom you feel comfortable; do not be afraid to ask questions!

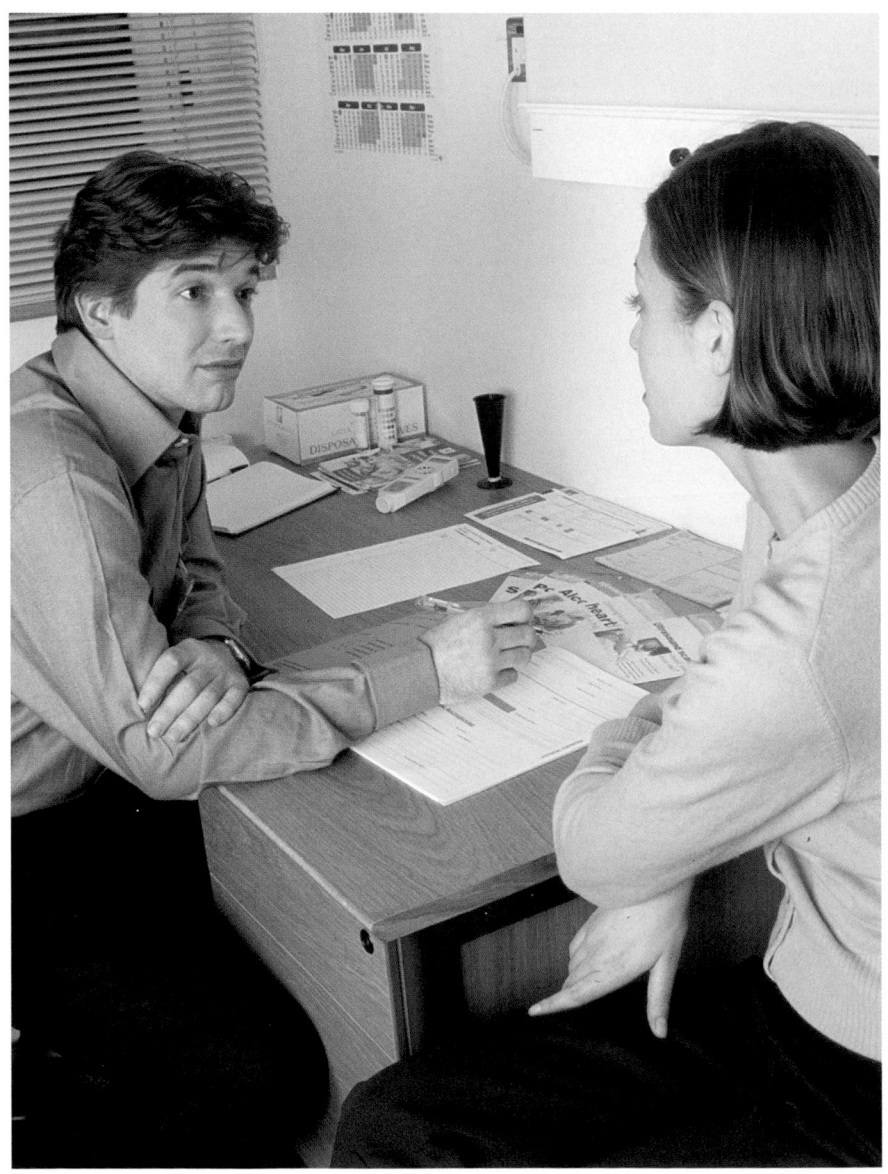

Your first antenatal checkup

Most women will have their first medical examination soon after they have discovered that they are pregnant, which may be six to eight weeks into the pregnancy. Your first visit will be the longest because your caregiver will want to establish a full medical history. You will be asked a lot of questions about yourself which will include: your age, past and present health status, whether you have had any operations, certain illnesses and previous pregnancies, stillbirths or miscarriages. You will be asked about your family's medical history, as well as that of your partner and his family. This is important in order to ascertain whether there are any diseases in either family that your baby could inherit. Your caregiver will also ask about your occupation to help form an overall picture of your needs. If you need special attention for any condition, it should be picked up at this early stage.

The physical examination

Once your interview is over, your caregiver may ask you to change into a gown for a physical examination. (Not done in all countries.)

An internal examination may be conducted during your first visit to confirm the pregnancy. This is done by feeling the cervix and assessing the size of the uterus. The doctor will gently insert two fingers into the vagina and at the same time press your abdomen firmly but gently with the other hand. Some doctors may

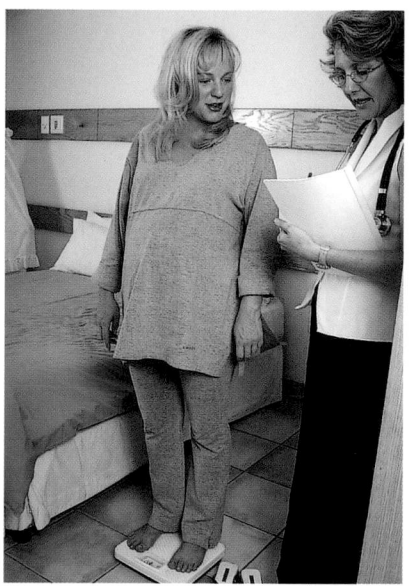

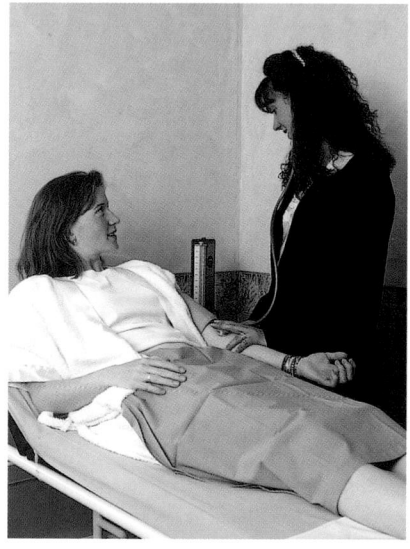

Top and above Your caregiver will check your weight and blood pressure at every visit throughout your pregnancy.

conduct an ultrasound scan instead of an internal examination. In most cases, you will not have another internal examination until 36 weeks into your pregnancy. (Many practitioners feel that an internal examination at the initial checkup is unnecessary.)

The following will be checked:

Weight Your weight will be measured to serve as the baseline for further comparison as your baby develops. You may be weighed at every checkup. (Not done in all countries.)

Height Your height will also be measured to estimate the size of your frame, and to form an idea of the size of your pelvis. This serves as a guide only and does not mean that because you may be small and short you will be a candidate for Caesarean section. Your shoe size may be asked for as well. (Not done in all countries.)

Blood pressure Your blood pressure will be taken at every visit. This is important because a change in blood pressure, especially if it becomes too high, can endanger your baby's life as well as yours. A low blood pressure can make you feel faint and tired.

Breasts Your caregiver may examine your breasts for lumps and check that you will not have any problems breast-feeding your baby. If there is uncertainty, visit a qualified lactation consultant! (Breast examination is not routine practice in the UK.)

Teeth and gums Your caregiver may examine your teeth and gums at this stage. You may need a calcium supplement, as your baby will deplete your body's supply.

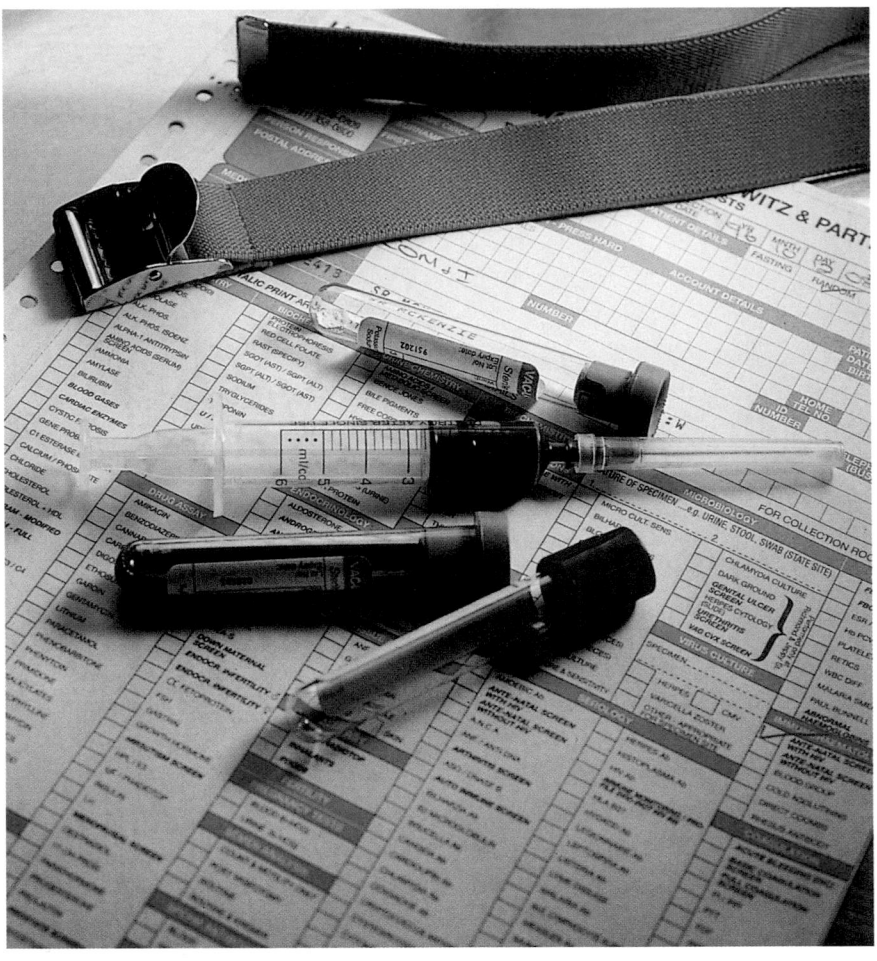

Blood tests

All blood tests require your consent; you must give consent for an HIV test. It is important that you understand the reasons for your tests and you may ask if they are all necessary, especially if cost is a factor.

Besides confirming your pregnancy, blood tests may also be conducted for the following reasons:

- to find out or confirm your blood group (A, B, AB, or O) as well as the Rhesus (Rh) factor (positive or negative)
- as a screening test for certain chromosomal disorders
- if gestational diabetes is suspected, you will be given a sugary drink and your caregiver will run a series of blood tests over a few hours. (Most hospitals now do a timed random blood sugar test as the first step in diabetes testing.)
- to test for the human immunodeficiency virus (HIV), which causes AIDS (*see* p29)
- to screen for viral diseases such as hepatitis B and rubella; sexually transmitted diseases such as syphilis can also be tested for and treated early, if necessary
- to test for anaemia – haemoglobin levels will be checked to ensure that the red blood cells, responsible for carrying oxygen and iron, have not decreased.

Urine test

A urine test will be done at every visit. Urine, like blood, can tell a lot about how your body is adapting to pregnancy. Your caregiver will inspect the colour of your urine and check for any deposits (blood and other particles that should not be passed through the kidneys); the pH (acidity) and concentration will also be checked.

The smell of urine can also indicate some conditions – an offensive smell may be due to pus caused by a major infection in the urinary tract, a 'fishy' smell is associated with a vaginal infection, and a 'fruity' smell is due to ketones (*see* opposite page).

You are usually asked to pass urine over a test stick, ensuring you wet the entire stick, or you may be asked to pass a small amount of urine into a glass container.

If your urine needs to be sent to a laboratory for analysis, your caregiver will ask you to pass a 'midstream' specimen into a sterile container. This means that you will need to pass a little urine into the toilet, allowing any bacteria sitting at the mouth of the urethra to be flushed away, stop the flow of urine and then pass a little more into the container. Replace the lid and give it to your caregiver. He or she will then send the labelled container to the laboratory for a full analysis of the urine.

The coloured blocks on the urine test stick can indicate the following:

1. Leucocytes (white blood cells) could indicate that you have a urinary tract infection.

2. Protein may show up in your urine as a result of a vaginal infection; it may also indicate kidney or blood pressure problems. If combined with swollen hands and ankles, and high blood pressure, the presence of protein may indicate a condition known as pregnancy induced hypertension (PIH) or pre-eclampsia (*see* p25). This potentially serious condition occurs more often in first-time pregnancies, usually toward the end of the pregnancy, but can start earlier. If you do have PIH, you will probably feel fine and, although most cases are mild, they still require observation. Depending on the severity, the treatment may require hospitalization or home bed rest; drugs are occasionally prescribed to lower high blood pressure.

3. Glucose or sugar may show a little from time to time but if it shows up repeatedly, you will be tested for diabetes. Some women develop a type of diabetes only during pregnancy known as 'gestational diabetes' (*see* p24). It must be controlled either by diet or insulin, and usually disappears once the baby is born. Further tests will be carried out if this is suspected.

4. Ketones are linked to diabetes and may show up if you are not eating enough or if you have been experiencing excessive vomiting. During excessive vomiting, the body loses vital minerals and salts which leads to an imbalance in the body, causing a state of ketosis. Ketosis occurs when food intake is inadequate, either by choice or illness.

5. Blood indicates infection and/or kidney disease; it may also be present in cases of pre-eclampsia and may show in the urine after sexual intercourse.

6. Bilirubin is a yellow-orange pigment in the bile. There may be an excessive amount of bile in the urine when jaundice is present. Bile may also be found in the urine in cases of hyperemesis gravidarum in pregnancy (*see* p27) – the mother is 'malnourished' because her body is not keeping food in her stomach long enough for absorption to take place.

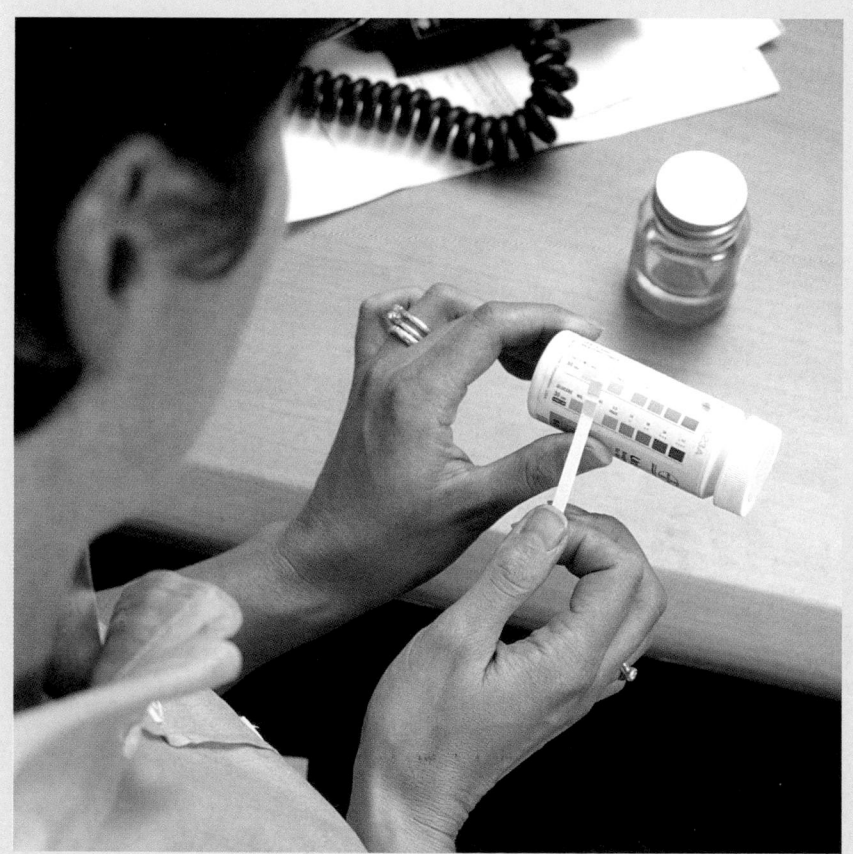

Left Your caregiver can tell a lot about the state of your health by testing your urine.

Routine checkups

Your antenatal visits will be once a month, depending on your circumstances, until about the seventh month and then every second week for the seventh and eighth months. In the last month before your due date, your visits will be once a week. Should you have any concerns between appointments, contact your caregiver immediately. (Note: there are usually variations to these schedules.)

Subsequent visits are quicker than the initial one. Your weight, urine and blood pressure will be monitored at every visit. Your caregiver will feel your abdomen to check the height of the fundus (top of the uterus), which will show the progress of your baby's growth.

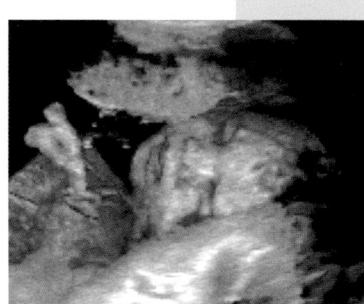

Right A three-dimensional scan in late pregnancy will show a clearer image of your baby.

Some doctors prefer to use the ultrasound and not to palpate the abdomen. He or she will listen to the baby's heartbeat; you may also be able to hear the sound of your baby's heartbeat if your caregiver uses a Doppler device (electronic heartbeat detector).

Having regular, good antenatal care is very important. Although it may be an effort, try to keep your appointments. Do not forget to include your partner as he may have questions of his own, and the baby will be more real to him if he sees the ultrasound scans. Pregnancy and birth may be stressful, but it is a natural process – you are not ill and

A guideline as to what a scan will show at various stages during pregnancy

Early scanning

WEEK 5 The pregnancy sac is visible.

WEEKS 6–7 The embryo is seen and the heart movement is visible.

WEEK 8 Early foetal movement. Twins can be confirmed at this stage.

WEEKS 9–10 The outline of the placenta is visible and the foetus can be measured to establish a due date.

Midway scanning

WEEKS 16–26 The organs are visible – the stomach, bladder, spine and the ex- ternal genitalia. The baby's head is measured to accurately date the pregnancy; the length of the femur (commonly called the 'thighbone') is also measured to determine the age of the foetus. The placenta is easily recognized from the rest of the uterus and the amount of amniotic fluid can also be assessed. A scan done between 18 and 24 weeks is the single most important routine scan because it gives an accurate assessment of the gestational age and permits detection of most major abnormalities in the foetus.

Late scanning

WEEKS 36+ The main reason for scanning at this late stage is to monitor foetal growth by measuring the circumference of the baby's head, the length of the femur and the size of the abdomen. If there is any concern regarding foetal wellbeing, a cardiotocograph (CTG), which measures foetal heart rate, will be done together with an assessment of foetal movement.

pregnancy is not a medical procedure but an extremely emotional and intimate event. This is one event you are not likely to forget.

Routine ultrasound scans

Ultrasound scans are useful for estimating the gestational age of the foetus and assessing the baby's wellbeing. They show the growth of the foetus and are often used for detecting birth defects. The machine utilizes high-frequency sound waves that are transmitted into the body. These waves 'bounce back' when encountering changes in density of different body structures (such as fat, muscle, fluid, body organs and bone). A picture is transmitted onto a screen via a hand-held transducer. The most commonly used scan is the 'real time' image, which provides a continuous picture of the uterus and its contents, enabling you to see your baby's movements as they happen.

Some caregivers perform a scan at every visit; others are more conservative and may not scan you as often.

Tests and scans

Although pregnancy is a time of great anticipation, many women are concerned about their baby's wellbeing. Tests can be done to decrease your anxiety, but some are not without risk and can seldom guarantee total reassurance. Tests are done to either rule out or diagnose problems.

It is important to note that although your doctor may recommend certain tests and scans, the decision to go through with them lies with you.

There are two kinds of tests that are recommended: screening tests inform a woman if she is at risk of having an abnormal baby (if a screening test is positive, a second screening test may be done or a diagnostic test considered), and diagnostic tests are done to confirm or rule out a suspected diagnosis of a rare condition.

Screening tests

Screening tests involve either blood tests or ultrasound scans, and the advantage is that they are noninvasive and will not harm your baby. The disadvantage is that they cannot tell you whether or not your baby has an abnormality – only diagnostic tests can.

Screening ultrasounds

The **nuchal fold test** is a screening test carried out at around 11–13 weeks and measures the amount of fluid beneath the skin on the back of the baby's neck which, in some cases, may suggest an increased risk for Down's syndrome (see Glossary). This test is over 80 per cent accurate, and if the test result turns out positive, your caregiver will suggest a diagnostic test such as amniocentesis or chorionic villi sampling (see p21) to diagnose the presence of Down's syndrome.

A positive test result can be very traumatic, and your caregiver will suggest counselling for you and your partner.

A **foetal anomaly scan** is performed at around 18–20 weeks, and tests for abnormalities that may be visible on screen such as anencephaly (congenital absence of most of the brain) and spina bifida (a gap in the vertebrae leaves the spinal cord partially exposed).

Below A radiographer will spread a jelly-like substance over your stomach and move the transducer across it to look at an image of your uterus and baby on screen.

Blood tests

The alpha-fetoprotein (AFP) test – a component of the triple test – is usually carried out at 15–18 weeks. It measure the major circulating protein (AFP) of the foetus and can calculate your risk of having a baby with Down's syndrome or an open neural-tube defect. The triple test (see Glossary) is slightly more accurate and also gives the risk factor for many other conditions, but it is not a routine test and you may have to ask for it.

Test results are expressed as a risk, e.g. 1:420, which means that for every 420 babies born, one will have Down's syndrome. If this is hard to grasp, rather look at the chances that your baby will not be affected – so for every 420 babies, 419 will be normal. If the screening test suggests that your risk is high, you may be offered a diagnostic test.

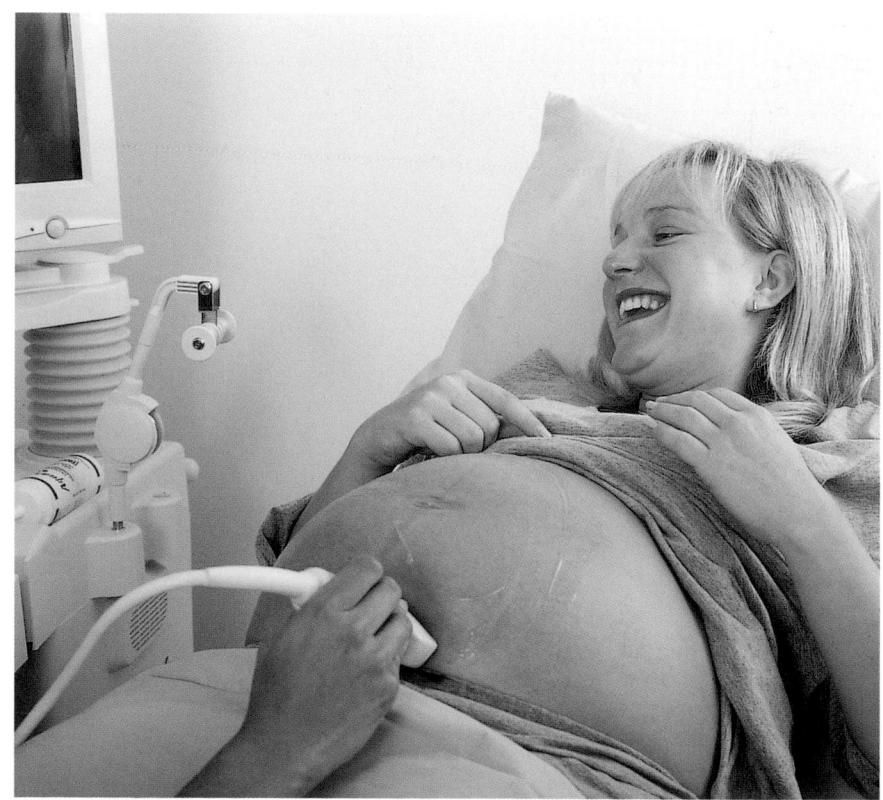

Diagnostic tests

Diagnostic tests are used extensively to diagnose particular abnormalities of the foetus, placenta and cord. While the diagnostic ultrasound is noninvasive, amniocentesis and chorionic villi sampling are invasive tests, and there are risks involved. Ask your caregiver about the risks and voice your concerns.

Diagnostic ultrasound

This scan is used to detect reproductive diseases and to:

- check that your baby's organs are developing normally and that everything is well
- locate the position of the placenta
- confirm the presence of twins or triplets
- estimate age and due date.

What to ask
- What information will the test provide?
- How accurate is the test?
- Are the results of the test essential in determining the course of care?
- Will enough be learned to justify exposing my baby to this test?

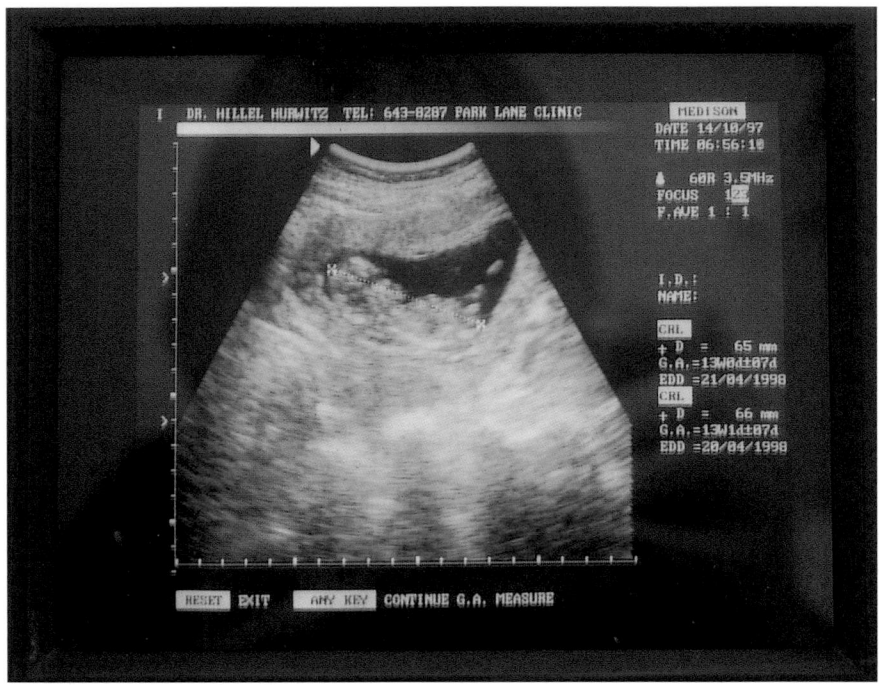

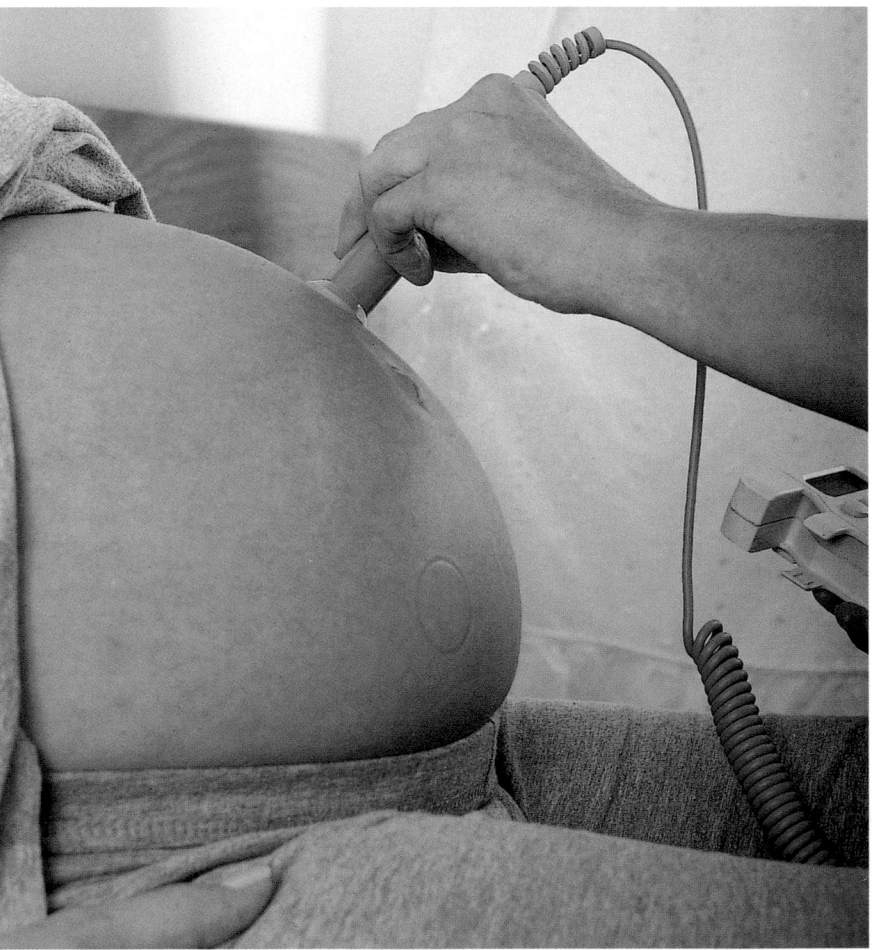

Above right An ultrasound scan is a window into the womb and can reassure you that your baby is growing well.

Right A diagnostic ultrasound is noninvasive and there are no risks involved; it will not harm your baby!

Chorionic villi sampling (CVS)

With this technique, foetal tissue can be gathered from the placenta from as early as eight weeks of gestation. A few villi are collected from the chorion which forms the placenta, and the sample is sent to a laboratory. There the sample is analyzed to diagnose or disprove the disorder.

This procedure is done under extremely sterile conditions: a sample of placental tissue is extracted through the vagina or the abdomen, and it takes about 10 minutes to perform. It is more common to extract the tissue via the abdomen. After the administration of local anaesthetic, the doctor guides the needle by ultrasound through the abdominal wall to the point where the placenta is developing. The mother will be advised to rest for about 30 minutes after the procedure and then be allowed to leave. She will feel tender for a few days after the procedure.

What it shows

CVS diagnoses some of the same conditions as amniocentesis. Diseases such as haemophilia and muscular dystrophy, Tay Sachs disease and sickle-cell anaemia can be detected in the first trimester. However, neural-tube defects such as spina bifida and anencephaly cannot be detected using this method.

Results

The results of this test can be expected within two to four days, and most laboratories will culture the cells for backup report within two to three weeks.

Early diagnosis means that a doctor can terminate the pregnancy in the early stages by inducing a miscarriage, which hopefully will reduce the emotional as well as the physical trauma for the mother.

Risks

There are complications involved such as infection, spotting for a few hours after the procedure and period-like pains. Risk of spontaneous abortion occurs in two to three per cent of cases. There is a possibility of disturbance in placental function.

CVS is performed earlier in the pregnancy than amniocentesis. There is a spontaneous foetal loss rate between 12 and 16 weeks (i.e. some babies are lost between 12 and 16 weeks even if no procedure has been performed). This spontaneous loss makes CVS appear much riskier than amniocentesis, however, when spontaneous loss is taken into account, the actual procedure-related risk of amniocentesis and CVS is about the same. This is a highly specialized procedure!

Amniocentesis

Amniocentesis is a fairly simple procedure and is considered an invasive diagnostic technique, which can only be carried out in the second trimester at about 15–17 weeks. The doctor will use an ultrasound scan to determine the position of the foetus and placenta. A long, hollow needle with a syringe surmounted to it is inserted into the womb, commonly under local anaesthetic, and a small amount of amniotic fluid is extracted from the amniotic sac. You may feel a 'popping' sensation when the needle enters the uterus, and some women feel pressure when fluid is withdrawn. This fluid contains cells from the foetus as well as substances from the pregnancy which can be tested. The procedure lasts for about five minutes and causes mild discomfort. Specially trained obstetricians carry out amniocentesis. Most hospitals with antenatal departments have their own unit; if not, you will be referred to the nearest available centre.

After the test, you will be advised to take it easy for a few days – avoid any exercise and do not lift heavy objects. It is normal to experience a 'tightening' feeling in your womb area, and you may feel a little tender the next day. If you have any concerns, contact your caregiver.

What it shows

Amniocentesis is used to detect chromosomal disorders – Down's syndrome being the most common. Other genetic disorders can also be detected but the laboratory will have to be informed about the history of these genetic problems, so that additional tests can be carried out.

Why it is done

You may be offered an amniocentesis if:

- you are over 35 years of age at the time of conception
- you have had a positive screening test, which indicated a higher risk of Down's syndrome or spina bifida
- you have already had a baby with certain problems or have a history of specific genetic problems
- you have had a previous pregnancy terminated for a genetic problem
- something unusual was found on an ultrasound scan that may be associated with chromosomal problems.

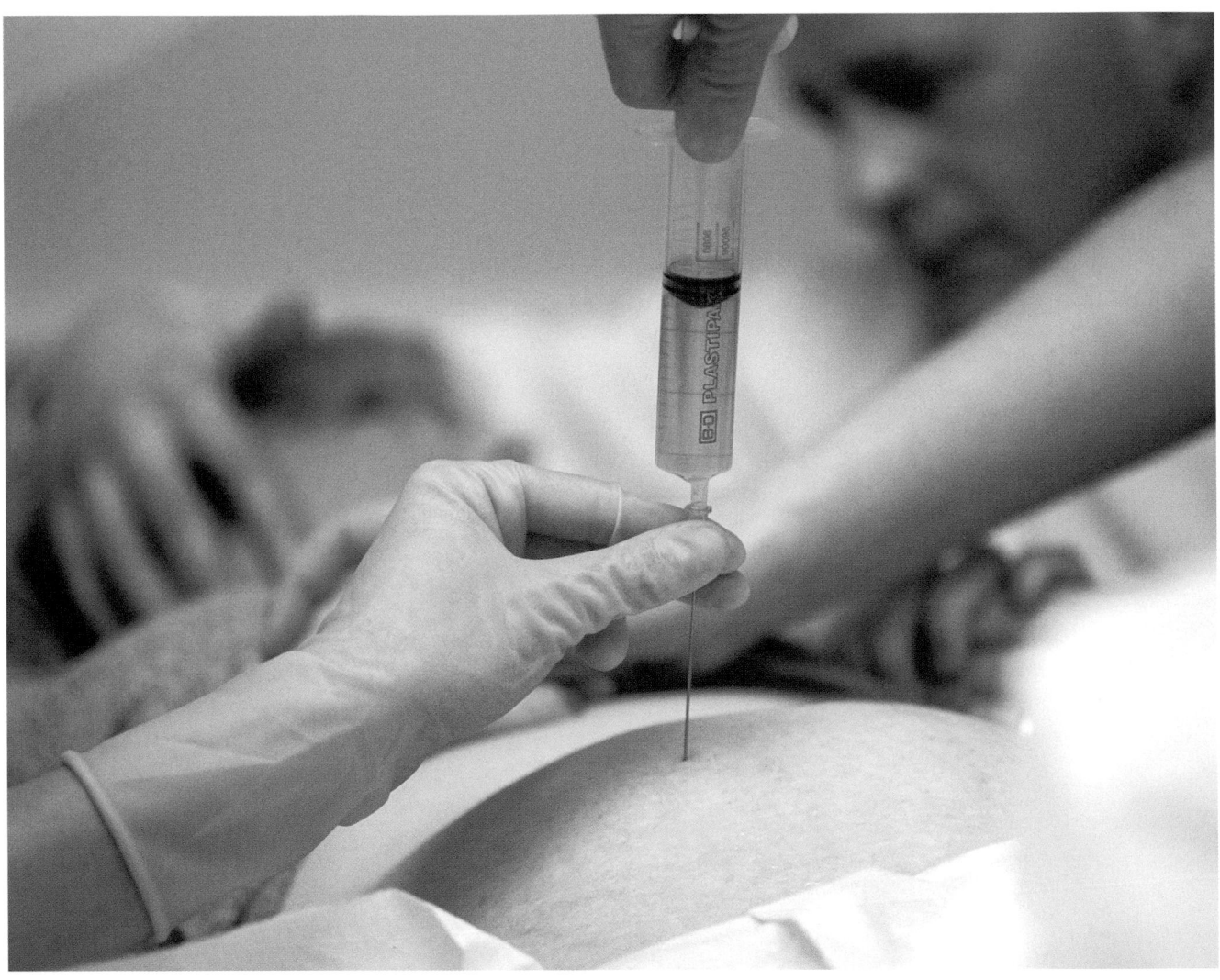

Above Amniocentesis is a simple procedure: a needle is inserted into the uterus, under local anaesthetic, and amniotic fluid is drawn. The cells shed by the foetus are separated from the rest of the fluid and cultivated in a laboratory for analysis.

Results

The test results for Down's syndrome are usually confirmed after two weeks because the cells have to be 'grown' in the laboratory. Your doctor will contact you to give you the results and, if necessary, you will be offered the opportunity to speak to a genetic counsellor.

Risks

Only one in every 150 women suffers a miscarriage associated with amniocentesis, making the overall risk rate 0.5 to one per cent. Placental puncture is the major risk, therefore the doctor uses ultrasound to locate the position of the placenta in the uterus before carrying out the procedure. If miscarriage is going to occur, it usually happens within 48 hours of the procedure. Do not be surprised if you feel tense and on edge for the two- to three-week waiting period before the results become available. It is completely normal to experience some anxiety. Talk to those closest to you or ask your caregiver to put you in touch with a genetic counsellor.

Note: Flourescent *in situ* hybridization (FISH) is now used to test for Down's syndrome and other chromosomal abnormalities. The results are usually available within two days.

Possible complications during pregnancy

Anaemia

Oxygen and other nutrients are transported around the body via the haemoglobin in our blood. This important substance contains iron and is found only in the red blood cells. When haemoglobin decreases it is known as anaemia – iron deficiency being the most common cause in pregnancy.

Nature will make sure that the baby is protected from the effects of anaemia and nutrients are actively absorbed across the placenta during the last few weeks of pregnancy – even if you do not have enough for yourself!

Symptoms

The following symptoms may indicate anaemia:

- feeling lethargic, weak and drained
- delayed healing, especially after delivery
- palpitations – a feeling that your heart is beating too fast (may occur if there is too much iron in the body as well)
- shortness of breath
- pale complexion
- recurring infections – at the first antenatal checkup most women will have a routine screening blood test for anaemia (if it does show up, your caregiver will conduct follow-up blood tests regularly).

Prevention

To prevent anaemia, change your diet as follows:

- eat iron-rich foods such as fortified breakfast cereals, peas, wholegrain bread, beans and lentils, and vegetables – especially dark green vegetables. Other food sources are raisins, dried prunes, apricots and figs, avocados, soya beans, carob and cocoa
- combine the iron-rich foods with calcium and vitamin C because these enhance the body's ability to absorb iron

- avoid alcohol, cigarettes, tea and coffee as these substances interfere with nutrient and iron absorption
- rest as much as you can
- exercises that improve circulation such as swimming, walking or cycling will make you feel more energetic.

Most caregivers will prescribe iron supplementation. It is better to take the ferrous rather than a ferric form which inhibits the absorption of other vitamins.

Iron supplements should normalize body stores within four to six weeks, but can cause nausea and constipation. Take your supplements after your evening meal to combat nausea and if constipation becomes a problem, increase your intake of fibre and roughage. If necessary, you may take a homeopathic laxative.

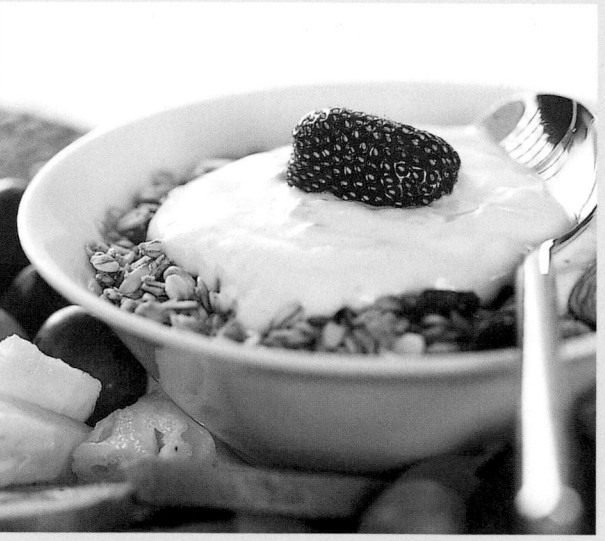

Above *Include fortified breakfast cereal in your diet to help prevent anaemia; it will also provide roughage to combat constipation.*

Gestational diabetes

Gestational diabetes mellitus (GDM) is a form of diabetes first recognizable after 28 weeks of pregnancy. It affects between one and two per cent of pregnancies. In the woman with gestational diabetes, the pancreas is unable to produce enough insulin to meet the increased demands of pregnancy. The consequence of this 'insulin deficiency' is that the blood sugar rises to abnormally high levels.

The abnormally elevated blood sugar crosses the placenta to the baby, causing the baby's pancreas to secrete more and more insulin which in turn causes excessive foetal growth. The development of a large baby is a complication of uncontrolled GDM, leading to difficulties with normal vaginal delivery. The good news is that, with the correct treatment, complications can largely be avoided, allowing the woman with gestational diabetes to deliver a perfectly healthy, normal baby.

Prevention

The aim is to maintain the blood sugar levels of the mother in the normal range as follows:

- eat a healthy diet – eliminate sweet foods and drinks
- go for high-fibre carbohydrates such as rice, pasta, whole-wheat bread, peas, beans and lentils
- regular, small meals are recommended – aim for a weight gain in pregnancy of 10–12kg (22–26 lb)
- regular exercise helps to control blood sugar.

These measures may be all that is required for control. If blood glucose remains high, insulin injections should be used on a daily basis. The insulin will not harm the baby because it does not cross the placenta.

In most cases, GDM disappears after delivery but it is more likely to recur in subsequent pregnancies. Women can reduce their risk of developing diabetes by maintaining an ideal weight through healthy eating and regular exercise, although this may not always be the case. If they are considering having more children, they should be tested early in pregnancy for the recurrence of diabetes.

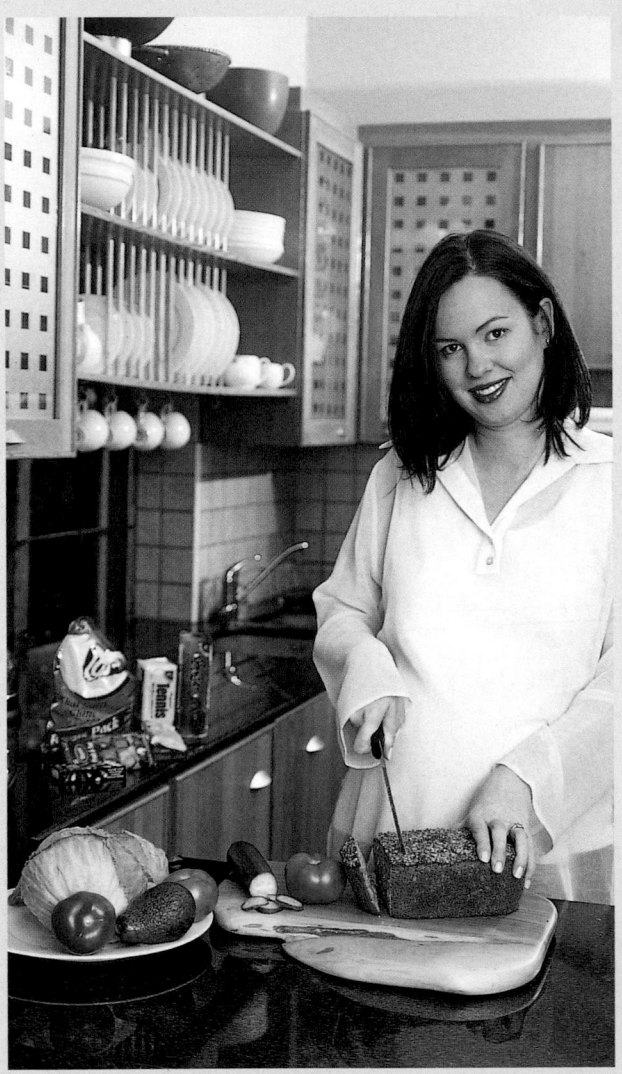

Above Opt for healthy foods such as fresh vegetables and wholewheat bread. Avoid sweet foods and drinks, especially if you have been diagnosed with gestational diabetes.

Pregnancy induced hypertension

(Also known as Pre-eclamptic Toxaemia or PET)

Pregnancy induced hypertension (PIH) is the term given for high blood pressure that occurs only in pregnancy. The blood pressure usually returns to normal within six weeks of birth. Protein is found in the urine after the 20th week of pregnancy and swelling (*see* p63) also occurs – there can be excess weight gain before the onset of PIH. Pre-eclampsia will affect approximately one in 10 pregnant women, and is more common in first-time mothers and women who are pregnant for the first time by a new partner.

There are many theories about the causes of PIH, but one possible explanation is that it is a disorder of the placenta that causes a partial failure of the blood supply, with serious knock-on effects for both mother and baby. Affected women often do not feel ill even if they have the classic signs of PIH – high blood pressure, protein in the urine and swelling of their hands, feet or face – but it is important not to miss any antenatal checkups. All pregnant women should have their blood pressure and urine tested at every visit.

Pregnancy induced hypertension reduces blood flow to multiple organs in the mother's body. If reduced blood flow occurs in the placenta, it may be fatal to the foetus. The good news, however, is that the risk of recurrence in the next pregnancy is small and if it does recur it is usually milder.

Symptoms

The following symptoms occur when the disease has progressed to a more serious stage:

- headache and visual disturbance – blurring and spots before the eyes
- vomiting
- upper abdominal pain
- reduced urination
- swollen hands, feet and face
- fits (seizures) – usually in severe cases; when it occurs it is called eclampsia
- reduced foetal movements or foetal death (due to impaired placental blood flow).

Treatment

Treatment depends on the severity of the disease, the duration of the pregnancy and the foetal condition. In some cases, the pregnancy may need to be terminated by stimulating birth, although the lung maturity of the foetus must be taken into account. The focus of the treatment is on the wellbeing of the mother and the delivery of an infant who will survive and develop normally. Delivery is therefore delayed, unless the maternal or foetal condition deteriorates.

Bed rest promotes a drop in blood pressure and improves placental blood flow and foetal wellbeing. Also, blood pressure-lowering drugs are useful in the short term to allow time for foetal growth. Steroids are given to the mother to stimulate the baby's lung maturity when the decision is made to deliver the baby.

Prevention

No major advances have been made in the prevention of PIH, but the following factors are important:

- high standards of antenatal care – regular checkups, monitoring weight, blood pressure and urine checks
- hospitalization if there is any early deviation from normal
- daily, low-dose aspirin in high-risk groups throughout pregnancy (there is no definite evidence that aspirin works)
- vitamin C is said to improve placental function, and generally helps to fight infections.

Left Citrus fruit is rich in vitamin C, which helps to build a strong placenta.

HELLP syndrome

HELLP syndrome, a combined liver and blood-clotting disorder, is one of the serious complications of pre-eclampsia and may occur any time from 17 weeks of pregnancy to six days after delivery. HELLP syndrome is more likely to occur in women who have already had children. Its name is derived from:

- **H**aemolysis (rupture of the red blood cells)
- **E**levated **L**iver enzymes in the blood (reflecting liver damage)
- **L**ow blood levels of **P**latelets (cells that are vitally important for blood clotting).

HELLP syndrome affects the mother rather than the baby, although the baby's rate of growth may be slowed. This is due to insufficient blood flow to the placenta. An early delivery is often necessary – this brings to the baby its own associated problems such as immature lungs which leads to respiratory problems.

Symptoms

The following symptoms are associated with HELPP syndrome:

- severe pain in the upper and middle abdomen, as well as to the right of the abdomen
- vomiting and headaches.

HELLP syndrome can be diagnosed with a series of blood tests to check for rupture of the blood cells, elevated liver enzymes and low blood levels of platelets. If left untreated, HELLP syndrome can lead to:

- severely disturbed blood-clotting function, which can cause heavy bleeding
- severe liver damage, which can lead to failure or even rupture of the liver
- severe kidney problems, including kidney failure
- breathing difficulties, which can become very severe
- a stroke caused by bleeding in the brain.

Because HELLP syndrome is life threatening and delivery of the baby is the only treatment, the baby is delivered as soon as the mother's condition is stable. After delivery of the baby, the mother will need to have treatment in ICU, as symptoms can become worse. Provided the mother has not suffered permanent damage, she should recover fully – often within days – although it can take up to three months.

Approximately one in 20 women who have had HELLP syndrome will suffer a recurrence in their next pregnancy. However, it is impossible to predict who is most likely to develop it again, so mothers who have had the condition in a previous pregnancy will be closely monitored. Low-dose aspirin, which acts as a preventative measure, is often prescribed in the next pregnancy.

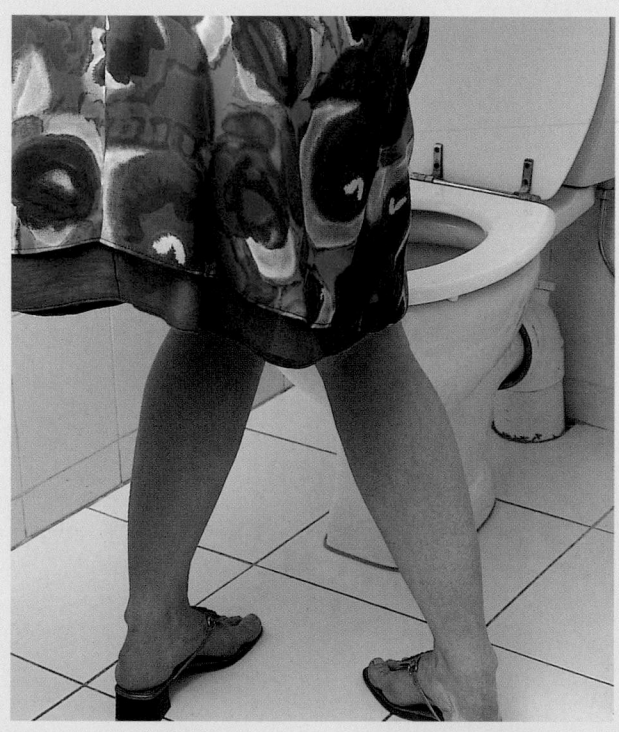

***Above** A woman who experiences persistent vomiting must report it to her caregiver, as it could be a symptom of a serious condition.*

Hyperemesis gravidarum

Vomiting that differs from morning sickness and continues throughout the day is called hyperemesis gravidarum. This may begin in the first trimester and can lead to severe weight loss and dehydration. Women who experience persistent vomiting must report it to their caregiver. Treatment may involve a short stay in hospital, where medication will be administered to relieve the vomiting and nausea, and correct the electrolyte imbalance.

Rhesus (Rh) incompatibility

The Rhesus factor (Rh) is an agglutinogen found on the surface of red blood cells. You are considered Rh positive if you have this substance, which most of the population does have. When the Rh factor is absent, the blood is classified as Rh negative. It is important to determine the Rh factor of a pregnant woman early on in the pregnancy. The presence of these antibodies is detectable through a routine blood test called a 'Coombes' test (see Glossary).

If the mother tests Rh negative and the baby is Rh positive, there is a possibility that the Rh factor from the baby could pass into the mother's bloodstream. Although the blood systems of the mother and baby are separate, blood from the baby may cross the placenta into the mother's bloodstream at the time of birth. If this is the mother's first pregnancy, it is unlikely that the foetus will be affected. If the problem was not treated, she may build up antibodies against the Rh factor. Therefore, if her subsequent pregnancy were Rh positive, there would be a strong possibility that the foetus could be harmed when the mother's antibodies cross the placental barrier into the foetus's bloodstream and cause jaundice, anaemia, heart failure and brain damage.

To avoid this, the Rh-negative mother would be given an injection of Rh immune globulin each time she delivered an Rh-positive baby. Even if the mother lost the baby through miscarriage or abortion, she would need to receive this immune globulin, as there is a possibility that the foetus could have been Rh positive.

If a mother is Rh positive, the amount of antibodies in her blood system have to be monitored throughout her pregnancy to check if she has become sensitized to the Rh factor. Depending on the outcome of the results, treatments will be decided upon and may vary from early delivery or, in some extremely rare cases, an intra-uterine blood transfusion.

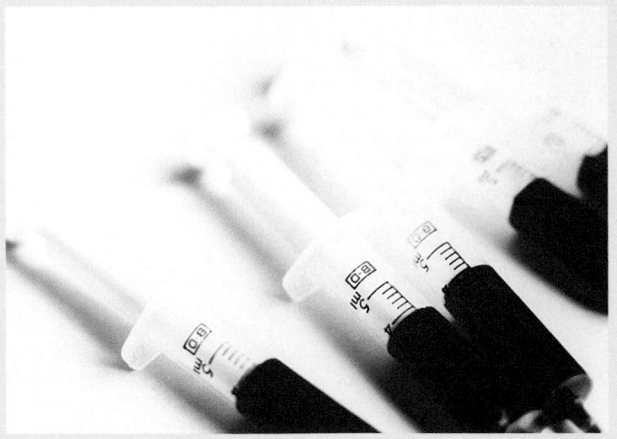

Above The Rhesus factor of both mother and foetus is tested for compatibility as part of the routine blood tests.

Multiple pregnancy

Any pregnancy where more than one foetus are present is considered a multiple pregnancy. If a history of twins exists in your family or if you have gained weight rapidly and your uterine growth has exceeded the normal rate, these would be signs of possible multiple birth.

The most common kind of multiple birth is twins, occurring about once in every 90 pregnancies. With multiple births, both the mother and the foetuses are at increased risk for certain problems. Early diagnosis is crucial and the mother's progress will be closely monitored. Routine checkups and ultrasound scans will be more frequent than usual. Proper eating habits and good nutrition are of prime importance. Preterm labour and delivery are more common, and the delivery options are limited due to complications associated with multiple birth (all depending on the position of the foetuses). There is a greater chance of a Caesarean birth.

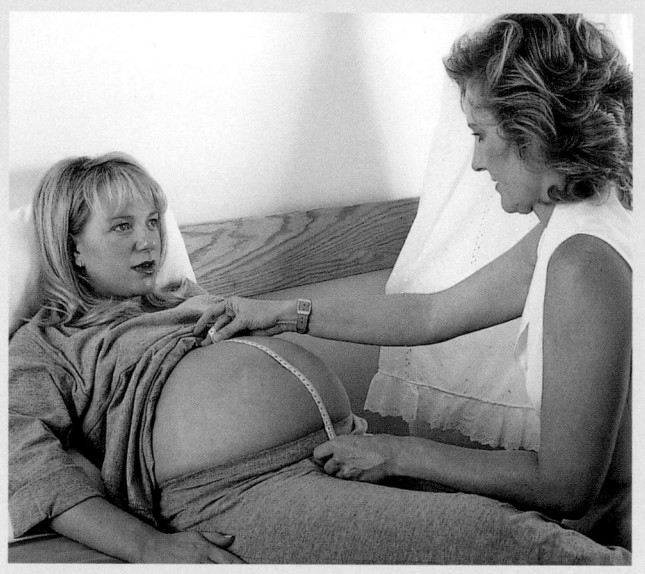

Above *When expecting multiples (twins, triplets, etc.), the rate of growth of the uterus will be faster than normal.*

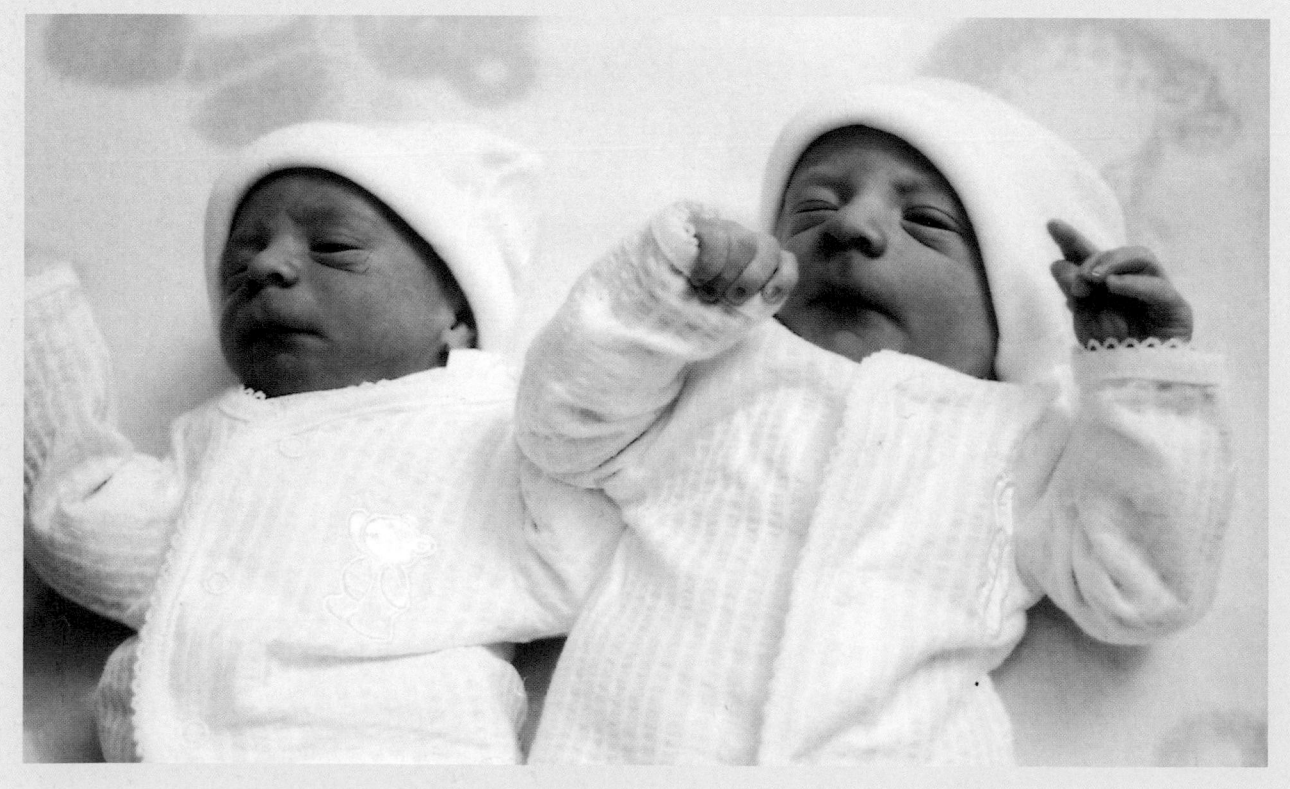

Sexually transmitted diseases

Sexually transmitted diseases (STDs) can affect a woman's chance of conceiving and, if acquired during pregnancy, can infect and even harm the foetus. STDs are more likely to occur if a woman has more than one sexual partner. If a woman suspects that she may have an STD, it is imperative that she seeks medical treatment as soon as possible. Her partner will also have to be treated. It is important to remember that the use of condoms and spermicides can lower the risk of contracting a sexually transmitted disease.

Syphilis

This is still a highly contagious and very dangerous disease that can cause tremendous damage to the foetus such as blindness, problems with the nervous system, skin, bones, liver, lungs and spleen. It is usually easier to detect in men, as a sore is likely to appear on the penis and is visible. With women, however, a sore may be inside the vagina where it remains unnoticed. Besides the sore being a sign of the disease, diagnosis can also be made from a blood test, which is routine in the antenatal period. Receiving treatment as soon as possible will decrease the chances of the baby suffering more damage, but may not reverse any damage that has already been done.

Chlamydia, Gonorrhea and Pelvic Inflammatory Disease (PID)

These are severe infections that start in the vagina and can spread to the cervix and the entire pelvic area involving the uterus, the fallopian tubes and the ovaries. Often women with these infections have no symptoms and will only be alerted to the problem when their partner is diagnosed; men will experience a penis that 'drips'. If the foetus is infected with chlamydia or gonorrhea during the birth, eye infections as well as other serious problems could result.

Herpes simplex virus

This virus causes genital herpes. Sores and blisters develop around the sex organs and the infection is transmitted through sexual contact with a person who has 'active' sores. Some people may be fortunate enough to experience only one outbreak, others, however, may have repeated outbreaks. Should a mother have signs of an active infection close to delivery, the doctor may consider a Caesarean birth, as this will avoid the chances of the baby coming into contact with the virus in the vagina. The foetus could suffer from skin infections, blindness, mental retardation and damage to the nervous system if it were to become infected.

Human Immuno-deficiency Virus (HIV) or AIDS

HIV causes AIDS and it is a huge concern for any sexually active woman, especially a pregnant one. HIV destroys the body's natural defence, the immune system, thereby leaving the body open and susceptible to very harmful infections that will eventually cause that person to die. The infection is there for life and in most cases it is fatal.

HIV is spread via body fluids such as semen and blood either through sexual contact or infected blood, as well as infected needles used for intravenous drugs.

The virus may spread to the foetus through the mother's blood during pregnancy, as the virus is able to cross the placenta before birth. It is also present in breast milk and a mother needs to know that she could pass the virus onto her baby should she become infected soon after the delivery.

If you have used intravenous drugs or had sexual contact with someone who has multiple partners, you are at risk of being infected with the HIV.

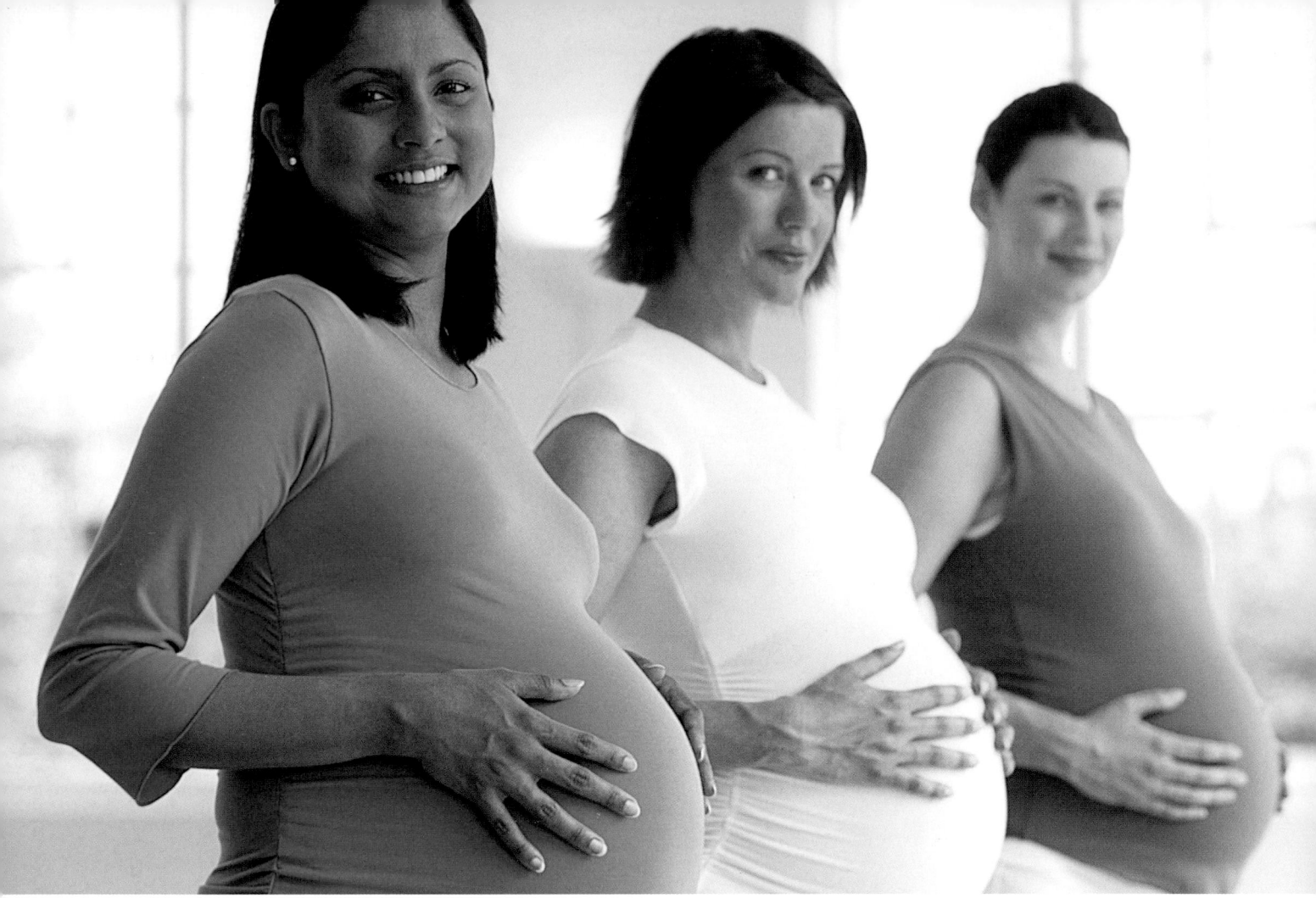

The trimesters of pregnancy

Pregnancy has a profound effect on a woman's body. The moment the egg and sperm fuse, the body swings into action to protect and nurture this life. The body changes in response to the pregnancy hormones, and the foetus develops from the union of two tiny cells into a fully formed baby within 280 days. Pregnancy is divided into three trimesters – doctors and mid-wives talk about the progress of pregnancy in 'weeks' while mothers talk about the 'months' of pregnancy. The first trimester is a vital phase as this is when your baby is developing. It is most vulnerable to harmful substances, as well as viruses and illnesses experienced by the mother.

WITHIN 280 DAYS, THE UNION OF TWO TINY CELLS DEVELOP INTO A FULLY FORMED BABY

The most critical time

The sperm and egg combine to form the zygote – the very first stage of human life. The most striking advances occur during the first two months. During this time, the developing human is called an embryo and the period is referred to as the embryonic period. At the end of this sensitive period, all the major structures are present.

The development of the embryo is most easily disturbed during the organogenetic period – the stage of formation and development of the organs – especially between days 13 and 60. Although the embryo is well protected in the uterus, certain agents called 'teratogens' (see p74) may cause congenital malformations. Each developing organ has a critical period during which it is highly sensitive (see pp32–33). We now know that the embryo is extremely vulnerable to radiation, viruses and certain drugs during the first trimester. Radiation tends to cause abnormalities of the central nervous system and eyes, and it causes mental retardation. The rubella virus, which is more commonly referred to as 'German measles', causes mainly cataract, deafness and cardiac malformation.

***Below** A brief representation of fertilization, cell division and implantation that takes place in the female reproductive system.*

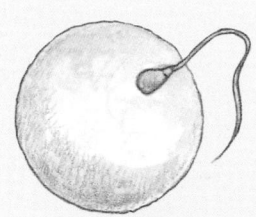

FERTILIZATION
One sperm out of millions reaches the egg, penetrates it and creates a barrier to all the other sperm. This is when fertilization takes place.

CELL DIVISION

Two cell
The fertilized egg is called a 'zygote' and the cell of the egg divides into two.

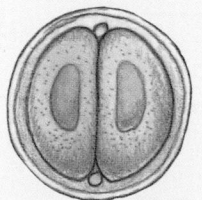

Four cell
The cells continue to divide and the cluster of cells is called a 'morula'.

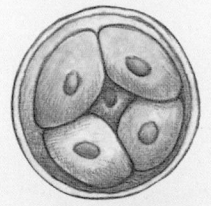

Sixteen cell
The cells continue to divide and form a ball, which develops into a blastocyst.

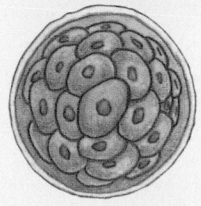

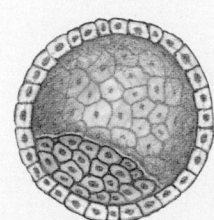

The cells of the blastocyst move to one side and a fluid sac is formed on the other side.

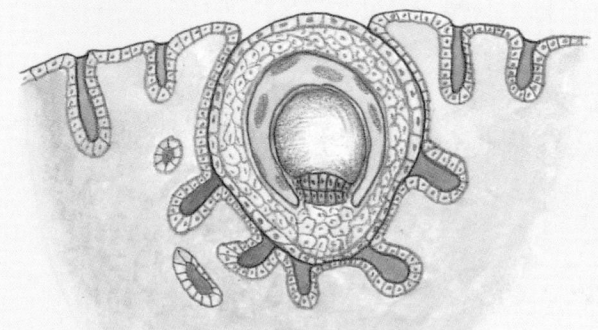

IMPLANTATION
The blastocyst moves down to the uterus and implants itself in the uterine wall, where it gets its nourishment and continues to develop from a ball of cells into a fully formed baby. Implantation occurs from day seven to day 12 after fertilization.

Sensitive areas in a developing embryo/foetus

The most sensitive period in a baby's development is in the first 12 weeks of its life. During this time, the baby's organs and brain are developing. After three months, fine-tuning of all these structures takes place, so it is important that a mother-to-be develops a good awareness of her environment, and also of what she eats, drinks and inhales during the entire pregnancy. The health of this future human being is decided during this time, so look after yourself in every way.

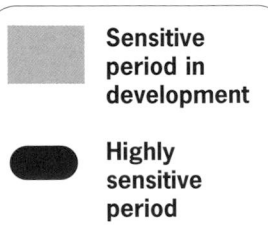

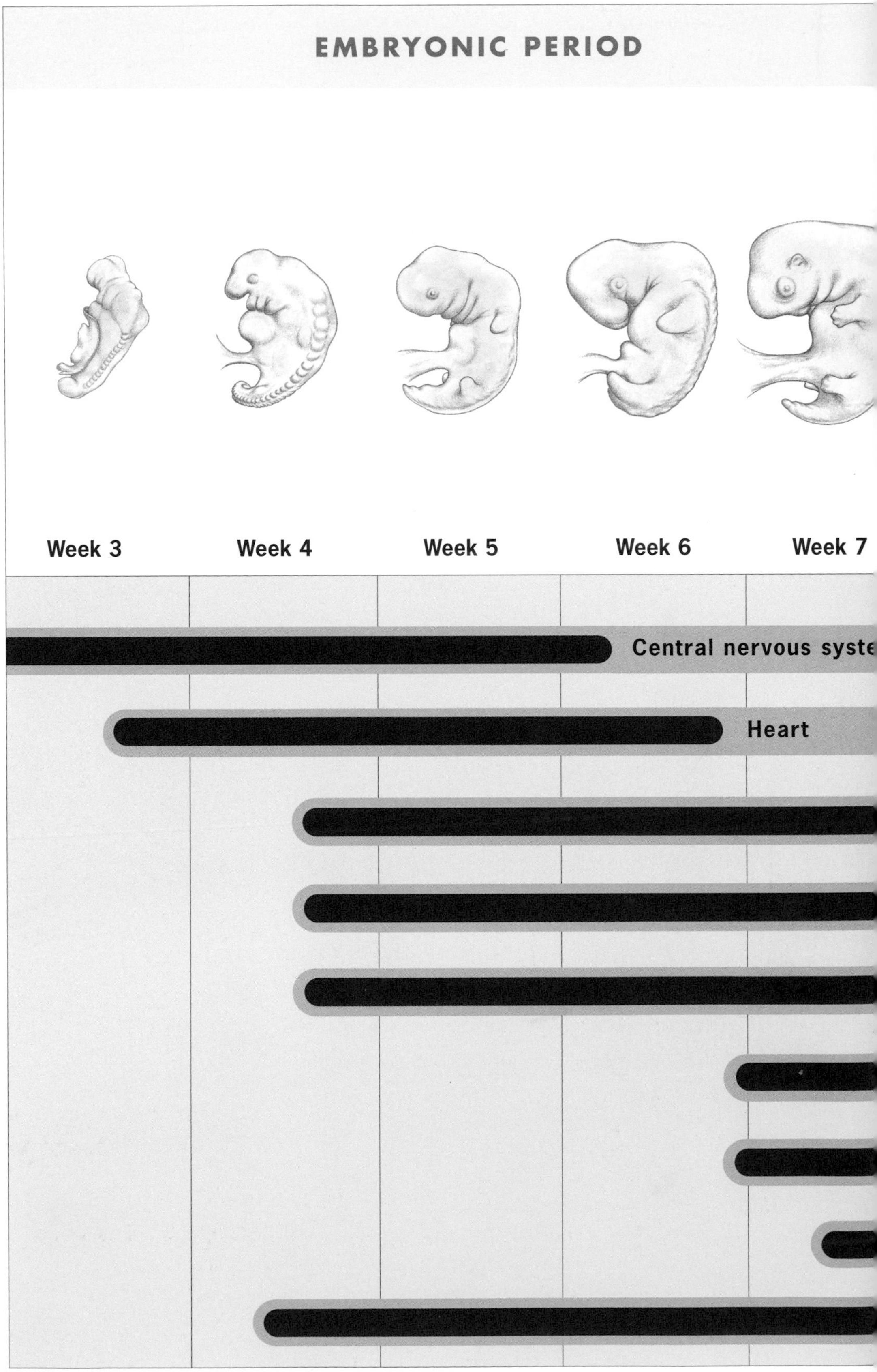

Sensitive period in development

Highly sensitive period

EMBRYONIC PERIOD

| Week 3 | Week 4 | Week 5 | Week 6 | Week 7 |

Central nervous syste

Heart

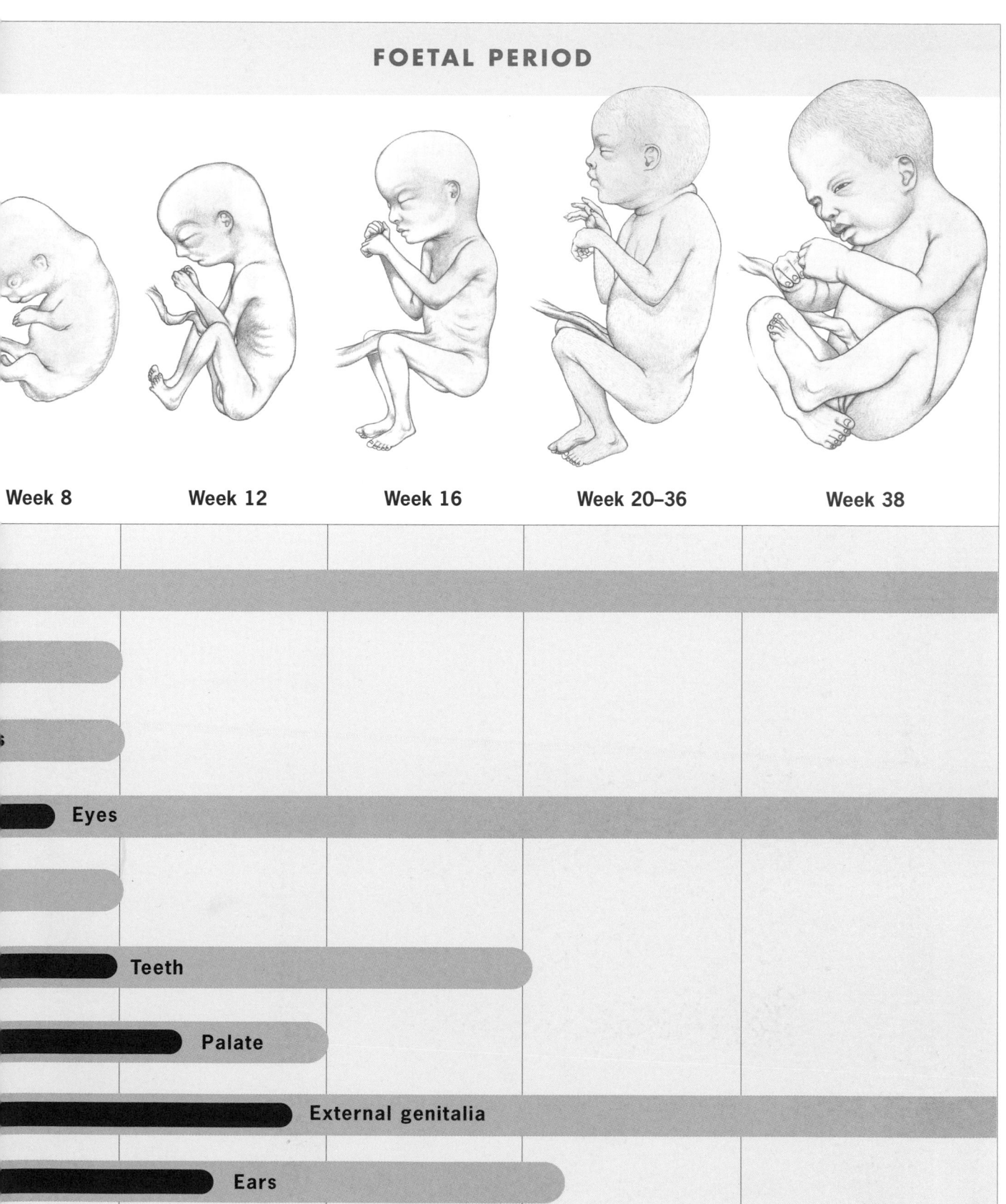

FOETAL PERIOD

| Week 8 | Week 12 | Week 16 | Week 20–36 | Week 38 |

Eyes

Teeth

Palate

External genitalia

Ears

Month one – weeks 0–4

Baby's world

In the first two weeks following conception, the fertilized egg becomes a ball of cells which resembles a bunch of berries and is called a 'morula'. These cells change continually in preparation for their individual functions. As this continues, the morula becomes a blasto-cyst which floats down the fallopian tube and implants itself in the lining of the uterus. Once implantation has taken place, the blastocyst divides into two groups of cells: one group will develop into the placenta and the other group into your baby.

Things are very different from the third week onward. The flat appearance of the one group of cells gives way to a tubular structure as the embryo takes on a different shape. The long groove of the neural tube opens up – this is where the spinal cord will develop. One side of the tube curves to form the brain and small clumps appear on either side of the groove where the vertebrae and the muscles will form.

In the fourth week, the two tubes of the heart fuse and by the 22nd day they will start to contract. During this week, the neural tube will 'zip' itself close – this is a crucial time because two of the most important organs are being fine-tuned. The arms and upper body develop faster than the legs. By the end of week four, the embryo weighs 0.4g (0.01oz) and is approximately the size of a grain of rice. In the first month, most women are not even aware of their pregnancy, although some may be suspicious.

rectum

uterus

developing baby

cervix

bladder

urethra

vagina

anus

Mom's world

Signs of pregnancy can appear within a few days of conception. If you suspect that you are pregnant, buy an over-the-counter pregnancy test or have your blood drawn at a laboratory or doctor's rooms for testing. A blood test is more accurate than a urine test if done very early; a urine test is most accurate after the first missed period. If you are

Left In the first month, although there are many changes occurring at cellular level in the mother's body, nothing is visible externally.

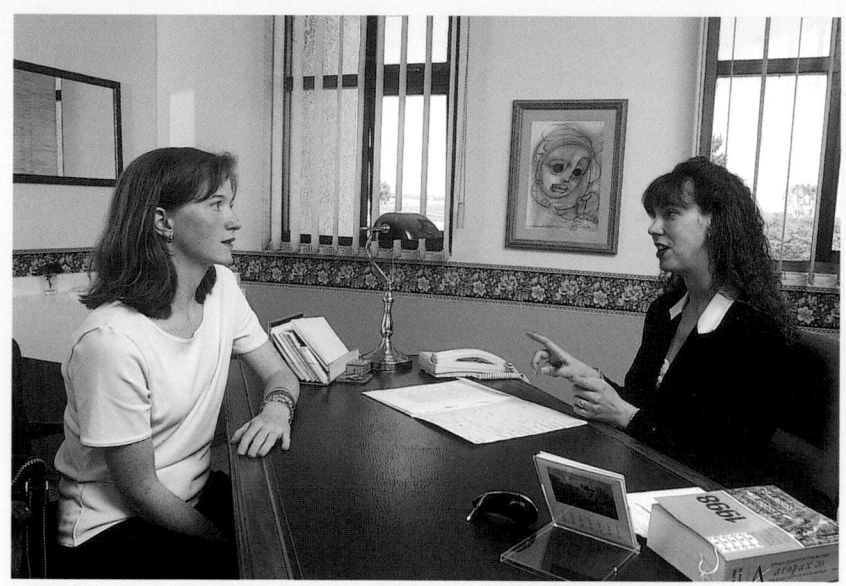

pregnant, you may begin to feel nauseous, tired, hungry and need to visit the toilet more often. Most women usually have their pregnancy confirmed six weeks after their last menstrual period (LMP).

Must do

- Book your first antenatal checkup.
- Slow down and start to take things easy, even though you may not 'feel' pregnant.
- Find out about maternity programmes.
- Watch what you eat, drink and inhale.
- Take a folic acid supplement.

Nice to do

- Speak to your mother about her experiences during her pregnancies.
- See what maternity clothes are available; do not buy any clothes just yet.
- Go through your wardrobe and find your 'biggish' clothes that you can use as maternity clothes in the later stages of your pregnancy.

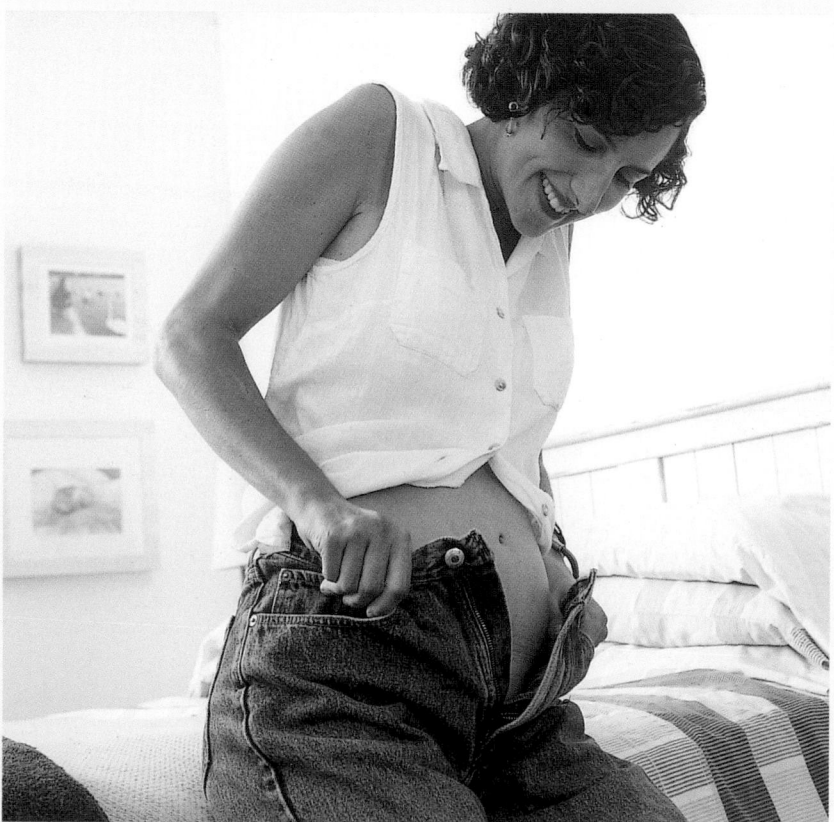

Above left It is wise to immediately book your first antenatal checkup when your pregnancy has been confirmed.

Left As you pass the four-month mark, you may find that your clothes start to become a little tight and uncomfortable.

Month two – weeks 5–8

Baby's world

During the second month, the embryo grows in size and will be about as big as an M&M or a Smartie. The arms and legs grow longer and slight curves appear where your baby's elbows and knees will be. Tiny 'fans' spread across the ends of the limbs where the hands and feet will develop. Cartilage forms from tissue for the fingers and toes, and the palate of the mouth is also forming at this stage. The embryo has gill-like structures that will become your baby's jaw, neck and face. Nerve channels and muscles link up and the tiny embryo starts to move. The primitive heart starts to bulge, and bone condenses out of tissue and is laid down over the cartilage.

The cardiovascular system is the first system to function. The development of your baby's heart is highly sensitive between the third and sixth week. At first, the heart simply pushes blood back and forth but by the 25th day, it is beating and moving the blood in one direction. Blood circulates between the embryo, yolk sac and the newly forming umbilical cord.

In the seventh and eighth week, the upper lip and nostrils develop on the face and the ears have now moved to the side of the head and are surrounded by a simple flap of skin. The eyes, while still set wide apart, move closer to the centre of the face and become pigmented. During this time, the rubella virus can affect the eyes.

The internal organs are becoming more defined and the sex organs are forming. It is still impossible at this stage to see if the embryo is a boy or a girl.

The arms, legs, fingers and toes become more defined, and the muscles in the neck and body begin to contract spontaneously, although the mother will not feel any movements. The embryo is now about the size of a two-peanut shell when measured from head to buttocks. The legs are still too short to be taken into this measurement. At the end of the second month, the embryo measures 8mm (0.31in) in length and weighs about 2g (0.07oz).

This marks the end of the embryonic period and also the end of the time when most birth defects are likely to occur.

The concern for most women is that this is usually when their pregnancy is confirmed and the baby's most vital parts have already developed. This is why pre-conceptual

Left The human embryo resembles a chicken embryo as the baby's tiny body starts to take shape.

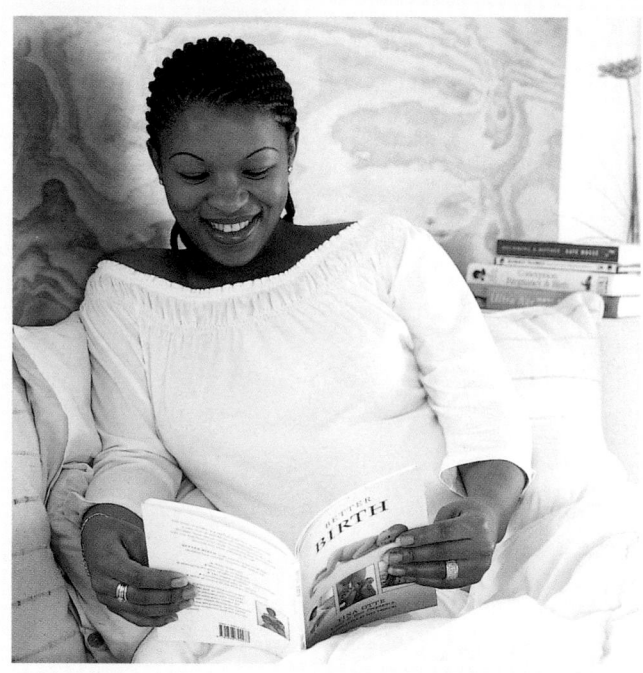

Above *Read books on pregnancy and birth to help you understand the changes your body is going through in preparation for childbirth.*

planning is so important. It allows you to be vigilant for any potentially harmful substances that could spoil your baby's chances of developing normally.

Mom's world

At this time, you should be noticing some subtle changes in your body. You may be feeling heavy and bloated – similar to the way you feel when you are expecting your period. Your uterus is about the size of an orange and your metabolism, breathing and heart rate increase due to the increased blood volume. Flatulence is a common complaint, but it can be a real problem in the first trimester – there is a tendency to swallow a lot of air in an attempt to relieve feelings of nausea. Your sense of smell may become more acute, and you may develop an aversion to certain foods and cigarette smoke. A scan at six to seven weeks will show the pregnancy sac and heart movement, and at eight weeks multiples (twins, triplets, etc.) would be identifiable.

Must do

- Consider what foods make you feel nauseous and avoid them.
- Go for your first checkup and enjoy seeing your baby on the ultrasound scan.
- Stop using tampons and notify your caregiver if you have any itching or burning in the vagina.
- Sleep whenever you can and take time out in the office to stretch; do this away from your desk.
- Talk to your doctor about tests that need to be conducted.
- Take brisk walks in the early evening or morning to increase your energy.

Nice to do

- Buy a book on pregnancy and birth.
- Dig out old toys and children's books, if you have any.
- Spend some time with your friends who have children.

The foetal period begins at about eight weeks after fertilization and ends at birth. This is a period of rapid body growth and maturation of the organ systems. The changes that occur in the foetal period are not as dramatic as those in the embryonic period, but they are very important. The foetus is less vulnerable to the teratogenic effects of drugs, viruses and radiation but these agents may interfere with normal functional development, especially of the brain.

Month three – weeks 9–13

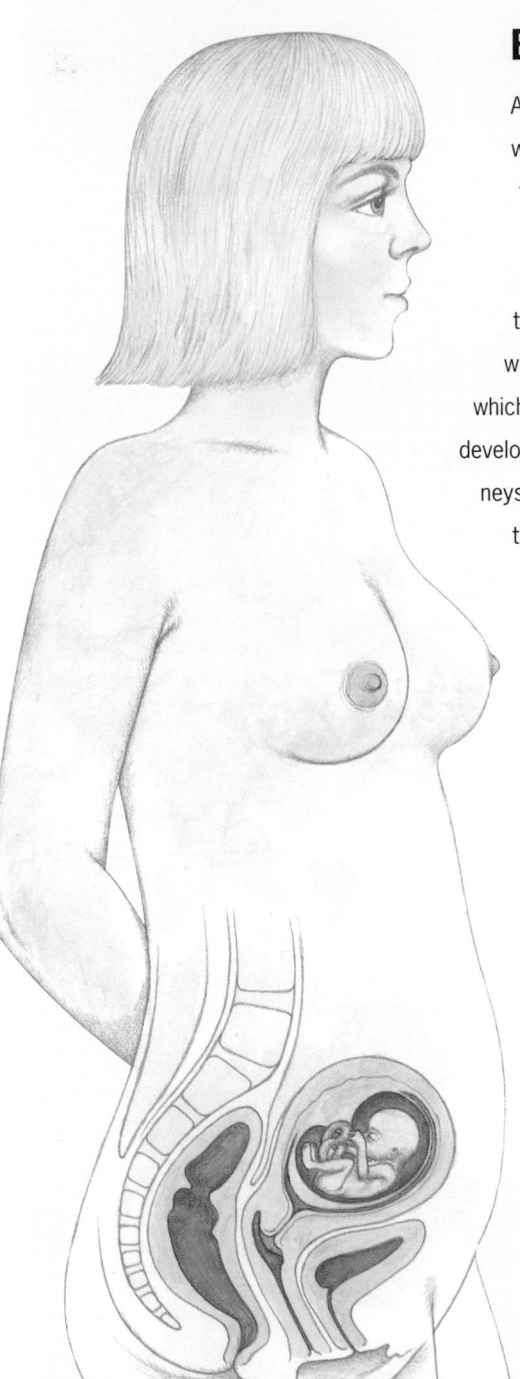

Baby's world

As the third month starts, the foetus is already floating in amniotic fluid (*see* Glossary) with its head bobbing and its tiny body bent forward. The umbilical cord connects the foetus to the mother as it grows and develops. The muscles of the neck become stronger and it pulls itself up a little straighter. The face is still forming: the eyes have some colour, the mouth has a tongue with taste buds developing on it (your baby can taste the amniotic fluid) and there are 20 buds in the gums for future teeth. The foetus will open its mouth and start to suck its fingers. The eyelids grow and cover the eyes, which are usually closed until sometime during the sixth month. The hands and feet are well developed at this stage, and the fingers and toes have soft nails by the ninth week. The kidneys are functioning and secrete urine into the bladder. Amniotic fluid flows into and out of the lungs, and the diaphragm begins to move in preparation for breathing. At the beginning of the third month, bone growth begins in earnest and the sexual organs are well developed, but it is still impossible to tell the gender of the foetus. By week 12, your baby starts to swallow amniotic fluid. The framework for all the organs, limbs, muscles and bones is already in place. The foetus weighs about 16g (0.6oz) and measures 9cm (3.5in) from head to rump.

Mom's world

You will notice that your abdomen is starting to swell slightly and your waistline will start to become a little less defined – you may have gained some weight. Your uterus is growing and moving outward above your pelvic bone, and your breasts are getting bigger. You may experience feelings of dizziness, as there is a drop in your blood sugar levels. You may feel hotter than usual and your hands are always warm due to the increase in blood circulation. Although you may be feeling less nauseous, your moods may not yet improve and do not be surprised to find yourself a little more emotional at this time. Rapid mood swings, irritability and feelings of ambivalence are very common, even if the pregnancy was planned.

Left Feeling lethargic is common as you approach the end of the first trimester. Outwardly, you may notice slight changes to your body but no-one else will.

Routine checks will once again be done at your 12-week appointment and a scan may also be done. If a Doppler device is used, you will hear your baby's heartbeat, which is much faster than yours.

Must do

- Get advice on diet and exercise. Pregnancy is not a time to lose weight, but weight control is an issue.
- Do not take any medication that has not been prescribed by your caregiver.
- Cut out alcohol and cigarettes.
- Avoid undercooked or raw eggs. Be aware that paté and ripe soft cheese can carry the risk of salmonella or listeria infection (see p74). Limit the amount of liver you eat as it contains large amounts of vitamin A (see p75).
- Ask about your rights at work and available maternity benefits.
- Give in to the messages from your body telling you to rest and put your feet up.

Nice to do

- Start planning the changes to your baby's room.
- Rest as much as possible – eliminate unnecessary chores and ask for help when you need it.
- Read a novel that has nothing to do with pregnancy.
- Have someone take a photograph of you now that you are at the end of your first trimester.

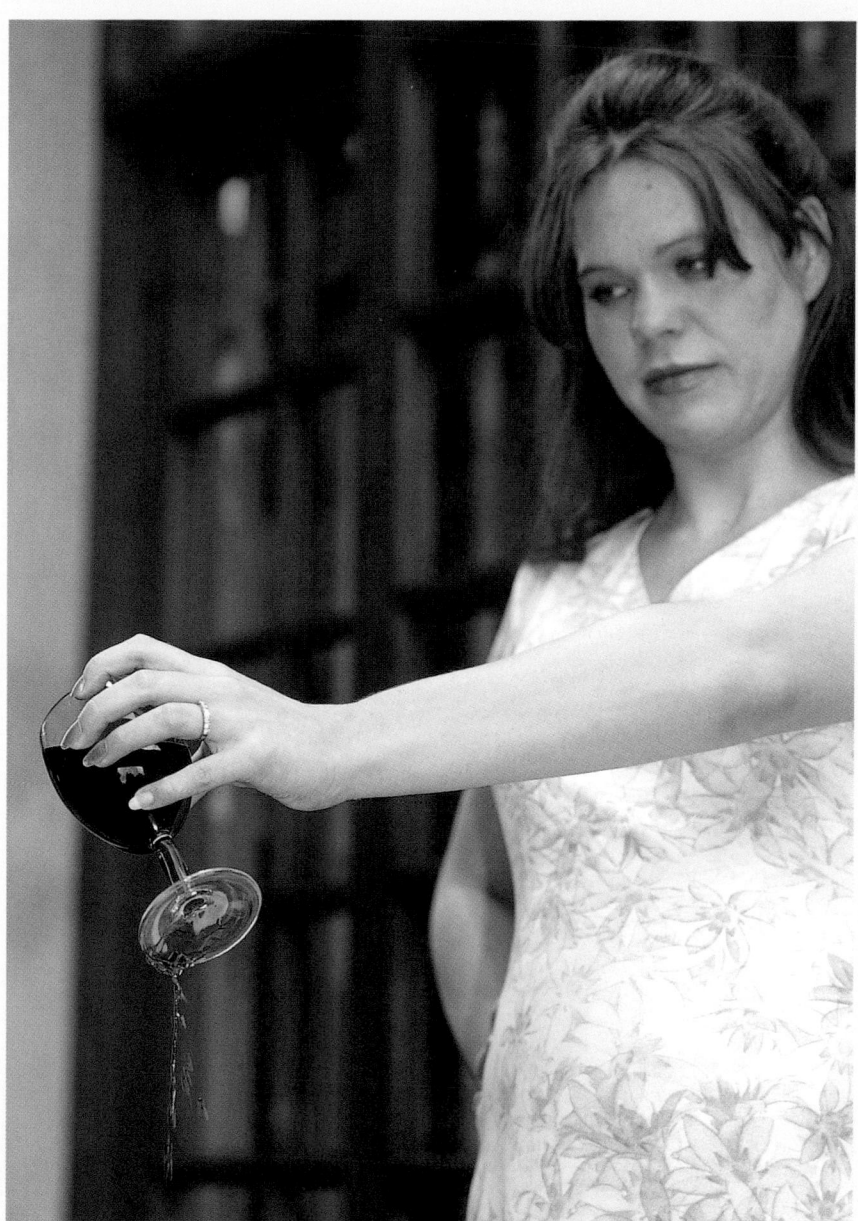

Above With alcohol there is no particular 'safe' limit and the most sensible approach is to avoid it altogether.

Month four – weeks 14–17

Baby's world

By now the risk of major malformations is over. The rate of your baby's growth during this month is rapid, but weight gain is slow. From the 12th to the 16th week, your baby's diaphragm moves up and down as if breathing, however, this is not the case; the movement will disappear until the third trimester. The nerve cells in the brain reach their maximum number and the heartbeat is very strong. The fingers are longer and become more tapered, and the skin is completely transparent and underlying blood vessels are visible. Complex movements of the lips, sucking and facial expressions are present. Fine hair called 'lanugo' is growing on your baby's upper lip and eyebrows. The legs will be longer than the arms at the end of this month. The organs start to round out the stomach, but the limbs are lean and lanky. The eyes and ears are now in their correct place on your baby's face and head respectively. The foetus measures about 25cm (10in) from head to heel and weighs approximately 227g (8oz) – just less than a small brick of margarine.

From about 14 weeks of foetal development, the epidermis will be invaded by melanocytes (a cell that contains melanin), which will determine your baby's skin colour.

Mom's world

Your pregnancy is becoming more obvious and you are probably wearing your 'big' clothes, but not yet maternity clothing. Your hormone levels should stabilize and you should find your energy levels picking up. Your hair may be thicker and have a healthy shine, and your skin may be better or worse than usual. Your nails may grow longer and be stronger than usual.

At your 16-week checkup, routine tests and observations will be done and a thorough scan is done to detect the presence of abnormalities. An AFP test (see p19) can be done in this month, which can indicate the risk of having a baby with spina bifida. You may notice an increase in your libido between now and the fifth month of pregnancy.

Left You may be looking and feeling 'fat' as you move into the second trimester, and your pregnancy will soon be obvious.

Must do

- Notify your employer of your pregnancy if you have not already done so.
- Make sure your working environment is safe to avoid accidents.
- Start thinking about the birth you would like. Although this may seem very early to do so, it is best not to leave things for the last minute.
- Enrol in an antenatal exercise class. This is great because everyone in the class is going through similar changes and experiences.

Nice to do

- Start playing soothing music in your car and at home. If possible, you could also play soft music at work.
- Have a facial or massage or even a foot massage. Your skin may be a little dry or perhaps oily.

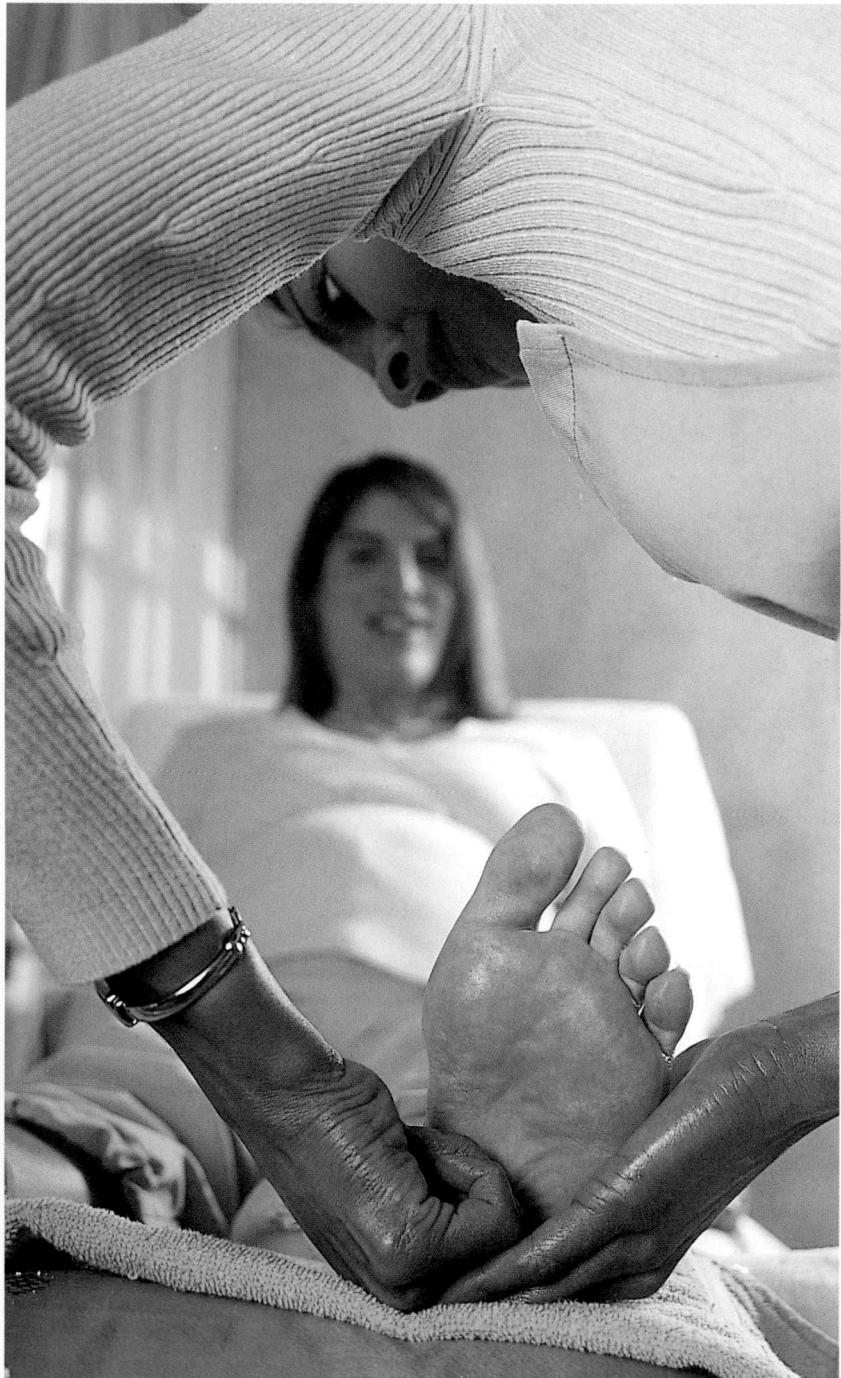

Right A professional foot massage or reflexology session can help alleviate many of the common 'niggles' of pregnancy.

Month five – weeks 18–21

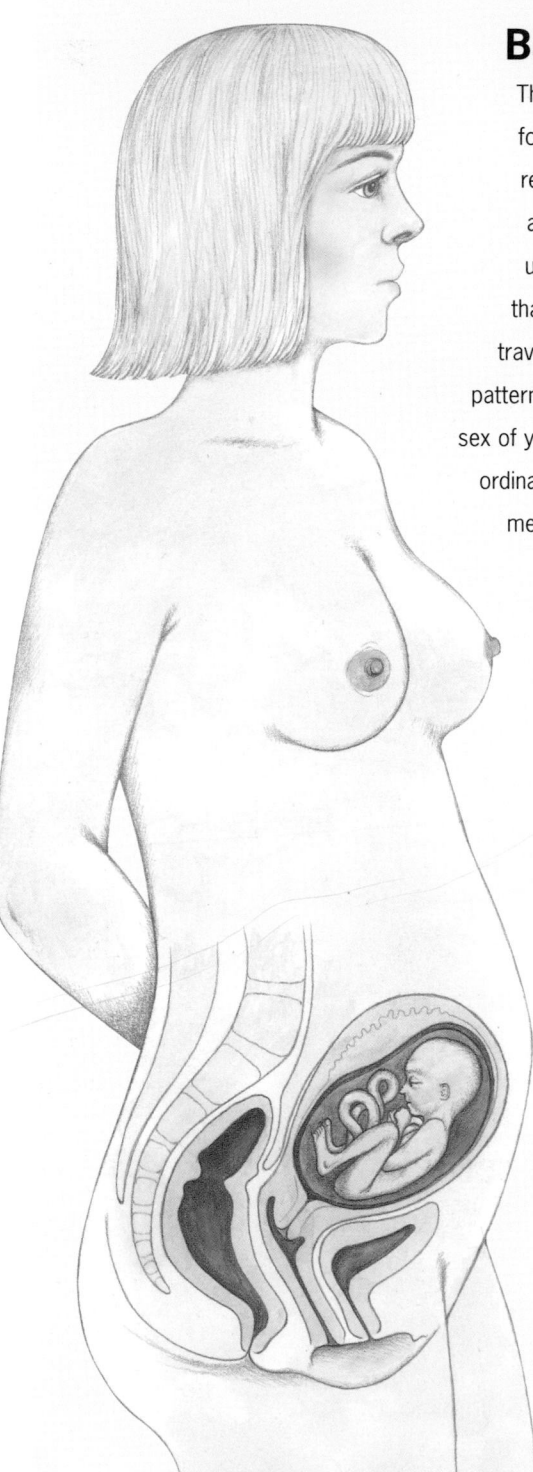

Baby's world

The sebaceous (oil) glands begin to function. Together with the dead skin cells of the foetus, they form the white cheese-like substance called *vernix caseosa*, which is responsible for making your baby 'waterproof' during pregnancy. The entire body is now also covered with lanugo. This is the midpoint of the pregnancy, and your baby continues to mature and gain weight. The baby adds brown fat, which is rich in cell structures that turn fat directly into energy. The brain is still developing furiously, and nerve signals travel faster on their trips to and from the brain. Your baby begins to acquire regular sleep patterns. Its own primitive immune system is developing. Your doctor may be able to tell the sex of your baby from a scan at this time. Your baby's movements are stronger and more co-ordinated due to a maturing nervous system. He or she weighs about 450g (16oz) and measures approximately 30cm (12in) from head to heel at the end of the fifth month.

Mom's world

You are now sporting a proper bump! Your breasts have undergone some changes: the areolae become darker and the nipples enlarged. The blood vessels under your skin are more prominent due to an increased blood flow, and you may have noticed that your gums and nasal passages are swollen and congested. These are common effects of the pregnancy hormones. A dark line known as the *linea nigra* may become visible in the area from your navel to your pubic hairline. Chloasma, often referred to as the 'mask of pregnancy', may appear. These are small, dark patches of pigmentation on the face and can be worsened by exposure to the sun. At the end of this month, you may feel your baby move for the first time and you will become aware of gentle contractions from the uterus known as 'Braxton-Hicks' contractions (*see* p64). In fact, the uterus contracts gently from the start of pregnancy but you only feel something from about 16 to 20 weeks.

Left At this stage, your doctor may be able to tell you the sex of your baby if you wish to know it.

Must do

- Schedule an appointment with your dentist if you have not already done so. Owing to the need for extra calcium, you are more likely to experience problems with your teeth.
- Note the date that you feel your baby move for the first time.
- Keep all your antenatal checkup appointments.
- Watch your posture (*see* p84) – bad posture can lead to back-ache which is common because your centre of gravity changes.
- Book into childbirth education classes.
- Investigate where you plan to give birth.

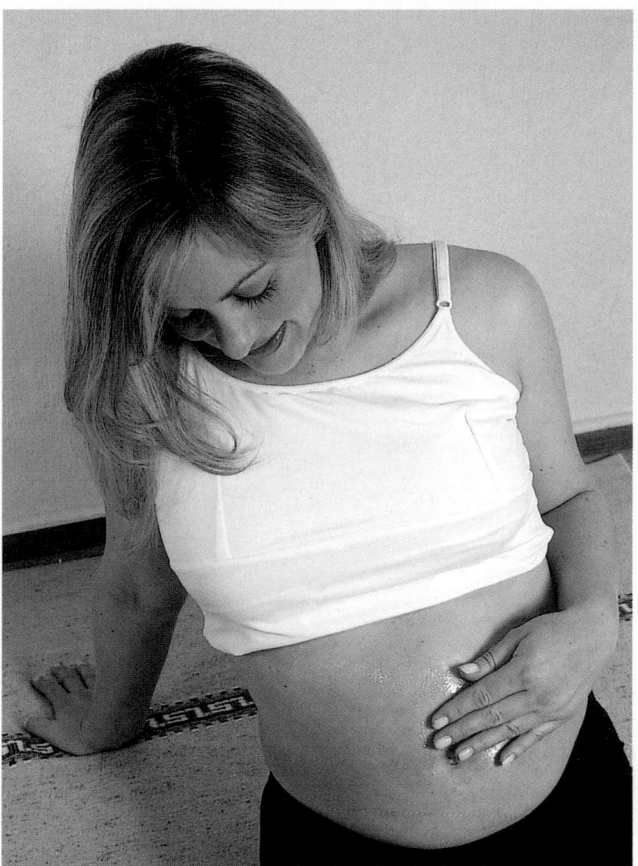

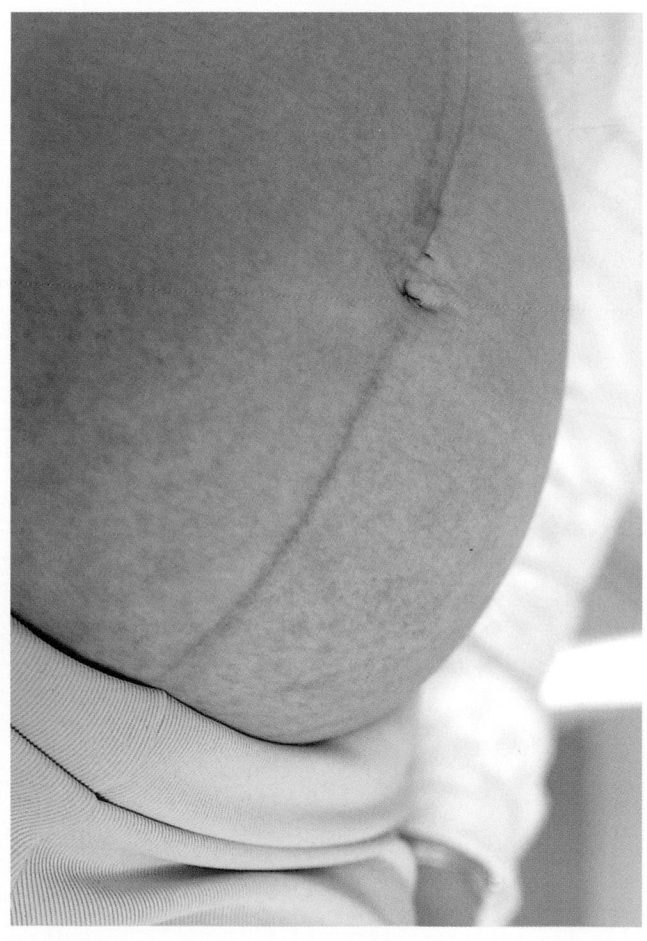

Above From the fifth month onward, you will most certainly feel your baby move – this is known as 'quickening'.

Left By the fifth month, you will notice a dark line running down from your navel to the pubic hairline called the linea nigra.

Nice to do

- Take your mom with you to an antenatal checkup.
- Start sorting photographs of yourself and your partner when you both were babies.
- Collect newspaper clippings of important events that occur during your pregnancy.

Month six – weeks 22–26

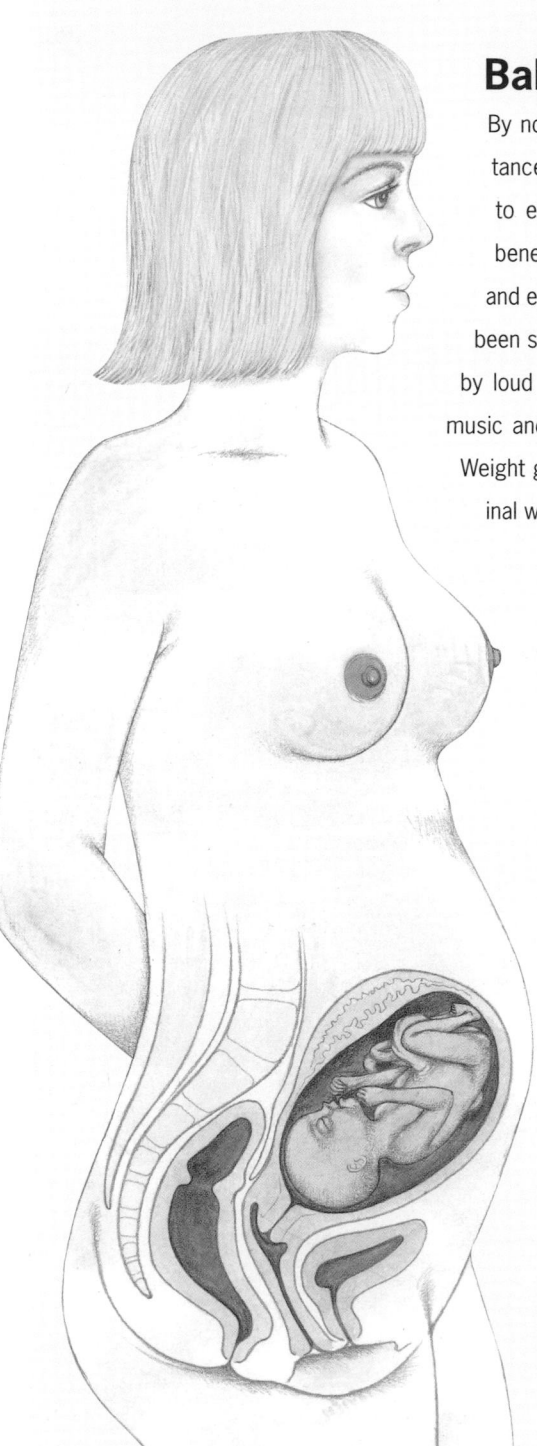

Baby's world

By now the foetus may be able to survive outside the womb (with a lot of medical assistance!). At 24 weeks, the lungs start to produce surfactant – a substance that helps them to expand and take in air – and display breathing movements. There is very little fat beneath the skin, so the foetus looks old and wrinkled. Hair starts to grow on the head, and eyebrows and eyelashes start to appear. Your baby is able to form a fist and many have been seen, on scan, playing with the umbilical cord. By this stage, most foetuses are startled by loud noises. Your baby is also remembering sounds and storing primitive memories of music and the sound of her mother's voice – more evidence of a maturing nervous system. Weight gain speeds up and different parts of her body will be identifiable through the abdominal wall. The foetus weighs about 500g (18oz) and measures about 35cm (14in) in length.

Mom's world

Your waistline continues to disappear as your uterus moves up even more. Your hands and feet may be swollen, especially at the end of each day, and leg cramps can be a problem. Your breasts may have started to leak a small amount of colostrum – a thin, milky secretion that precedes and follows lactation – and you may also have noticed that your pelvis feels a little 'loose'. This is due to the softening effect of the pregnancy hormones on your joints and ligaments. You may find that you have gone up a shoe size. Your navel starts to flatten and pops inside out, and the skin on your abdomen starts to itch as it stretches. Your 24-week checkup includes routine observations.

You are now more than halfway through your pregnancy and you will, at this stage, be far more aware of your baby's movements, and sleep and wake cycles. For some women, the second half of pregnancy may seem very much longer than the first.

Left Your baby's sense of hearing is well developed at this time. Start playing some classical music in your car or environment to stimulate this sense.

Must do

- Buy safe and soothing aromatherapy oil and get a professional foot and hand massage to help ease the swelling.
- Keep your skin well lubricated and hydrated because stretch marks can occur from now. This should be a part of your daily routine whether you are pregnant or not.
- Put your tired, hot feet into some cool water every day.
- Drink water according to your level of thirst. Rather sip small amounts so that your body absorbs the fluids, instead of letting it just pass through your system.
- Do not drink fluids with too much sugar or fizz.

Nice to do

- Get advice on your baby layette before spending a fortune.
- Start planning your baby's nursery in more detail.
- Go to a relaxation class.
- Get a photograph taken as you complete the second trimester.

Right Apply mosturizer to your whole body; pay special attention to the hips, thighs, abdomen and buttocks.

Month seven – weeks 27–30

Baby's world

Your baby's expanding brain begins to wrinkle to allow even more grey matter into the skull. The foetus can, at this stage, regulate her body temperature and spends 70–80 per cent of her time in REM sleep – equivalent to our dream-state sleep. Her eyes, ears and other organs are stimulated: the eyes open and close and develop the ability to focus. The sense of hearing also grows. Your baby's heart rate and blood pressure changes. More fat is being laid down, smoothing out and filling out wrinkly skin. Tetracycline treatment during the second and third trimesters of pregnancy may cause minor tooth defects and yellow or brown discoloration of the teeth, and distortion of bone growth. Her total weight at this stage is about 2kg (4.4 lb) and she has grown to a length of approximately 40cm (16in).

Mom's world

You may be feeling more breathless because the expanding uterus pushes up against your diaphragm. Backache is more likely to plague you now, so concentrate on good posture and regular exercise (*see* pp78–87). You will have trouble sleeping comfortably and Braxton-Hicks contractions become more intense and really get your attention. Take this opportunity to relax, breathe with awareness and release any other tension (*see* p93) in your body.

Left The sense of touch is a very dominant sensation and you should rub your abdomen and massage your unborn baby.

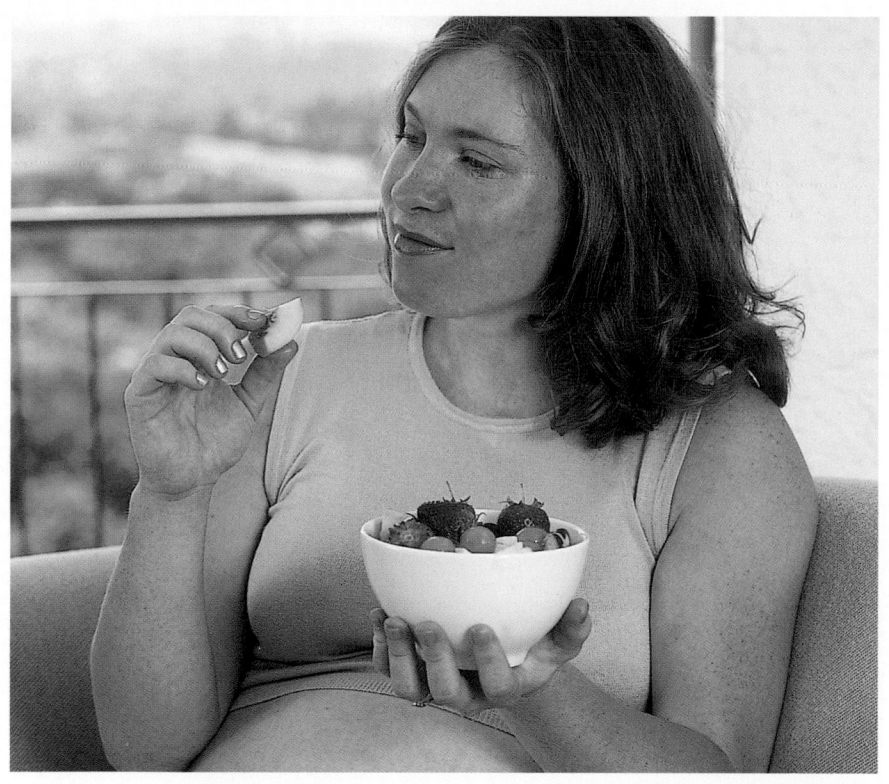

Must do

- Your appetite may be ferocious. Be sure to eat good-quality foods, but do not 'eat for two'. Do not eat more than usual.
- Start your childbirth classes. These educational classes will give you an opportunity to explore your feelings about birth and parenthood.
- Continue to read books on childbirth and get informed.
- Go about your day as normal but try to rest whenever you can.
- Sleep as often as you can.

Nice to do

- Write down those wild dreams you are having and add them to your pregnancy journal if you are keeping one.
- Enjoy an outing with a good friend and talk about your pregnancy.

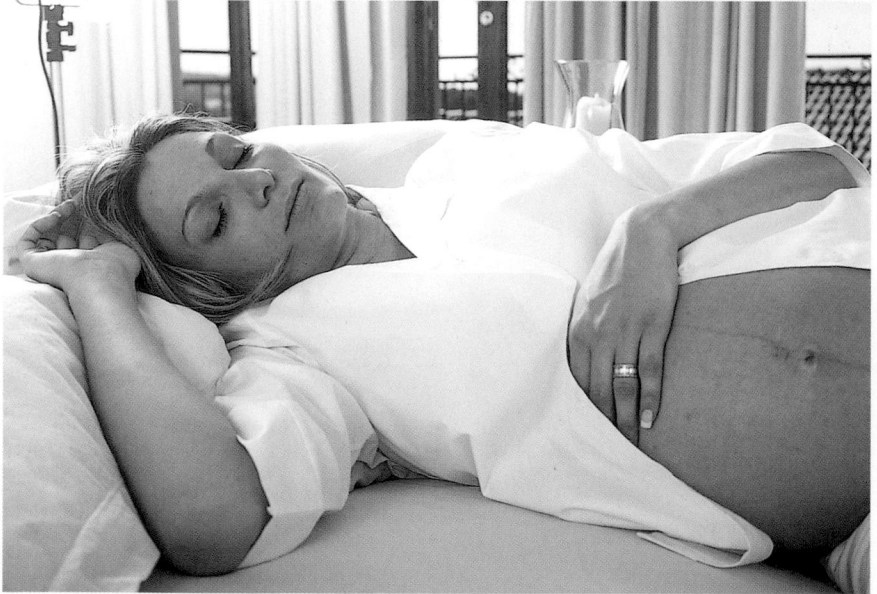

Above left Opt for fresh fruit if you feel the urge to snack between meals.
Left Try to get as much sleep as possible before your baby is born.

Month eight – weeks 31–35

Baby's world

Final touches start as work is completed on all major body systems. Your baby's central nervous system is developed enough to direct breathing motions and other reflexes such as narrowing the pupils in response to light. Fluid passes through his kidneys and contributes to the production of amniotic fluid. The immune system is still immature and he continues to receive antibodies. A fair amount of fat has been laid under the skin and his skin is pink and smooth. Babies born to dark-skinned parents will have light skin at birth as melanin is only produced with exposure to sunlight. Meconium, the first stool the baby will pass, is being produced in the bowel. He now weighs approximately 2.5kg (5.5 lb) and measures about 45cm (18in).

Mom's world

By now your navel has flattened out completely and you are experiencing Braxton-Hicks contractions frequently, which is the uterus's way of preparing for labour. You may also experience 'stitch-like' pain on one or both sides of the lower abdomen, which could be due to the straining of the round ligaments that support the uterus. You may find that you are more forgetful as the endorphin levels (*see* p114) in your body increase and there is more blood going to your uterus than to your brain. Breathing may become a little easier as your baby moves down into the pelvis, but now you may feel heaviness in the pelvic area. Your energy levels are dropping and you may feel apathetic and listless.

Left Your baby's eyes are able to change focus and blink, but his vision is not well developed before birth and, in fact, is the last sense to develop fully.

Must do

- Practise your breathing in response to your 'practice' contractions.
- Continue doing pelvic floor exercises.
- You may start doing perineal massage in order to prepare your pelvic floor for birth (see p129).
- If you intend to stop work at the end of this month, make sure that all your work is in order. It is advisable to take some time off before the baby is born.

Nice to do

- Fill in your baby's family tree.
- Connect with family and friends.
- Write a letter to your baby about how you are feeling.

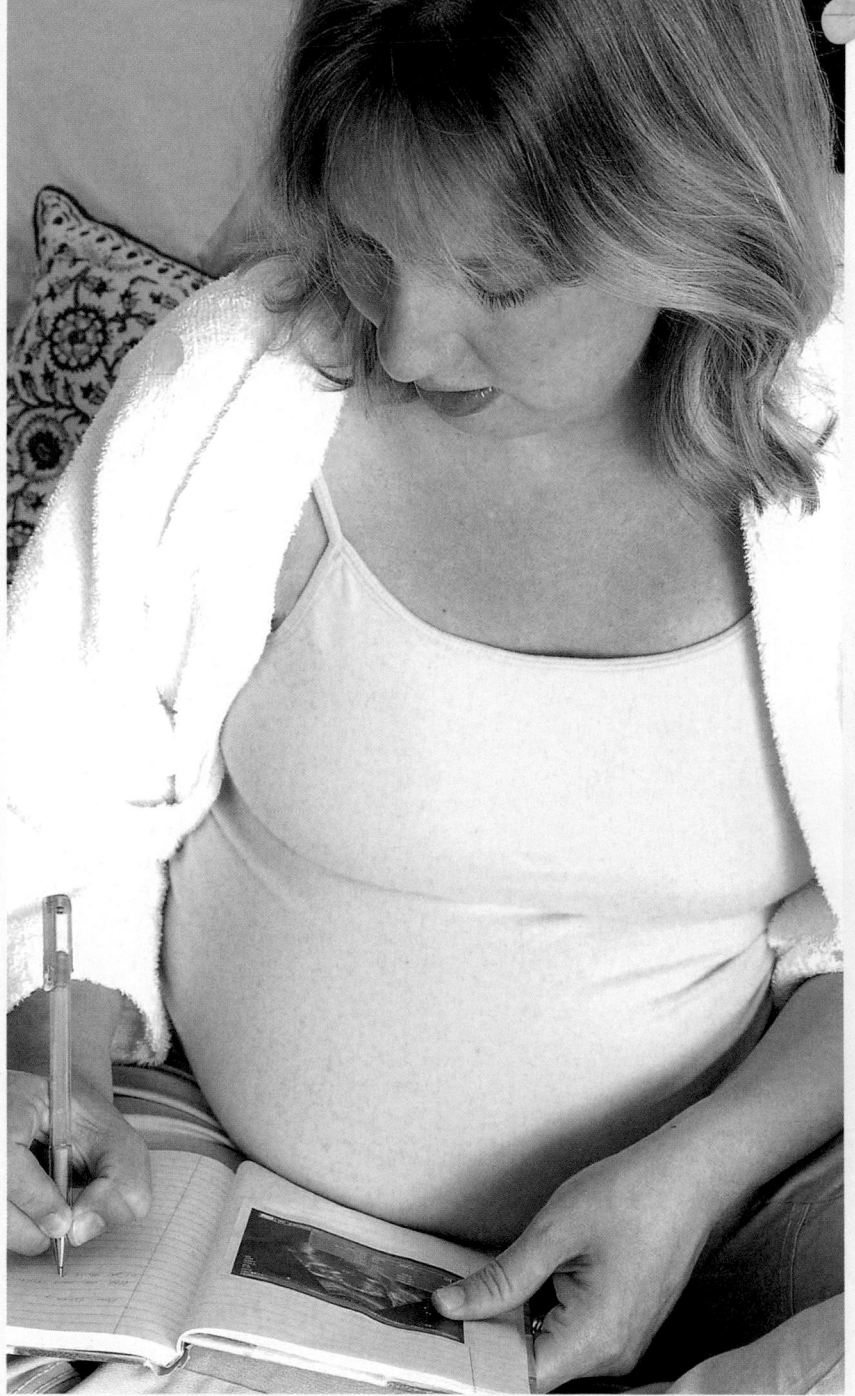

Right Write a letter to your baby and keep a journal of events leading up to the 'big' day.

Month nine – weeks 36–40

Baby's world

It is almost time for the birth; both baby and mother are reaching their limits. Your baby gains about 30g (1.05oz) of fat daily in order to cope with the lower temperatures after birth – the rate of your baby's weight gain slows down closer to the birth. Her lungs continue maturing. The lanugo and vernix are being shed and swallowed by the baby, and it then accumulates in her bowel. This forms part of the soft, green-black meconium. Most babies 'head down' into the pelvic cavity as they prepare for the contractions that will nudge them out into the world. Your baby will practise breathing, sucking and swallowing. She measures approximately 50cm (20in) and weighs about 3.3kg (7 lb).

Mom's world

Your baby starts to move snugly into the pelvis – this is known as 'lightening'. You are able to breathe with more ease, although now your bladder takes all the strain as the heavy uterus puts pressure on it, causing you to visit the toilet more often. Your final blood volume is 50 per cent greater than before you were pregnant. You may feel hot all the time because your body is working hard to accommodate all the changes and postural shifts.

You may feel emotionally vulnerable because the changes your body is going through do affect your body image and possibly your self-esteem. At the same time, you may be excited at the thought of meeting your baby for the first time or apprehensive about the approaching labour.

Braxton-Hicks contractions become more intense. You will know that you are in labour when contractions become stronger, longer and closer together.

Left During this month, it is normal for the baby to make her way down into the pelvis as she gets ready for her entrance into the world.

Must do

- Have a quiet romantic dinner with your partner and discuss how you wish to raise your child.
- Pack your hospital bags (one for you and one for the baby) and check the shortest route there in traffic. Many nervous dads have lost their way, even when they know the route very well.
- Finish the final touches to your baby's nursery.
- Delegate and leave the hard work for others to do.
- Rest and 'tune out' as often as you can. Mental preparedness is as important as physical preparation.
- Tie up any loose ends and make a list of people you have to phone to announce the good news.

Nice to do

- Have your hair washed and styled at your favourite hair salon.
- Buy something special for the baby.
- Enjoy your daydreaming; it happens for a reason.
- Keep positive (do not wish your baby out too soon).

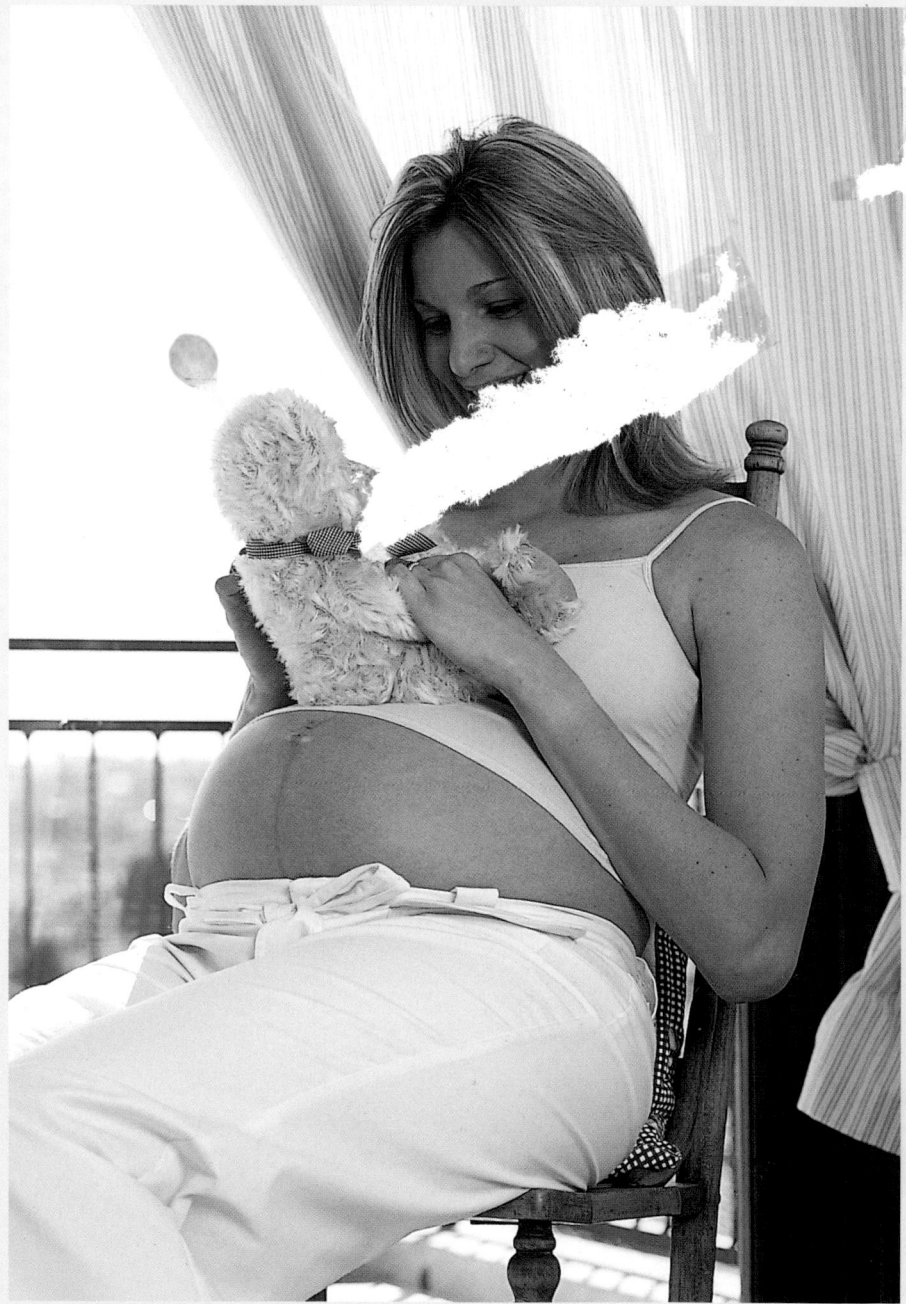

Above *Buy something special for your baby. If it is a toy, remember that it has to be safe and appropriate for his age.*

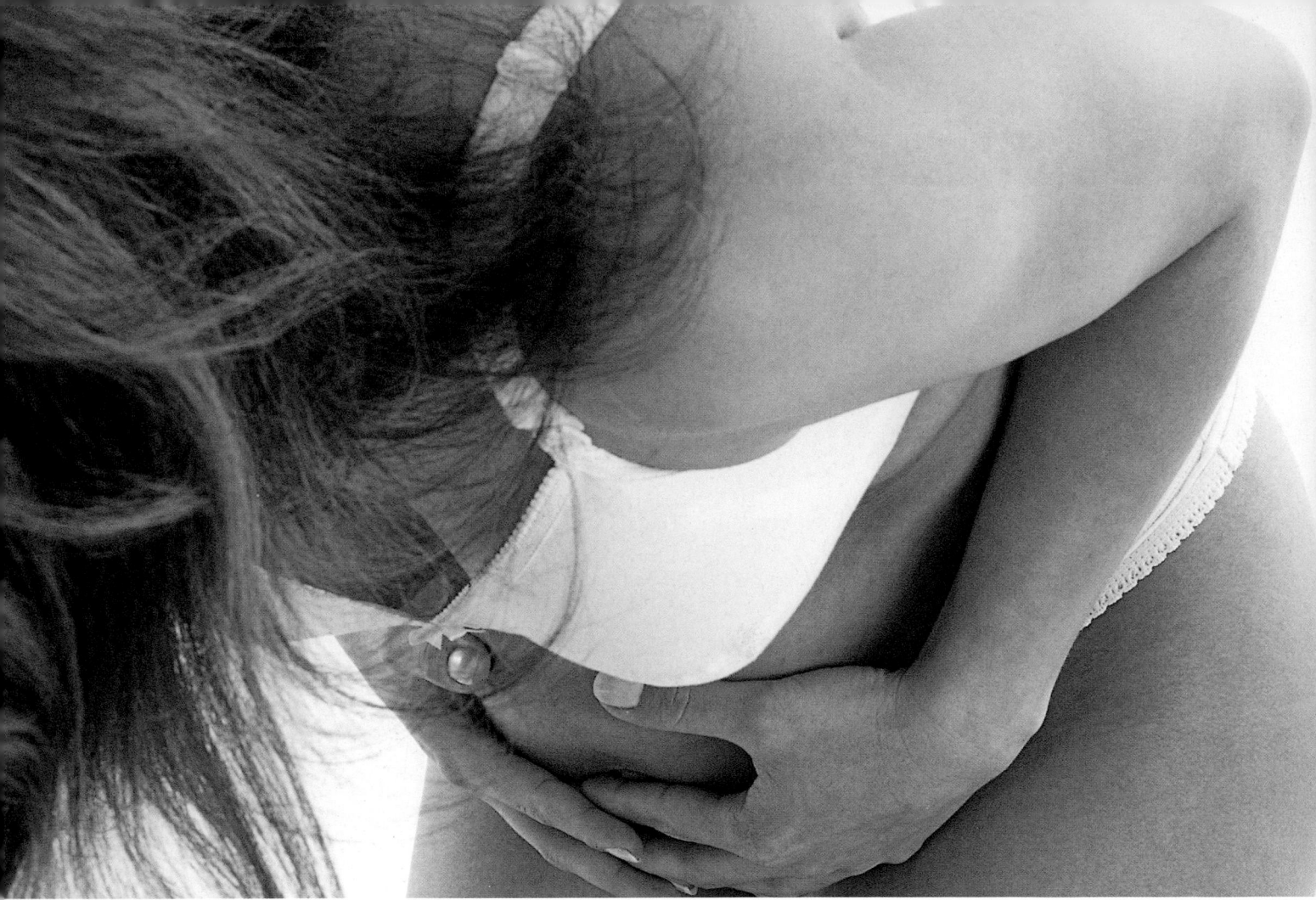

Growing pains

Although pregnancy is a natural process, your body is in an 'altered state' and it has to adjust to cope with the extra load. You will get constant reminders that nature is indeed performing a miracle. It is easy to complain about the not-so-subtle clues, but pregnancy aches and pains are reminders that your body is doing something amazing, and there is a reason for everything that happens. If, however, you experience severe pain or if the pain does not feel 'normal' and you are concerned about it, contact your doctor or caregiver immediately and have him or her tend to it as soon as possible.

PREGNANCY ACHES AND PAINS ARE REMINDERS THAT YOUR BODY IS DOING SOMETHING AMAZING

Abdominal pain

Just about every pregnant woman feels some kind of abdominal discomfort and, because it can be quite disconcerting, it is worth mentioning in a separate section. Understanding that a certain amount of discomfort is normal will go a long way in reassuring you that all is well.

Location	Possible causes	What to do	Cause for concern
A sharp pain on the side of the abdomen or in the groin area that lasts for less than two minutes. (Usually felt in the first and third trimester.)	The round ligament holding the uterus in place in the pelvis may be in spasm.	Bend at the waist toward the pain, relax and breathe deeply and slowly.	If the pain is accompanied by a rigid abdomen, nausea, vomiting or dizziness, or it lasts for more than two minutes, it may indicate an emergency with the placenta or uterus.
Pressure or a pulling sensation felt in the lower region of the abdomen. (Usually felt only in the third trimester.)	This could be due to the increasing weight of the uterus caused by the placenta, amniotic fluid and your baby.	Exercise and use positions that shift the weight of your baby off your lower abdomen. You may want to wear an abdominal support belt, especially if your job calls for you to stand a lot.	Should you have a watery, pinkish vaginal discharge along with this pressure, consult your doctor immediately – it could mean the start of premature labour.
Sensitivity in the abdominal wall. (Usually experienced in the third trimester.)	Strain on your abdominal muscles may cause them to separate and the tissue above them to feel 'thin' and weak.	Do the appropriate exercises, under supervision of course, to help strengthen your abdominal muscles (see p86).	If the separation of the muscles becomes severe, you could experience acute backache.
A sharp, burning pain in the pubic bone/groin area. (Usually felt in the third trimester.)	The pelvic ligaments become relaxed and loose due to the softening effect of the pregnancy hormones, which cause movement and discomfort at the symphysis pubis joint (see Glossary).	Take small steps and try to keep your knees close together when sitting (do not cross them). Avoid awkward movements, especially when getting in and out of bed. Do not lift heavy objects. Wear a support belt.	If this pain is severe and stops you from walking normally, ask your caregiver to refer you to a physiotherapist.

Backache

The changes in your body cause a shift in your centre of gravity, which affects your posture. The expanding stomach 'pulls' the abdomen forward, and your spine assumes a greater curve than normal. The abdominal muscles elongate and stretch up to 20cm (8in) to accommodate the expanding uterus. The recti muscles (*see p86*) separate down the middle, and the back takes more strain. A weak pelvic floor and tight hamstrings also contribute to backache.

Hormonal changes cause your body's tissue to soften and the ligaments around the joints become lax. You may feel pain in the buttocks and down your legs as the sacroiliac joint of the pelvis moves and sometimes traps a nerve.

Helpful hints

- Become aware of your posture. When walking, your chin should be pulled back, and the shoulders and ribcage raised and pushed back. When standing, try to tuck your bottom in so that you feel your abdominal muscles working to support your spine.
- Do not lift heavy objects! When lifting an object from the floor always squat, keep your back straight and bring the item close to your body.
- Place a hot-water bottle or heated buckwheat pillow against the affected area to increase blood circulation and release the spasm.
- Sleep on a firm mattress.
- When working, occasionally rest your head on your desk and stretch the back of your neck.
- Moderate, regular and gentle exercise will strengthen all the postural muscles of the body.
- Wear a bra that fits properly and offers good support.
- Avoid wearing high-heeled shoes.
- Ask your partner to massage your back while you sit on a stool or a chair, or lie on your side on a bed. Massage releases endorphins, which are the body's natural painkillers. Use a natural oil that will keep the skin supple and soft.
- Keep a small pillow or rolled-up towel in the car to place in the small of your back when driving.
- Take warm baths with safe aromatherapy oils or vigorous showers.

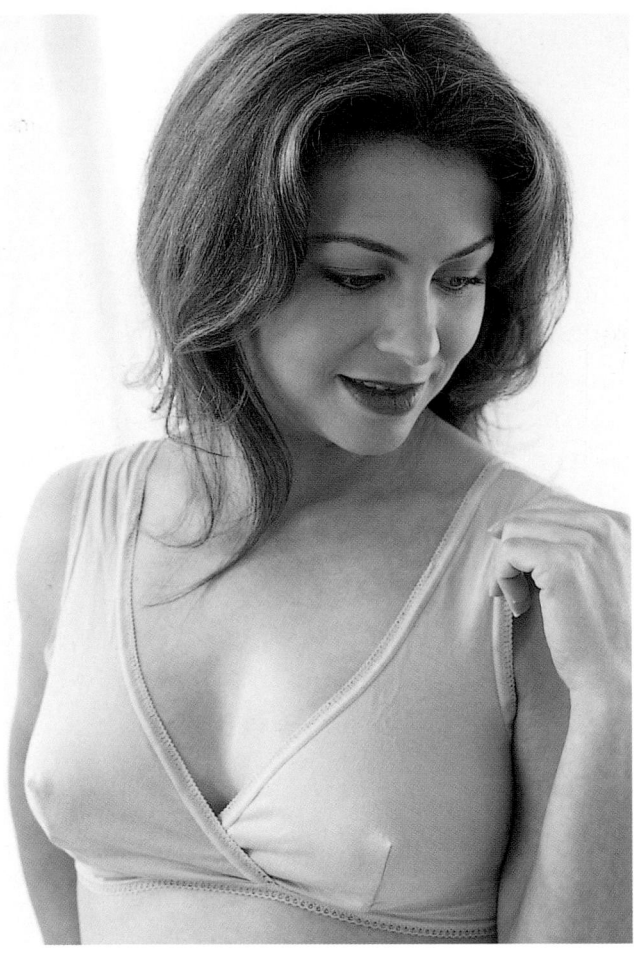

Above Your breasts become fuller and heavier as pregnancy progresses – wear a good support bra to help ease backache.

Below Relaxing in a warm foam bath does wonders for backache; rest your head on a rolled-up towel for added head and neck support.

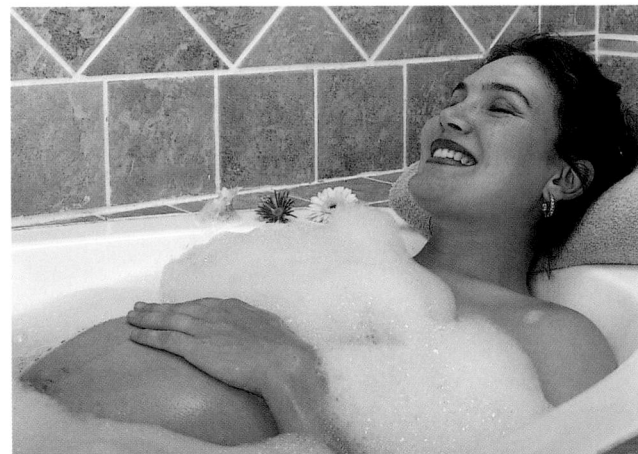

Bladder discomfort

(FIRST AND THIRD TRIMESTER)

In the early part of pregnancy, you are likely to experience the need to pass urine more frequently because your uterus starts to swell and it presses onto the bladder.

During the third trimester, you are most likely to be troubled by frequent trips once again because your body produces more urine as it gets rid of waste for the baby as well. Your kidneys are working harder than ever before, as your blood contains about 40 per cent more fluid. This extra urine means that your bladder fills up more often and the weight of your baby pressing against it means that it cannot hold as much as before.

Owing to the softening effects of the pregnancy hormone, relaxin, the ureters (see Glossary) become 'kinked' and urine is more likely to get caught up in these kinks, which can cause an infection. If your urine has a sharp smell, is very concentrated or causes a burning sensation, tell your caregiver. It may be an indication of a urinary tract infection, which is common in pregnancy.

Helpful hints

- Be sure not to limit your intake of fluid as you will then be more likely to develop bladder infections and other problems.
- Instead of drinking large glasses of water at a time, sip small amounts throughout the day. Your body will absorb more water that way, and you are therefore less likely to keep running to the toilet.
- Exercise your pelvic floor daily.
- Do not allow your bladder to fill up to the point where you need to run to the toilet.
- Do not lean forward on the toilet, as this may stop you from emptying your bladder completely.
- After you have urinated, always wipe from the vagina back toward the anus and not the other way round. This will prevent bacteria from the anus spreading to the vagina and causing infection.
- Avoid drinking too much tea or coffee because they are bladder irritants.

Breathlessness

(LATE PREGNANCY)

During pregnancy, you need to inhale more oxygen and exhale more carbon dioxide. Also, your growing baby is pushing your abdominal organs up toward your chest, and your lungs 'disappear' under your armpits. Your diaphragm (the plate-like muscle that separates your chest cavity from your abdominal cavity) also moves up by as much as 4cm (1.5in). As your baby continues to grow, your lungs will not be able to expand to their full capacity because your diaphragm has less space to work, hence the feeling of breathlessness.

In the late stages of your pregnancy, the ribs are stretched outward in order to provide enough room for your diaphragm and abdominal organs. Now they can only just function in an already stretched-to-maximum position.

Helpful hints

- Avoid slouching in your chair or while you are standing.
- Avoid taking up aerobic exercise during pregnancy, unless you are already accustomed to it.
- Practise deep-breathing techniques. Take some quiet time out to focus on your breathing, and breathe with awareness.

Sitting deep breath

This exercise increases your lung capacity and reduces tension and fatigue. Sit with your legs comfortably crossed in front of you – do not cross your ankles and make sure you keep one foot in front of the other. Clasp your hands and place them under your chin, keeping your elbows pointed downward. Inhale slowly, bringing your elbows up to ear height or higher. Exhale slowly, extending your head back as far as possible. Inhale, bringing your head forward again. Exhale as you bring your elbows back down to the starting position.

Below Sit in a comfortable, upright position and practise deep breathing daily.

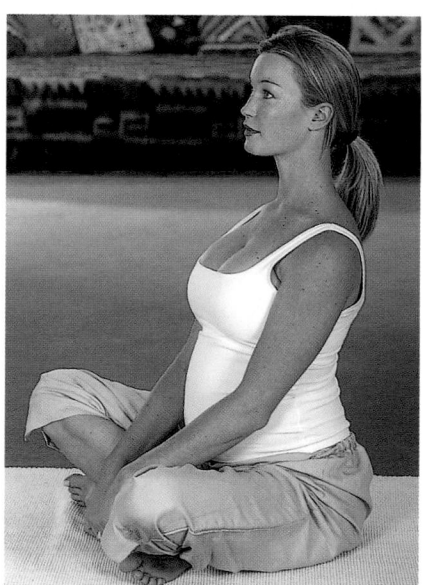

Constipation

(SECOND HALF OF PREGNANCY)

Constipation is usually caused by a slower rate of digestion, by pressure on the intestines or by lack of moisture. Other causes may be irregular eating habits, changes in your environment, stress or a lack of calcium and iron in your diet. Some medicines, too little exercise or not enough fibre may also contribute to the problem.

Helpful hints

- Start your day with warm liquids to stimulate intestinal activity and drink plenty of water (six to eight glasses).
- Eat plenty of wholegrains and raw fruits and vegetables – do not peel them!
- Drink chamomile tea with a little fresh ginger to help stimulate intestinal activity (it also eases heartburn; and if you are feeling nausea, the ginger should help).
- Drinking 125ml (0.8oz) of prune juice every night will ensure a system that is raring to go every morning (it causes no cramps and you will not feel bloated).
- Take a 30-minute, brisk walk several times a week to help revitalize your system.
- Exercise regularly – ensure that the activity allows your abdominal muscles to 'massage' your intestinal tract.
- Massage your abdomen in a clockwise direction every night before going to sleep – use massage oil that allows your hands to glide over the skin.
- Swallow a tablespoon of linseed oil with water twice a day. Two tablespoons of molasses in warm milk before bedtime may also help.

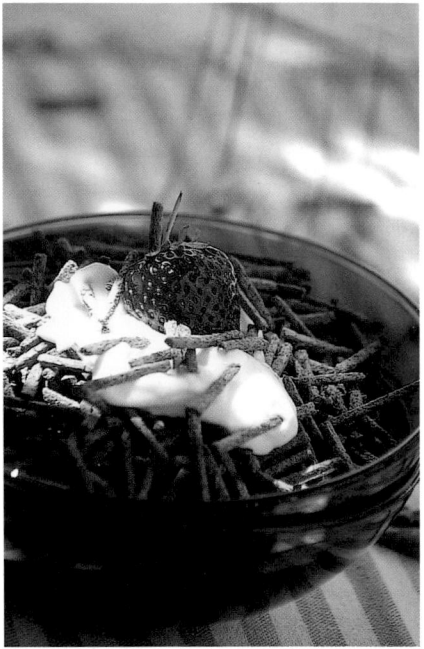

Above Fibre helps to prevent constipation, aids the digestion process and is vital for the absorption of nutrients from food.

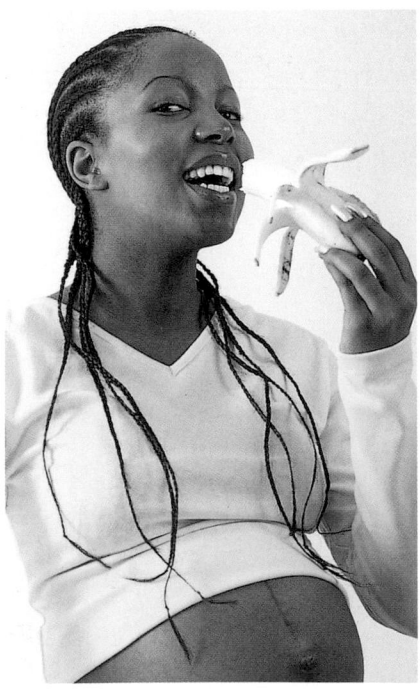

Left Bananas are the best natural source of magnesium; they are also a source of folic acid.

Muscle cramps

(SECOND HALF OF PREGNANCY)

Cramps usually affect the legs, feet and toes, and often strike during the night. No-one is sure why cramps occur in pregnancy, but lack of magnesium and poor blood supply to the affected area may be possible causes. Most pregnant women find that cramps are worse on waking in the morning.

Helpful hints

- Stand with your bare feet on a cold floor; this may help to relieve a cramp.
- If you experience a cramp in your calf muscle, flex your foot by pulling the toes toward the shin to relieve the pain.
- Ask your partner to gently rub the affected muscle but not while you are experiencing the cramp.
- Exercise regularly – brisk walking will help improve your blood circulation.
- Eat food rich in calcium and magnesium; taking daily supplements may also help, but speak to your doctor first.
- Soaking in a warm bath before bedtime may prevent muscle cramps.

Dizziness and fainting

(ANYTIME DURING PREGNANCY – BUT MOSTLY IN THE LAST STAGES)

Because of hormonal changes, the blood vessels have greater capacity and reduced tone in order to accommodate the increased blood volume. When you rise or move quickly, your vascular system takes a little time to adjust, which is the reason why you may feel a little 'light-headed'. Fainting, on the other hand, ensures that your body moves to the prone position, so that blood can flow to the brain. Low blood pressure may also be a factor.

Helpful hints

- Make sure you rise and change positions slowly. Have your caregiver check your blood pressure if you experience dizziness often.
- High-sugar snacks will worsen the situation (if you do crave sugar, opt for fruit juice diluted with water).
- If you feel dizzy when lying on your back, move onto your left side. This ensures that you are not lying on the major blood vessels supplying the brain.
- Avoid standing or sitting in one position for too long.
- Exercise your calf muscles or elevate your legs.
- If you feel hot or clammy, place a cool, wet cloth on your forehead or the nape of your neck. Run cold water over your wrists; it may also help.

Fatigue

(FIRST AND THIRD TRIMESTER)

Fatigue is just another aspect of pregnancy. Tiredness in the first trimester is understandable because it is the most important developmental stage of your baby's life. The lethargy that you feel is nature's way of slowing you down.

In the latter part of your pregnancy, fatigue will once again creep up on you, this time for a different reason: as your baby gets heavier, your body is carrying around between nine and 11kg (24 lb) of extra weight.

Other causes of fatigue include anaemia, a lower blood pressure and shortness of breath, poor nutrition, low iron reserves, and stress and tension.

Helpful hints

- Regular physical activity is your best weapon against fatigue. Enrol in an antenatal exercise class.
- Eat generous amounts of protein, carbohydrate, fruit and vegetables.
- Take an iron supplement as prescribed by your caregiver, and eat iron-rich foods.
- Practise relaxation and meditation to relieve stress and tension.
- During your workday, take time out to stretch and do foot circles as well as upper and lower back stretches.
- If you are comfortable doing so, lie with your feet elevated above the level of your heart for about 15 minutes. This will improve your blood flow and you will feel energized.
- Avoid taking stimulants or medications to increase your energy.
- Avoid excessive amounts of caffeine.
- Try not to 'push yourself' beyond your capabilities. Be reasonable and do not feel guilty saying NO to extra work.

Below Antenatal exercise classes are ideal for pregnant women who want to enjoy the social aspect of a group workout.

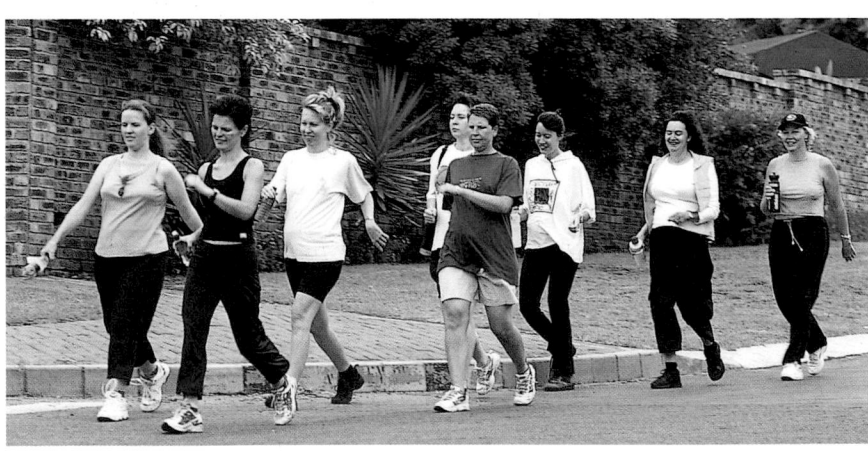

Headaches

(MAY OCCUR THROUGHOUT PREGNANCY)

Pregnancy may curb your headaches or exacerbate them. If you suffer from headaches, you already have your own way of dealing with them. If you are one of those people who 'pop a few pills', think twice before you reach for them; you now have an unborn baby to consider!

Although hormones do play a role in causing headaches, they are not the only factors. Many are related to food and stress – or your work or home environment may cause stress or physical problems such as tired, sore shoulders or back strain. Bad posture is a BIG culprit.

Eye and ear strain (loud or constant noise) can also bring on a headache, as can lack of sleep or constant worry.

Helpful hints

- Stretching exercises are very beneficial.
- Learn how to relax. Pamper yourself and enjoy your pregnancy. Practise the relaxation techniques you will learn in your childbirth classes. Listen to soft music that makes you feel good. Correct bad postural habits.
- Check that your mattress is not too soft or too hard. Your pillow should be at the correct height to support your neck.
- Work through any issues that may be worrying you, and share these concerns with your partner, doctor, childbirth educator or a friend.
- Develop a better body awareness all round. Remember to unclench your jaw as it can cause major tension of the face and neck.

- Massage is a wonderful stress reliever.
- A warm (not hot) bath with a little aromatherapy oil in the water may ease your throbbing head. Use any of the following: a few drops of peppermint, neroli, chamomile, rosemary or grapefruit oil.

Migraine sufferers

All of the tips given for headaches apply here in addition to these.

- Place an ice pack against your head and neck. Do not apply moist or dry heat to your head when you have a migraine.
- Avoid stress, late nights, flickering lights and loud noises.
- Do not skip meals.
- Avoid trigger foods such as wine, cheese (any food containing tyramine), chocolate, caffeine and artificial sweeteners. Explore substitutes to some of these foods.
- Read food labels: anything containing preservatives may be a trigger.
- Try to eat fresh food as much as possible.
- Try to increase your calcium intake.
- Dissolve 20 Mag Phos (a tissue salt) tablets in a little warm water. This will help normal headaches as well as migraines.

Below If you do suffer frequent migraine attacks, your doctor or a qualified practitioner can prescribe medication that is safe to take during pregnancy.

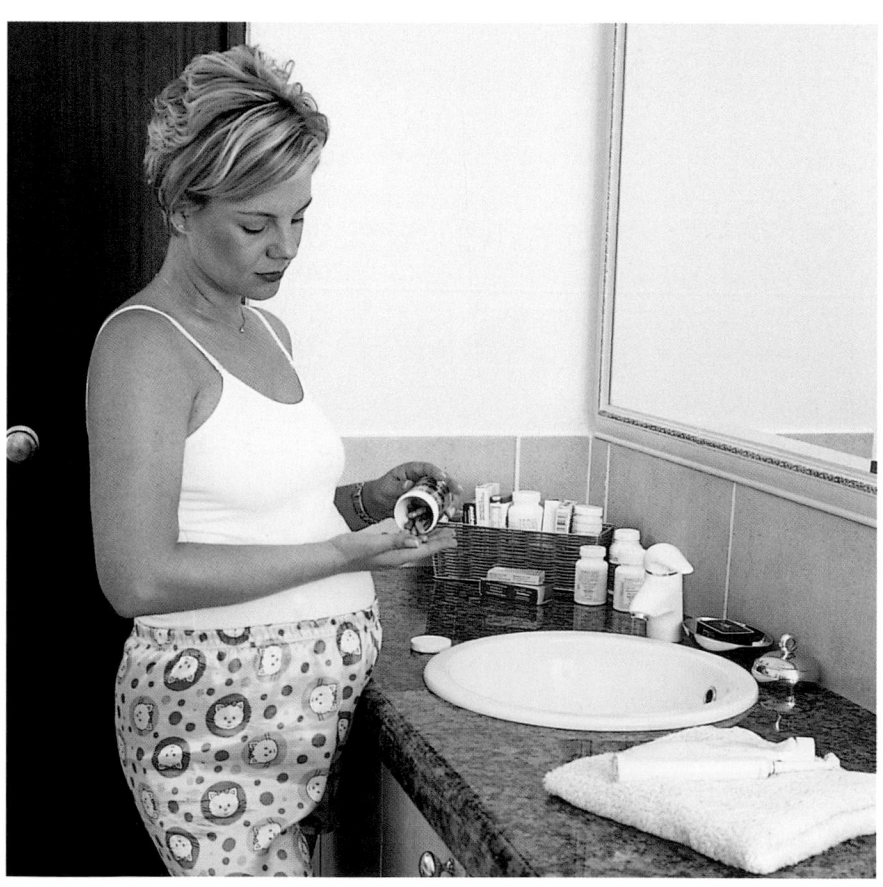

Heartburn

(SECOND TO THIRD TRIMESTER)

Heartburn is felt mostly in the second half of pregnancy, and it can be extremely uncomfortable. The valve between the stomach and oesophagus becomes soft and relaxed due to the pregnancy hormone, progesterone. As a result, stomach acids move up into the oesophagus; this causes a strong burning sensation that is felt in the chest area close to the heart. Progesterone also causes the stomach to empty more slowly so that as many nutrients as possible can be absorbed from the food you eat. So the next time you experience heartburn, know that your body is furiously absorbing nutrients from the digestive tract as a whole, and nature has planned this so that your placenta can do its job unhurried. Long periods between meals can make heartburn worse.

Helpful hints

- Eat smaller meals more frequently. Do not eat before going to bed!
- Eat slowly. This gives more time for the enzymes in your saliva to break down the food before it gets to the stomach.
- Do not overeat! Heartburn is more likely to become a problem if you do, especially if your meal includes a large amount of carbohydrates.
- Avoid spicy or acidic foods, overheated oils and fats, and coffee.
- Sit up straight when you eat.
- A glass of milk may relieve heartburn, especially at night.
- Some commercial over-the-counter antacids may help, but can also make the problem worse. Check with your doctor or pharmacist if it is safe for you to take an antacid.

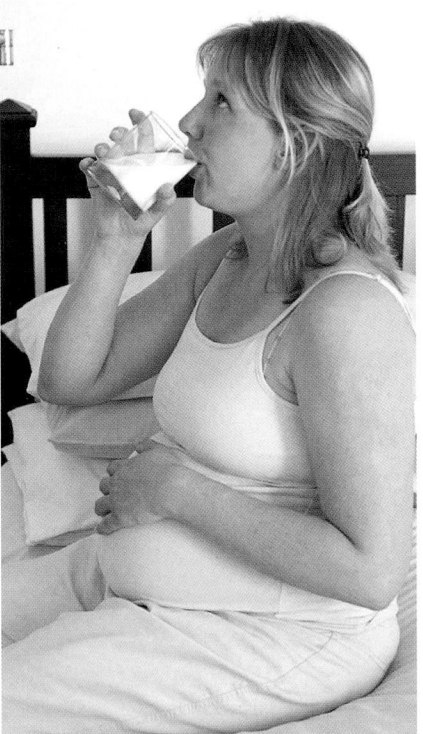

Above *Drinking a glass of milk before going to bed may relieve heartburn.*

Insomnia

(THIRD TRIMESTER)

Sleep patterns vary throughout pregnancy. In the first trimester, you may feel overwhelmingly tired and exhausted after doing virtually nothing. It may take a great deal of will and effort just to make it through dinner without falling asleep. These feelings often disappear during the second trimester, only to return in the seventh or eighth month when the added weight and stress hit a peak. At this time, even though you are tired, other pregnancy related changes may keep you from sleeping. You will not feel rested and life becomes hard to cope with as you feel irritable and have no zest for the day. This is nature's way of preparing you for what is to come!

Helpful hints

- It may be difficult but try to have regular sleeping and waking times.
- Avoid stimulants such as caffeine four to six hours before bed.
- Warm milk works wonders.
- If you are hungry before bed, eat something small and nutritious.
- Do not smoke!
- Do not watch television just before going to sleep.
- Keep your bedroom dark, quiet and cool, and make sure that there is enough air circulation. Pregnant women often experience night sweats.
- If after 15 minutes you have not yet fallen asleep, get up and read a book or do something else.
- Invest in good pillows and adequate bed linen for the season.
- Learn relaxation and breathing techniques.
- Choose sleeping positions that are comfortable for you. Try placing pillows at various places around your body until you feel totally supported.
- Sometimes taking a warm (not hot) bath with candles and calming aromatherapy oil before bedtime helps. (Lavender is especially powerful.)

Joint pain

(THIRD TRIMESTER)

One of the most common complaints of pregnancy is pubic bone pain. For some women, it is just uncomfortable but for others, even slow walking is difficult. This is very common in subsequent pregnancies. The pelvis has a joint in the front that is supported and held together by strong ligaments. During pregnancy, the ligaments soften causing the joint to become less stable in order for the pelvis to widen so that the baby can pass through easily during labour. Pain is usually felt low down over the symphysis pubis joint, in the hips, lower abdomen and groin. It is often worse when rising from a sitting or lying position and, for some women, simply walking is almost unbearable.

Unfortunately, there are no quick fixes and you just have to be patient; things will improve gradually.

Helpful hints

- If climbing stairs hurts, take the lift.
- Avoid walking long distances and standing for long periods of time.
- Sit on a high stool whenever you can. Try to take the weight off your pelvis.
- Do not cross your legs when sitting, and keep your knees together when rising from a sitting position.
- You may have to purchase an abdominal support belt.
- Physiotherapy will give some pain relief; it is worth going for a few sessions.
- Elevate your feet whenever you can.
- An operation can be performed to fuse or plate the symphysis pubis together. This is only done in extreme cases!

Nausea and vomiting

(MAY OCCUR THROUGHOUT PREGNANCY – MOSTLY FIRST AND THIRD TRIMESTER)

Although experts are not entirely sure what causes morning sickness, most agree that it is due to the high levels of HCG (see p11). This hormone stops the breaking down of the lining of the womb and can be measured in the blood eight to nine days after conception. The rate of secretion rises rapidly to reach a maximum at about seven to nine weeks after conception, and then decreases and stabilizes at a relatively low level at 16–20 weeks. This may explain why nausea is usually an early sign of pregnancy and why in most women it tapers off after three to four months.

It became known as 'morning sickness' due to the fact that many women felt worse nausea when rising in the morning and not having anything in their stomach.

For a small percentage of women, this feeling persists throughout the day and some women even experience nausea throughout their entire pregnancy.

Helpful hints

- Report persistent vomiting to your caregiver (see p27).
- Keep a few dry biscuits next to your bed and eat them before you get up. Try to start your day with warm water instead of tea or coffee.
- Ginger helps to alleviate nausea. Make a pot of ginger tea and keep ginger beer in the fridge. Ginger biscuits and ginger essential oil also help.
- Avoid smells and foods that make the feeling of nausea worse.
- Carry peppermint sweets in your handbag or try drinking mint tea.
- Do not go for long periods without eating. Low blood sugar makes nausea worse.
- Drink plenty of water.
- Try some reflexology: use a practitioner who is experienced with pregnancy.

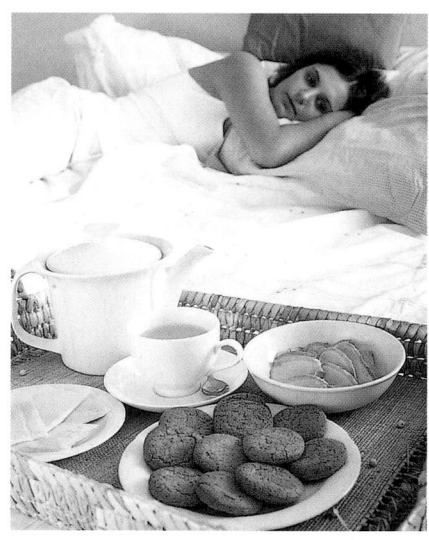

Above *You can ease 'morning sickness' by drinking a cup of ginger tea and eating dry ginger biscuits.*

- Avoid spicy, fatty and fried foods.
- Deep breathing calms the body. Stress will make nausea worse.
- Make flavoured ice popsicles or ice cubes to suck on when nausea strikes.

Oral problems

(SECOND AND THIRD TRIMESTER)

The pregnancy hormones cause the mucous membranes of the mouth (gums) to become engorged and soft, which will lead to bleeding gums. Food becomes trapped more easily and you may be at risk of developing gingivitis – an inflammation of the gums that may weaken the supports of the teeth.

Helpful hints

- Use a softer toothbrush than normal and do not brush too vigorously.
- Floss daily. Use a mouthwash if brushing toward the back of your mouth makes you nauseous.
- Ferrum phos (tissue salt No. 4) and Buso drops act as anti-inflammatories and promote healing of any mucous membranes in the body.
- Visit your dentist at least once during your pregnancy.
- Increase your calcium intake.

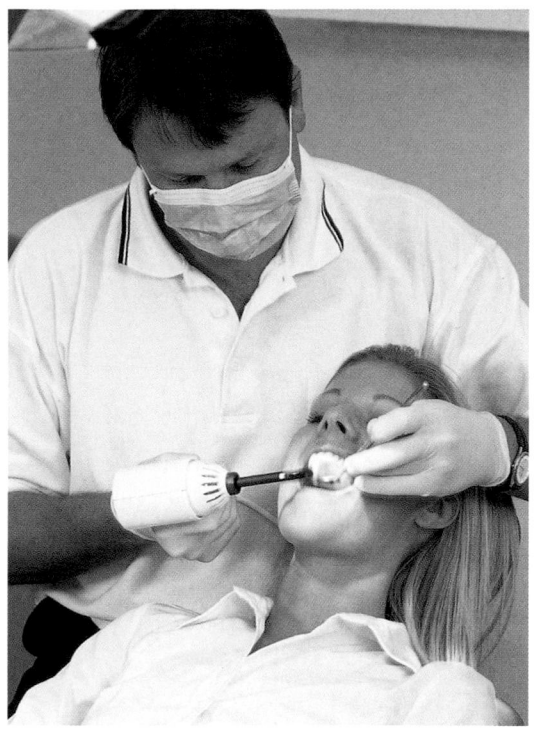

Right It is essential that you visit your dentist at least once during your pregnancy.

Varicose veins

(THIRD TRIMESTER)

Whether or not you have a history of varicosities in your family, you are more likely to develop varicose veins in pregnancy.

A varicose vein occurs when blood has difficulty flowing out of an area of your body and back to the heart. The added weight of pregnancy plus the increase in the volume of fluid in your bloodstream forces the valves to work harder and the blood does not always flow smoothly.

Helpful hints

- 'Put your feet up' as often as you can during the day and avoid standing for long periods at a time.
- Try to take a brisk walk when you can during the day. Walking and swimming are good forms of exercise to get the blood flowing and it really does work wonders.
- Stationary cycling is an excellent activity to help increase the blood circulation in your legs. You can watch your favourite television programme while doing it.
- If you are suffering and uncomfortable, you may wish to wear support hose.

Haemorrhoids (Piles)

(THIRD TRIMESTER)

Haemorrhoids develop in the same way as varicose veins do in the legs, and can be extremely uncomfortable and painful.

As your pregnancy progresses, the pressure on your pelvic region increases, making it more difficult for blood to flow in and out of that area freely. Haemorrhoids may be internal or protrude through the anus; they may cause bleeding, itching and pain. In some women, they show no symptoms at all.

Helpful hints

- Drink plenty of fluids and eat whole-grains and raw fruit and vegetables.
- You can avoid constipation by eating lots of fresh fruit and vegetables.
- Practise the Kegel (pelvic floor) exercises as often as you can (see p85).
- For temporary pain relief, sit in a bath of warm water or soak cotton-wool balls in witch hazel and apply this to the rectum.
- Homeopathic preparations and the tissue salts Calc Fluor and Nat Mur will help. Check with your caregiver before using commercial preparations.

Skin changes

Itchy skin Mild itching is common because of the increased blood flow to the skin. Toward the end of your pregnancy, the skin on the abdomen becomes very stretched and this is often the cause of itchiness around the stomach. Itching can also be a sign of a more serious problem; if it becomes severe or unbearable and you develop a rash, advise your caregiver immediately.

Rash A pregnant woman may develop a rash that may or may not be associated with pregnancy. The most common rash is called miliaria, or prickly heat, which results from a combination of dampness, friction and heat. An irritating red rash is likely to develop where one part of your body constantly rubs against another.

Stretch marks Stretch marks occur as a result of weakening or breaking of the elastic fibres deep in the skin. They usually appear on the lower abdomen, breasts, thighs and buttocks and tend to radiate outward from the centre of the body. These marks occur as a result of weight gain and, in some instances, due to hormonal changes.

Chloasma Pregnancy hormones affect your skin colour by causing melanin (the substance responsible for freckles and suntans) to be deposited in certain areas of your body. The most annoying skin change for many women is the appearance of dark patches across the forehead, cheeks and nose. This is referred to as chloasma or, more commonly, the 'mask of pregnancy'.

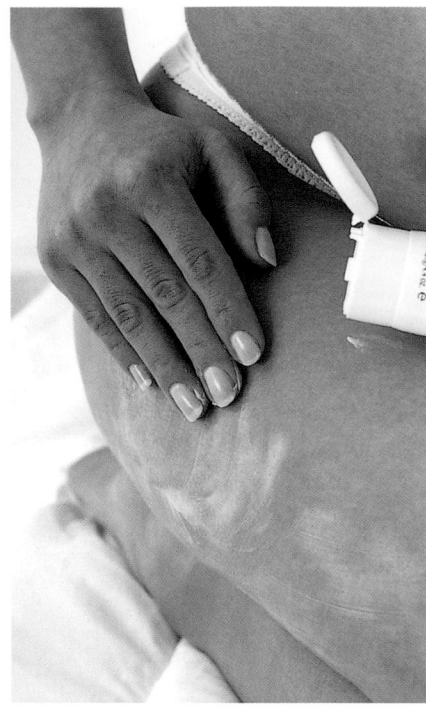

Above *Apply moisturizer to your skin daily; it will not prevent stretch marks, but it will improve the overall condition of your skin.*

Sunlight intensifies the dark spots, but they usually disappear or become less noticeable after birth.

Oily skin Pregnancy can work wonders for the complexion, clearing up blemishes and pimples, and reducing blackheads. But it can also cause blemishes and pimples, because the hormonal changes make sweat glands and sebaceous glands work overtime.

Helpful hints

- Apply a good-quality cream or oil for stretch marks.
- Do not scratch your skin if it itches.
- By strengthening the muscles under the skin of the abdomen, hips, thighs and

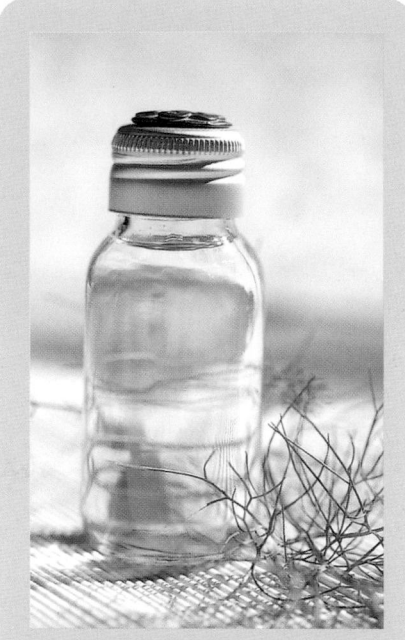

Make up this essential oil blend and rub it gently into your skin after taking a bath or shower:

- *30ml (1oz) almond oil (carrier oil)*
- *15ml (½oz) wheatgerm oil (carrier oil)*
- *10 drops borage seed oil (essential oil)*
- *5 drops carrot oil (essential oil)*

Shake the oils together in a glass container and apply regularly to the abdomen, hips, thighs and buttocks.

buttocks, you may prevent at least some of the breakdown of elastic fibres that occurs during pregnancy.

- Regular exercise may help.
- Wear a good support bra, as your breasts become heavier and pull on your skin, contributing to the severity of stretch marks.
- Try to avoid rapid weight gain, although stretch marks may appear even if your weight gain is normal.

Swelling

(THIRD TRIMESTER)

Some swelling is normal during pregnancy. A certain amount of fluid retention is necessary but too much can be uncomfortable, and could lead to certain health problems such as high blood pressure.

Each woman retains fluid according to her body's needs during her pregnancy. A woman who is overweight during pregnancy will retain more fluid than an underweight woman. Even women who show no signs of swelling carry an increased amount of fluid in their bodies.

You may well have noticed that in most women swelling is more evident in the legs, especially around the ankles and the wrists. This is because the pressure of the growing baby, together with the increased blood volume, makes it more difficult for the blood to return from the arms and legs to the heart. In the legs, however, both gravity and the weight of the uterus on the veins slow down the return flow, making swelling worse in the legs than the arms. Your caregiver will check your wrists and ankles at every antenatal appointment.

Helpful hints

- Elevate your legs and hips for about 15–20 minutes during the day, so that gravity can do its job.
- Lie on your left side when sleeping or resting; this will relieve the weight of the uterus off the large blood vessels that return blood to the heart.
- Moderate exercise three to four times a week will improve blood circulation.
- Do not sit with your legs crossed, as this puts more pressure on your blood vessels.
- Drink plenty of water to keep your kidneys and bladder functioning effectively.
- Do not eat spicy foods. Watch your salt intake especially.
- Place your feet in cool water at the end of a long day.
- The tissue salts Nat Mur and Nat Sulph (one of each) sucked every four hours help to distribute body fluids evenly. (Note: The names of these tissue salts are long and not easy to remember, so we have used the abbreviated versions. On the actual packaging of these products, the abbreviated versions are almost always used.)

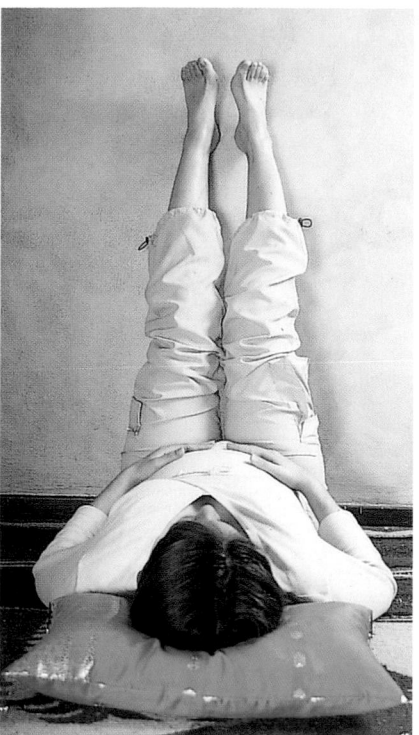

Above *To relieve the swelling in your legs, place them up against a wall to allow blood to flow back to your heart. Use pillows to support your neck and lower back.*

Vaginal discharge

(CAN OCCUR THROUGHOUT PREGNANCY)

During your pregnancy and while you are breast-feeding, you will not have your menstrual cycle, so it is usual to experience an increase in vaginal discharge as a result of hormonal changes. It is usually thin, colourless and watery. There is no need to be concerned unless it burns or itches, is a colour other than white or clear, or if it has an offensive smell. Report this to your caregiver immediately, as it may be the start of an infection.

Helpful hints

- Do not use tampons during pregnancy.
- Use sanitary towels or panty liners if it will make you feel more comfortable.
- Wear cotton underwear, especially if you live in a hot country.
- Do not use feminine sprays or talc.
- Avoid using bath oils or foam bath.
- You may add a few drops of tea tree oil to your bath.
- Use a mild, fragrance-free bath soap. Harsh soaps are acidic and, if used close to the vaginal area, increase discharge.

Warning signs and symptoms

Vaginal bleeding

Vaginal bleeding is not normal and it could be a life-threatening condition. It can however be of a less serious nature, but to be on the safe side and avoid complications, check with your caregiver, especially if you are feeling pain and rigidity in the abdomen.

In early pregnancy (before 16 weeks), bleeding could be an indication of an ectopic pregnancy (a pregnancy outside the womb) or threatened miscarriage.

Miscarriage can occur as a result of infection, uterine abnormality, rhesus incompatibility (see p27) or other medical condition. Unfortunately, in the majority of cases the cause is unknown.

If bleeding occurs after six months, a low-lying placenta or placenta praevia (placenta lies over the cervix) could be the problem.

Placental abruption (see p130) is a serious condition where the placenta detaches from the uterus, and may threaten the life of the mother and baby. It may be mild, moderate or severe but should never be ignored. Your pulse may be raised and your blood pressure could be very low or very high.

Excessive swelling (Oedema)

About 40 per cent of women experience some swelling toward the third trimester and it usually improves with rest. If excessive swelling persists and you experience other signs such as excessive weight gain, blurred or disturbed vision, severe and sudden headaches, high blood pressure, and if you are urinating less and the urine is more concentrated, notify your caregiver immediately as you may need to be hospitalized.

This condition can be life threatening to mother and baby because it can affect the normal functioning of the placenta. High blood pressure, which occurs with this condition, can affect the brain, liver and kidneys. This is most likely to occur in first pregnancies after the 30th week, but it can occur any time after week 20. Cardiac disease, renal disease and malnutrition may also be causes of oedema.

Bladder infection

Pain and burning when passing urine or cloudy urine with a strong odour are signs of bladder infection and definite cause for concern. Other signs include sudden pain in the lower abdomen or tenderness and rigidity in this region.

In most cases, infection is detected early and with the correct treatment will not be too troublesome. In some instances, bladder infection can develop into a more serious condition known as pyelonephritis (inflammation of the kidneys and renal pelvis).

Vaginal fluid loss

If a pale, straw-coloured fluid escapes from the vagina during pregnancy, it is cause for alarm. There is a high risk of infection, as well as the risk of prolapse cord (the umbilical cord moving down into the vagina in front of the baby).

Fluid loss from the vagina could also mean a rupture or 'tearing' of the amniotic sac. If this occurs close to your due date, it could indicate the start of labour. If this occurs earlier during pregnancy, it may be the start of premature labour and your must notify your caregiver immediately.

Contractions

The uterus contracts mildly throughout pregnancy. Most women become aware of the contractions, referred to as 'Braxton-Hicks' contractions, in the second half of pregnancy. They are sometimes intense but not usually painful. If they cause extreme

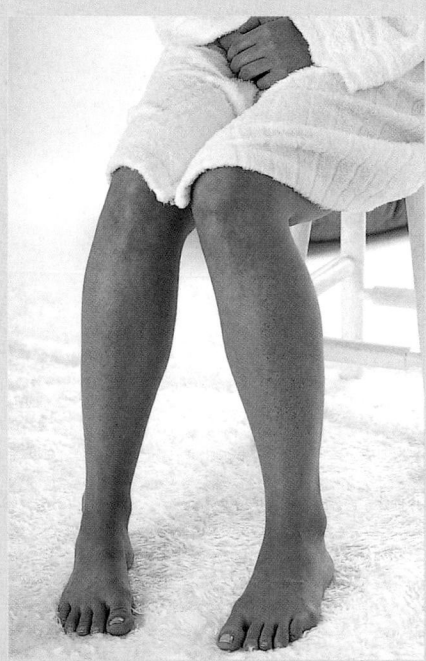

Above Vaginal bleeding is serious, especially if accompanied by abdominal pain, and a doctor must be notified immediately.

discomfort, this could indicate something more serious than just 'practice' contractions.

Painful contractions of the uterus may mean the start of labour. Sometimes if the mother has had a busy day and been on her feet for long periods, the uterus may become 'irritable'. It is a good idea to inform your caregiver if you are concerned that these contractions feel different from the usual. Having a warm relaxing bath may be all that you need.

Decreased foetal movement

Each foetus differs in the amount of movement. Ten to 12 movements in 24 hours are considered normal. It is usual for your baby to quieten down close to your due date. If you notice a dramatic change in the amount of times your baby moves in a day, it could be due to placental problems, too little or too much amniotic fluid, or you may have high blood pressure. Notify your caregiver immediately! Food makes your baby move: after eating, lie down on your left side for an hour. If your baby does not move, there is cause for concern.

Severe abdominal pain

Do not ignore severe abdominal pain during pregnancy. In the case of a fall or accident, or if the pain persists and does not improve with bed rest, seek medical advice.

Severe pain may indicate placental abruption or pre-eclampsia, both serious conditions

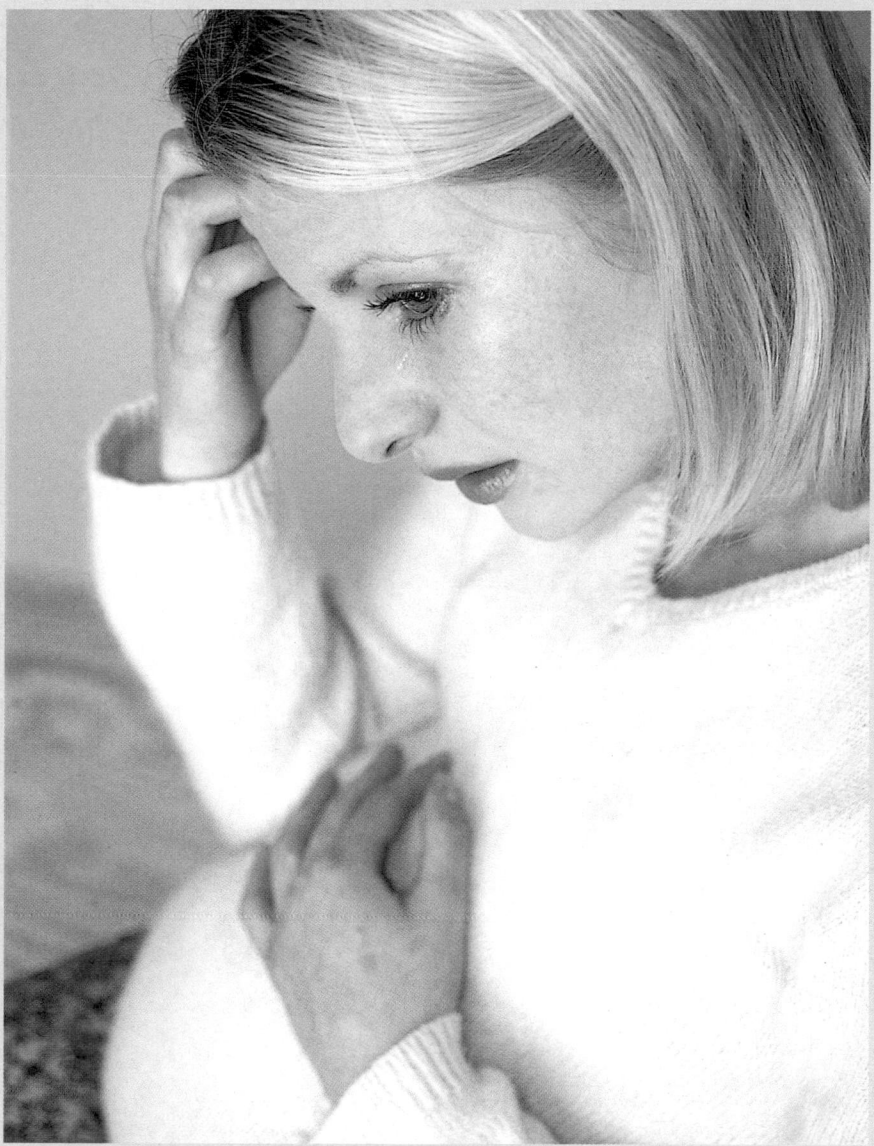

that need immediate medical attention. Severe abdominal pain may also be an indication of one of the following conditions: severe urinary tract infection, the start of labour or a strained round ligament (in which case, the pain is usually felt more to the sides of the abdomen).

Above If there is a dramatic change in the frequency of the foetus's movements, notify a medical practitioner at once!

Sexual intercourse

Some women note a decline in sexual interest throughout their pregnancy while others feel more responsive, particularly in the second trimester.

During the first trimester, major changes occur in your body, which take their toll on your energy levels and you may not feel very 'sexy' when you are experiencing morning sickness. The initial lethargy felt in the first trimester may make it difficult for you to become aroused or even vaguely interested in sex. It is important for your partner to realize that this is completely normal and usually does not continue throughout the entire pregnancy.

Many couples report that the second trimester is the best time of their sexuality during the pregnancy. The mother is not feeling cumbersome, as she is just starting to show, her energy levels have picked up, and nausea and vomiting have usually toned down or stopped altogether at this stage.

In the third trimester, feelings of tiredness and fear of labour can once again lower a woman's libido. This is the time for some creative ideas for lovemaking. As a rule of thumb, any position should leave a woman free from pressure on her stomach and breasts.

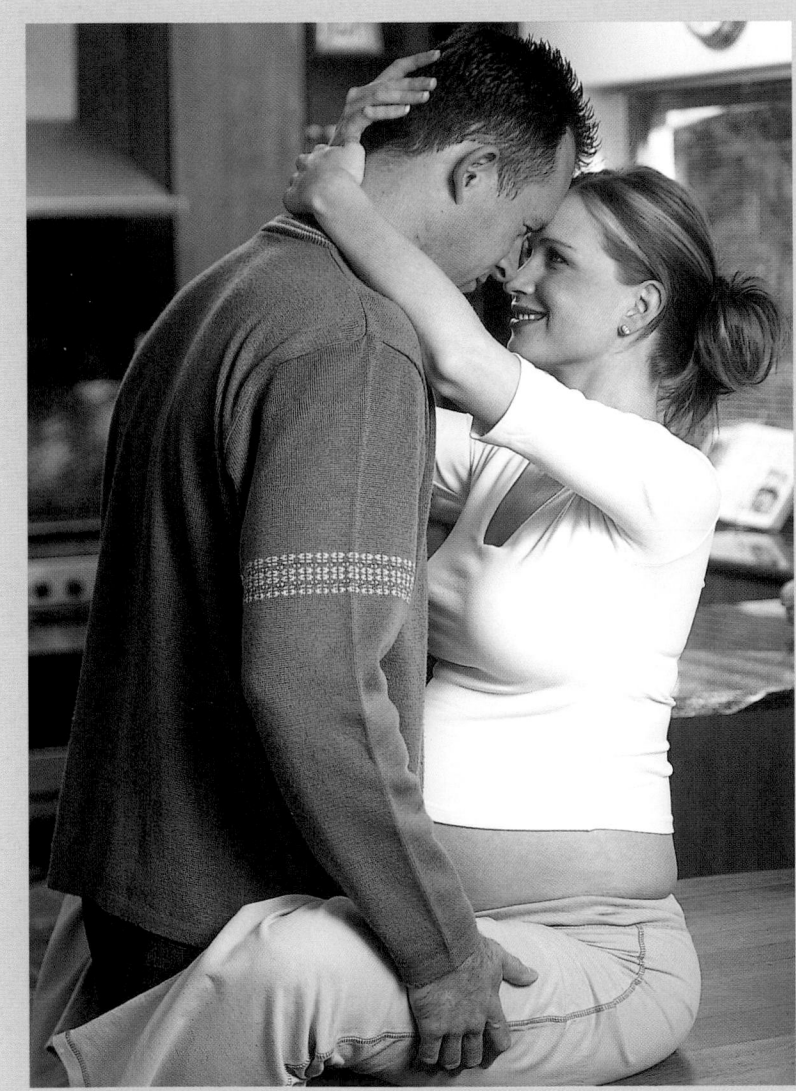

Does sex interfere with the baby?

Many couples worry that sex can hurt the baby, but be assured that this is not the case. The baby is well protected by the walls of the uterus, as well as the cushioning effect of the amniotic fluid. There is a thick mucus 'plug' that seals the opening of the uterus (the cervix), so there is no risk of injury to the unborn child. If your doctor is at all concerned about miscarriage or premature labour, he will discuss this with you. No studies have shown conclusively that sex in early pregnancy contributes to miscarriage. The contractions felt during arousal and orgasm are not powerful enough to start labour unless, at the time, the mother was 'on the edge' and about to start spontaneously.

Your doctor may advise you to refrain from penetrative sex if you have a low-lying placenta or placenta praevia. Once your membranes have broken, it is not advisable to have sexual intercourse. Always consult your doctor if you are not sure.

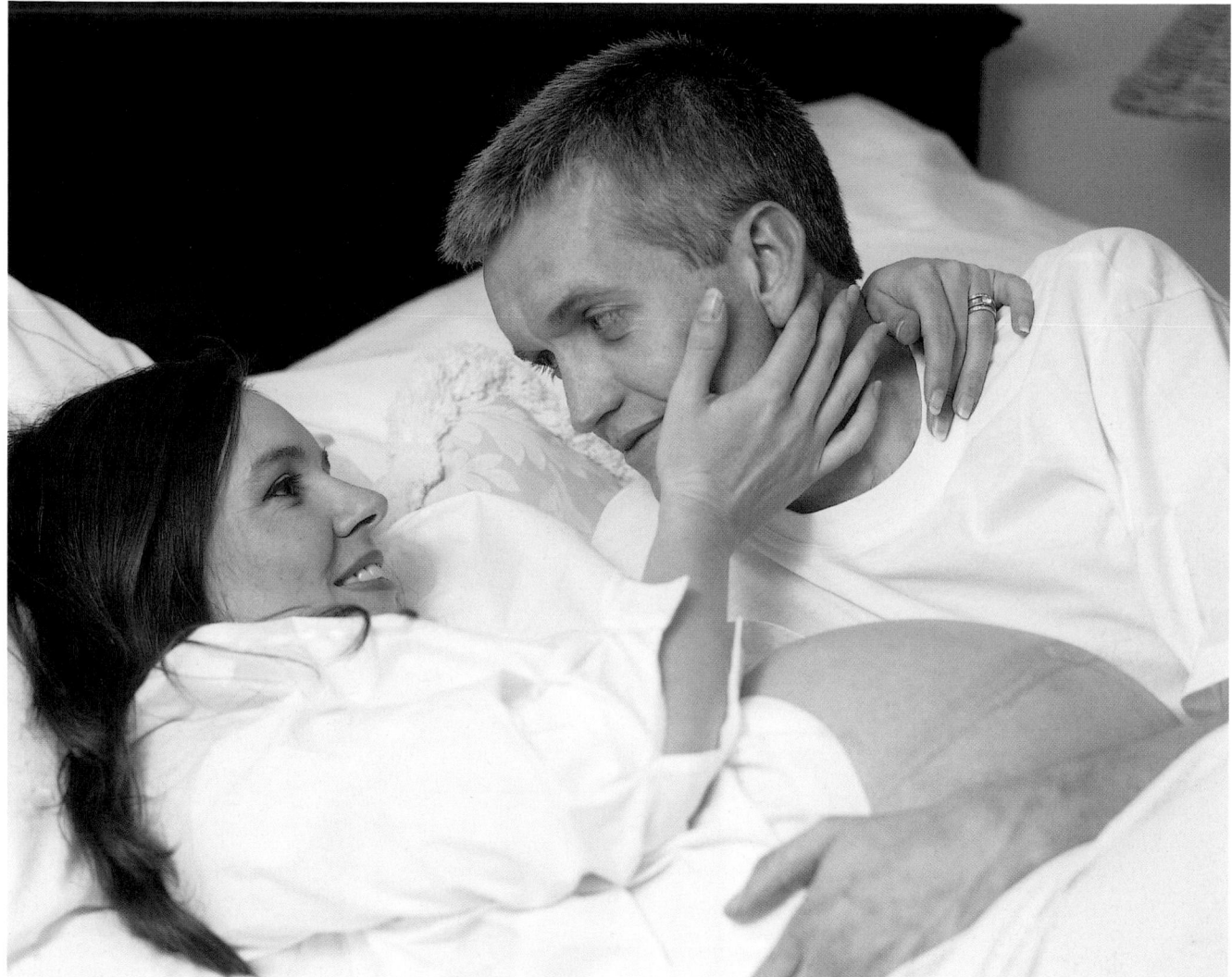

Dedicated to dads

While all these changes are occurring in a woman's body, her partner definitely has a part to play in how she sees herself and how she feels about her changing body.

Men are often left out of the pregnancy equation, which can lead to frustration and resentment. Some men are 'turned on' by their partner's pregnancy, and changing body, while others are not. Men have different concerns, other than possibly hurting the mother and the baby. Emotions and impending responsibilities of parenthood may decrease their libido as well.

What to do

An important consideration of any relationship is intimacy, and this can flourish as you both become aware of the new life that you have created together. Pregnancy is a perfect opportunity for you as a couple to share the unique process and remain close. Comfort and safety should always be a

Above Take time to discuss with your partner the feelings, or even anxiety, you may be experiencing about intimacy during your pregnancy; work through it together.

concern and, for most couples, sexual intercourse can continue throughout pregnancy. If you feel reluctant, share your feelings and reasons with your partner. Good communication is paramount at this emotional stage in your lives, and it will do much to prevent misunderstanding and resentment.

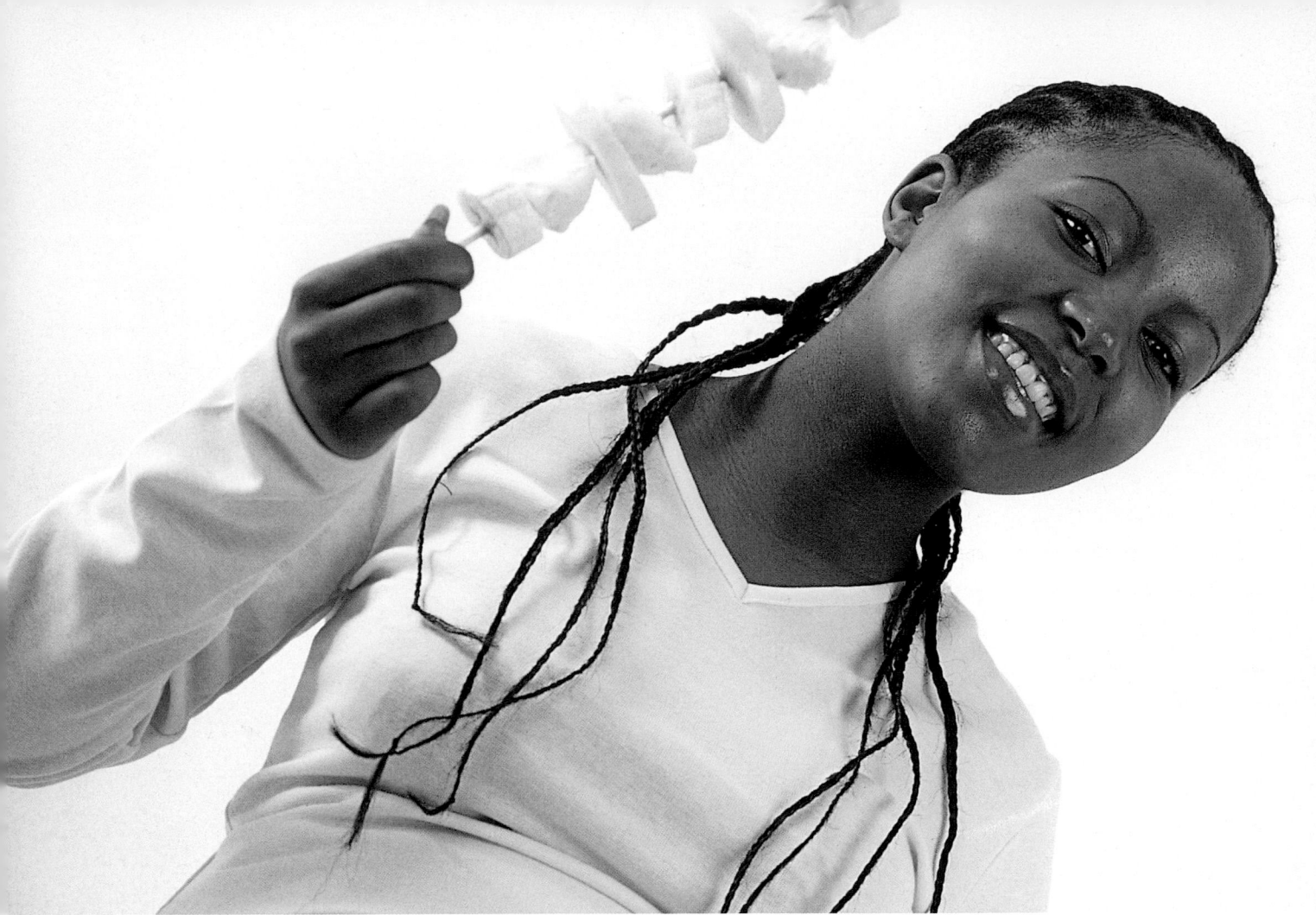

Building a healthy baby

Never before will nutrition play as vital a role as it does during pregnancy. Eating intelligently makes all the difference for you and the baby you are 'building'. It takes 80,000 calories to grow a baby, and it will be created from the nutrients supplied by and through your body, so it is important for you to obtain the essential building blocks, which include protein, vitamins and minerals. While you strengthen and improve your own body, remember that you are also building the body of a brand-new person. Pregnancy is a time when your nutritional reserves will be raided, so it is important to have good eating habits prior to conception.

EATING INTELLIGENTLY MAKES ALL THE DIFFERENCE FOR YOU AND YOUR BABY

Nutrition

The quality of food consumed is just as important as the quantity, and a pregnant woman's nutritional requirements increase dramatically during pregnancy. Satisfy your appetite with healthy food; avoid sugar, sweets, fatty foods, cold drinks and refined cereal products. These foods contain insufficient nutrients in terms of protein, minerals, vitamins and fibre. Consuming more fresh vegetables and fruit, unrefined cereals and milk will provide you with the extra fuel as well as the extra nutrients without causing weight gain.

You will need to check your weight and it is best to make the necessary adjustments during the preparatory or pre-conception phase. Do not use appetite suppressants to attain your goal weight! Pregnancy is NOT a good time to go on a diet. You should enter your pregnancy at a comfortable weight for your frame, with good eating habits and a stable metabolism. If you need guidance in this area, contact your caregiver or consult a nutritionist or registered dietitian. There are also groups such as Weight Watchers that can assist you in making permanent, healthy changes to your eating habits.

Weight gain

The timing of your weight gain is as important as the amount of weight you 'put on'. The foetus gains most of its weight in the last trimester, so you must not cut down on calories at this time, even if you have gained a fair amount already. If this is the case, seek advice on what food to eat to supply nutrients and fuel for your baby, but less fat for your body reserves. Weight gain equal to 20 per cent of your normal weight is acceptable, so based on an average weight of 55–75kg (121–165 lb), an increase of 11–15kg (24–33 lb) would be fine (*see* p70).

Weight distribution in pregnancy

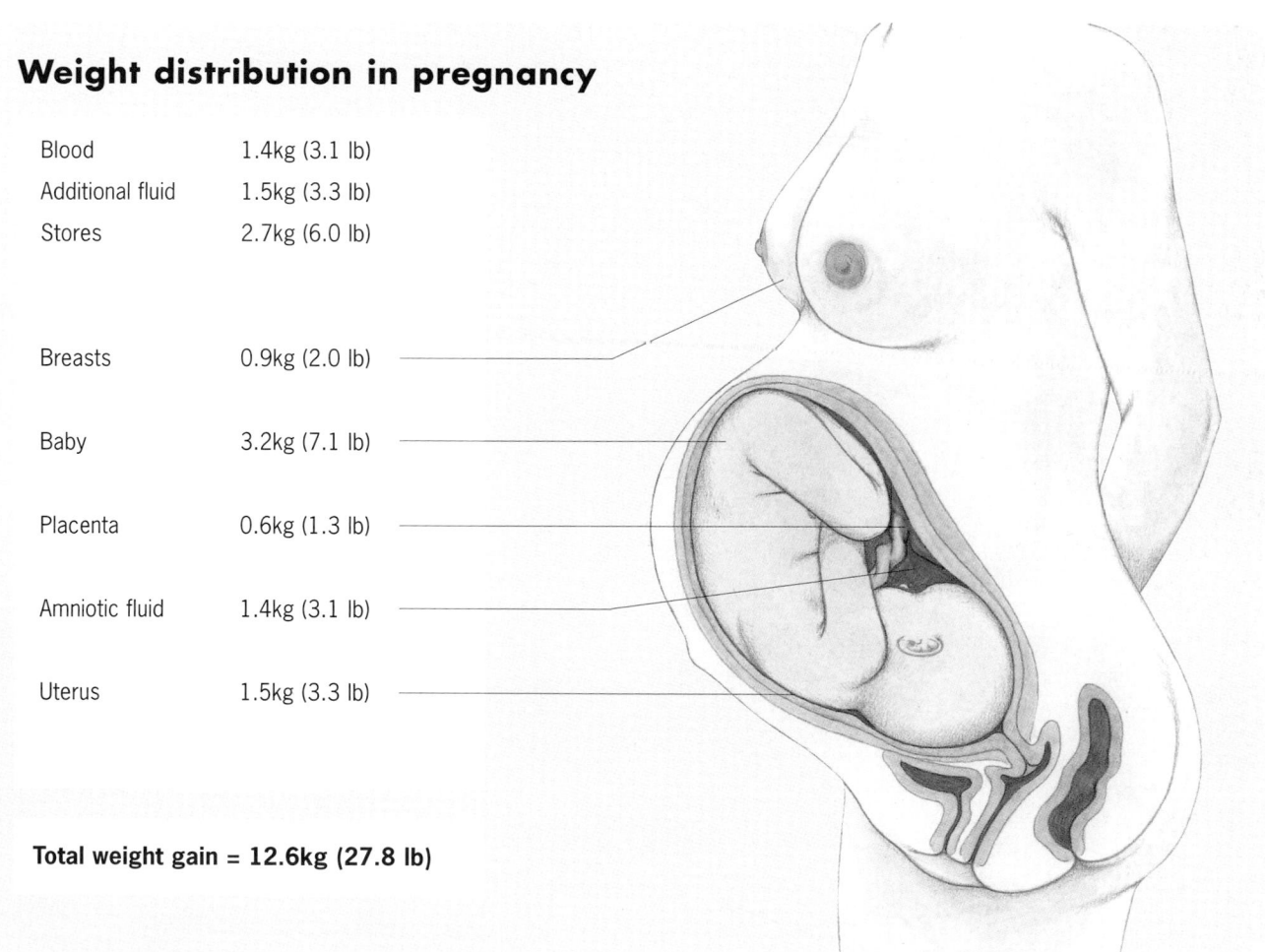

Blood	1.4kg (3.1 lb)
Additional fluid	1.5kg (3.3 lb)
Stores	2.7kg (6.0 lb)
Breasts	0.9kg (2.0 lb)
Baby	3.2kg (7.1 lb)
Placenta	0.6kg (1.3 lb)
Amniotic fluid	1.4kg (3.1 lb)
Uterus	1.5kg (3.3 lb)

Total weight gain = 12.6kg (27.8 lb)

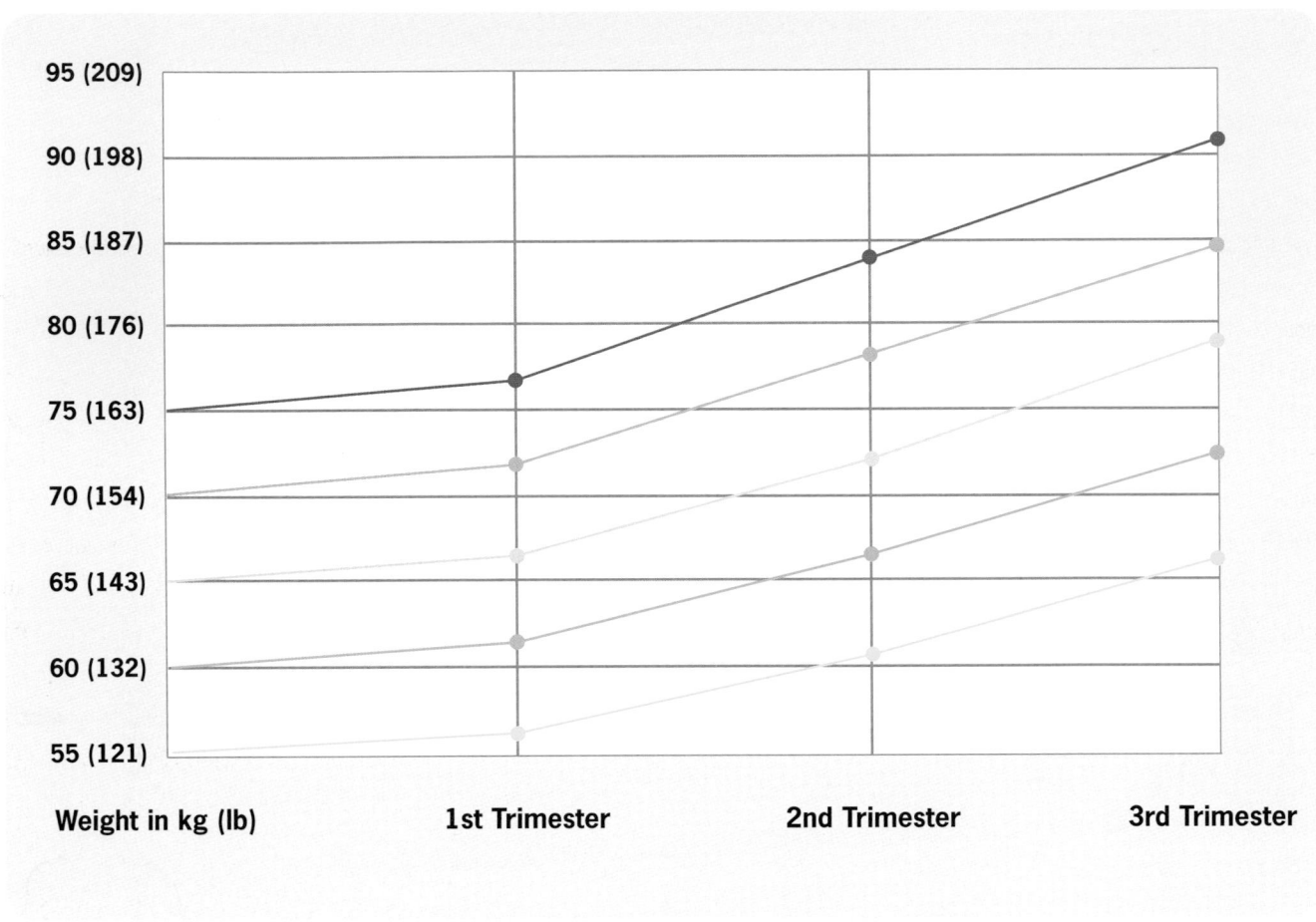

The graph: y-axis labeled in kg (lb): 95 (209), 90 (198), 85 (187), 80 (176), 75 (163), 70 (154), 65 (143), 60 (132), 55 (121). X-axis: Weight in kg (lb), 1st Trimester, 2nd Trimester, 3rd Trimester.

Above The graph gives an indication of normal weight gain in different weight categories during pregnancy.

Bear in mind that the foetus, placenta, enlarged uterus, stored nutrients, the milk glands and fat constitute the total weight in pregnancy. The increase in blood volume and cellular fluid also contribute to your weight. When assessing your weight gain, you need to take into consideration your height and build.

First Trimester

The body's need for specific nutrients varies according to the stage of your pregnancy. Research shows that a mother's diet at the time of conception can affect her baby's health throughout its life. What you eat in the first trimester is important because it is the time when cells differentiate and develop into the baby's organs. So, whatever is lacking at this critical stage cannot be made up for later.

WEIGHT GAIN There should be a small weight gain of 0.7–1.4kg (1.5–3 lb).

Second Trimester

In the second trimester, the foetus needs calcium because of the abundant and rapid bone and cell formation.

WEIGHT GAIN 0.3–0.4kg (0.6–0.9 lb) per week is acceptable.

Third Trimester

In the third trimester, your baby really starts to gain weight and doubles in size. Adequate nutrients, including carbohydrates, are vital to supply the huge energy demands made by the foetus. Protein is essential for the manufacture of new tissue during the last 10 weeks of pregnancy.

WEIGHT GAIN 0.3–0.4kg (0.6–0.9 lb) per week is acceptable.

Vital nutrients

What you eat influences your baby's growth and development, and each food group plays a vital role in cell development. This chapter shows you which foods provide the different building blocks that will 'construct' your baby's body. You will, however, need to take additional supplements as advised by your caregiver.

A healthy diet can boost your baby's immune system so his body is better able to fight off infection once he is born. Research in the UK has found that vitamins C and E may reduce the risk of a mother developing pregnancy induced hypertension (*see* p25), a condition characterized by abnormally high blood pressure, which occurs only during pregnancy.

Folic acid

The discovery that folic acid, taken before conception and during pregnancy, reduces the risk of neural-tube defects must surely be the most significant breakthrough of recent times. Folic acid is a naturally occurring B vitamin that is vital to the proper growth of cells. A deficiency of folic acid at the time cells around the spine of the baby are dividing and growing can result in a neural-tube defect, such as spina bifida.

Folic acid is found in all leafy green vegetables, bananas, cheddar cheese, yeast extract, nuts, eggs, oranges, haddock and salmon. The average daily intake is only half the ideal intake for a woman planning a pregnancy, and it is therefore recommended that a woman take a daily 400mcg supplement of folic acid, 12 weeks before conception until 12 weeks into her pregnancy. Folic acid may also reduce the risk of premature labour and cleft palate.

Carbohydrates

Carbohydrates provide most of the calorific content. These are fuel foods that provide energy and if taken in excess, they will be stored in the body as fat. Carbohydrates are necessary for the growth of the foetus, placenta and maternal tissues. Bread, cereals and grains ensure good bowel function.

Wholewheat pasta, brown rice, wholewheat bread, unrefined cereals, fruit, milk and dairy products, honey, sugar and many vegetables are all sources of carbohydrates. Breads and cereals contain no more calories per gram than meat, and contain far less fat.

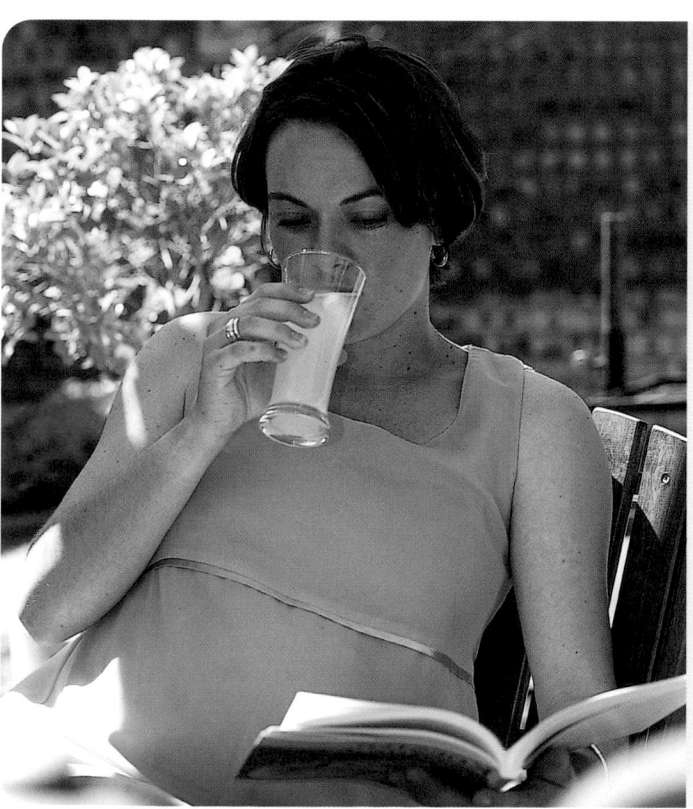

'Baby boosting' foods

- Wholewheat bread provides plenty of fibre and iron.
- Unsweetened, pure orange juice and fresh oranges are good for vitamin C.
- Oily fish, such as salmon and sardines, boosts eye and brain development and helps to prevent premature birth.
- Yoghurt is a good source of calcium.
- Lean red meat provides a good source of iron.
- Fortified bran flakes also provide iron, fibre and vitamins.
- Lentils, dried apricots, beans and chickpeas are great foods to add to your diet.

Left Drink a tall glass of freshly squeezed orange juice for a boost of vitamin C.

Vitamins and minerals

These substances are required in minute quantities but are essential. They work with other nutrients in thousands of combinations.

Minerals

- **Iron** is needed for the formation of blood. The foetus starts to store iron from about five months of gestation. Iron prevents anaemia and is found in organ meats (e.g. liver, kidneys, etc.), eggs, green leafy vegetables, iodized salt and wholegrains.
- **Calcium** is needed for the formation of bones and teeth as well as muscle function. It is required to synthesize vitamin D, and is found in cheese, milk, yoghurt, broccoli, spinach and sardines.
- **Phosphorus** together with calcium hardens bones and teeth. Fish, eggs, cheese, milk and green leafy vegetables are all sources of phosphorus.

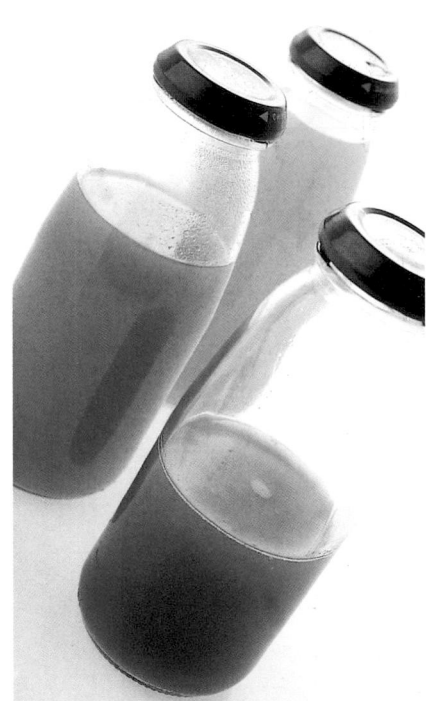

- **Sodium** (salt) is needed to maintain water balance in the body and for the formation of plasma, bone, muscle and the brain. Sodium should always be used in moderation.
- **Magnesium** is important for the growth of bones, teeth and muscle. It is found in wholegrain cereals, legumes, nuts, meat and milk.
- **Zinc** repairs damaged cells, aids growth, and boosts the immune system. It is found in meat, fish and wheatgerm.

Vitamins

The most important vitamins for the pregnant mother are vitamins A, B, C, D and K.

- **Vitamin A** is a fat-soluble vitamin that is necessary for cell development and tooth-bud formation. Food sources include green and yellow vegetables, butter and cream. Excessive amounts can lead to birth defects (see p75), so check with your caregiver before taking supplements.
- **Vitamin B** is a group of water-soluble vitamins of which B_1, B_2, B_{12} and folic acid are important. B vitamins are required for growth of the nervous system and muscles, formation of blood and they also help with protein metabolism. They are found in wholewheat bread, yeast, certain vegetables, lean meat, dairy products and eggs.
- **Vitamin C** is water-soluble and is required for skeletal development of the foetus. It enhances the absorption of iron and calcium and is found in citrus fruit, broccoli and green peppers, as well as green leafy vegetables (the darker, the better), melons, mangoes and jelly.

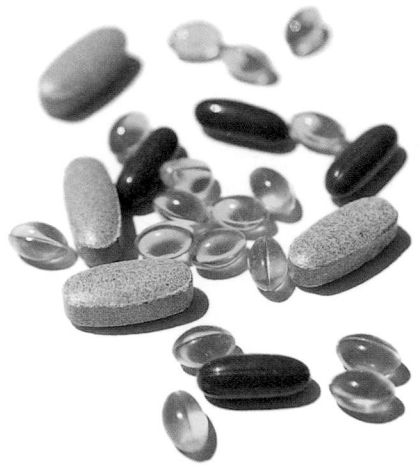

Above Your caregiver may prescribe supplements according to your body's needs.
Opposite Ensure that your diet includes foods from all the food groups.
Below left Diluted fruit juice is a healthier alternative to fizzy drinks, tea and coffee.

- **Vitamin D** is fat-soluble and essential for calcium absorption and balance. It is found in milk, margarine and butter and, of course, sunlight.
- **Vitamin K** is a fat-soluble vitamin that is needed for the coagulation of blood, which is an important consideration at the time of birth for mother and baby. It is found in cabbage, lettuce, carrots, milk and butter.

Essential fatty acids

Essential fatty acids must be present for the absorption of fat-soluble vitamins A, D, E and K and they also contain vitamins A and D, which enhance the absorption of calcium. These fatty acids prevent dry skin and are found in avocado, nuts, meats, vegetable oils, olive oil, butter, cheese, and oily

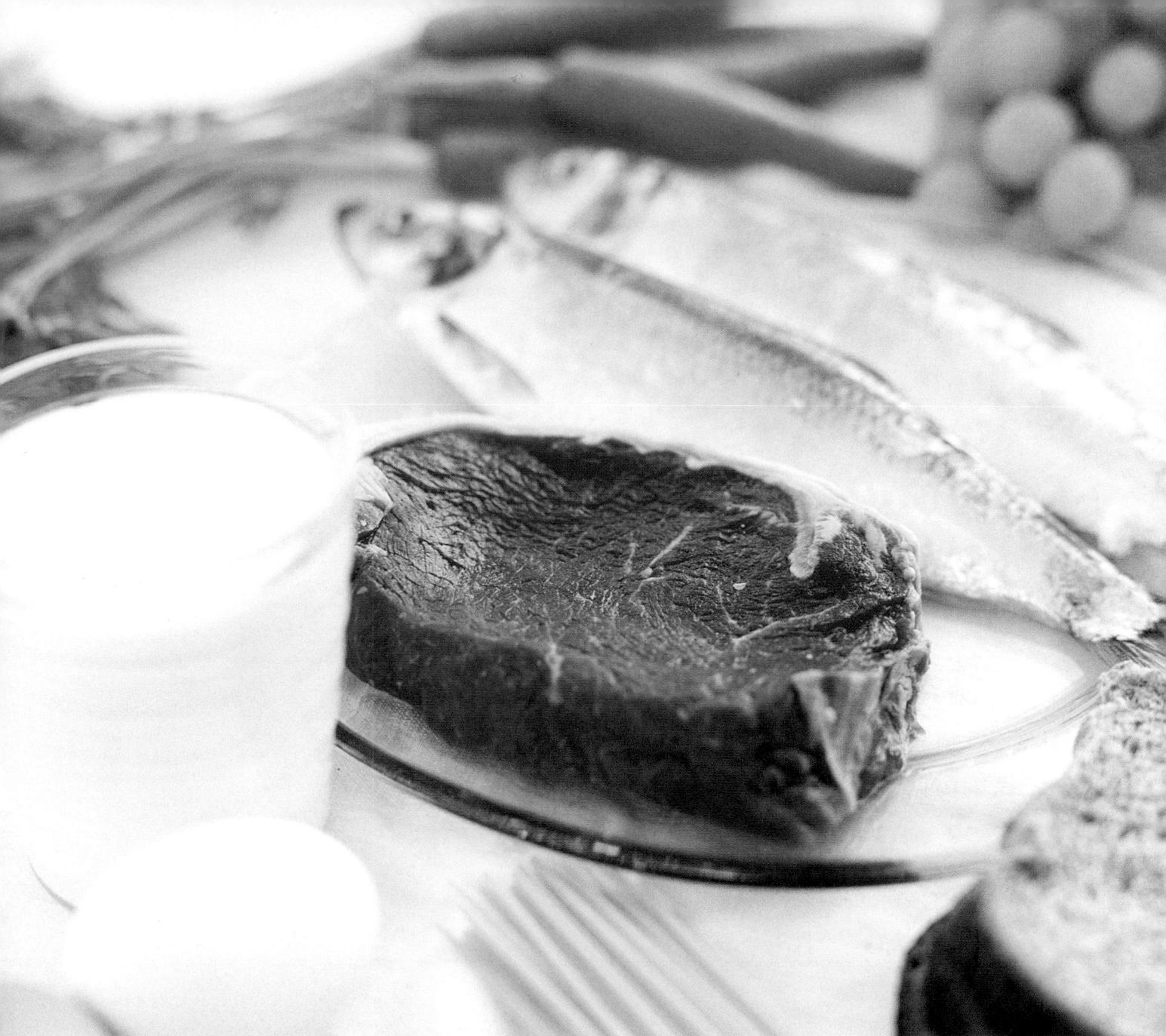

fish such as salmon and sardines. Note: use low-fat yoghurt or low-fat buttermilk instead of oil as a base for salads.

Protein

Protein is found in every cell in the body and it is the only substance from which the baby's body tissue can be built. It helps repair cells and organs, and supports the placenta, the growing baby and the increased blood volume. If you are carrying twins, you need to eat even more protein than if you were carrying a single baby.

First-class proteins or adequate proteins are found in eggs, milk and other dairy products, fish, poultry, meat, and nuts, seeds and soybeans. Second-class or incomplete proteins include legumes (peas, beans, lentils and peanuts), vegetables, sprouts and grains.

Milk and dairy products

Essential for healthy bones and teeth, milk and its products supply many of the required vitamins, proteins and fats for pregnancy. Food sources include fat-free, low-fat or whole milk, cheese, yoghurt, custards, puddings, cottage cheese, milk powder and ice cream.

Dangerous substances

These foods are the so-called teratogens – substances that cause malformation in the foetus. They may contain bacteria and toxins and should be handled with care.

Salmonella

Most of these bacteria are killed by stomach acid, but some can reach the small intestine where they start to reproduce. The bacteria release a toxin that is responsible for the symptoms – nausea, fever, abdominal pain and vomiting – experienced by the infected person. To avoid salmonella poisoning do the following:

- cook meat thoroughly
- do not eat an egg that has a cracked shell
- use pasteurized milk and dairy products
- store cooked meat, poultry and other leftover food in airtight containers and refrigerate immediately
- buy prepackaged fish and shellfish and check the expiry date.

Listeria

Even though listeria usually causes mild illness with fever as the only symptom, it can still affect your unborn baby. Unlike other food-contaminating bacteria, listeria can grow in the refrigerator. You can prevent food poisoning by:

- cooking meat all the way through
- eating only freshly prepared foods and fresh cheeses
- avoiding ready-to-eat seafoods (smoked fish and mussels) and foods that have been refrigerated for more than a day

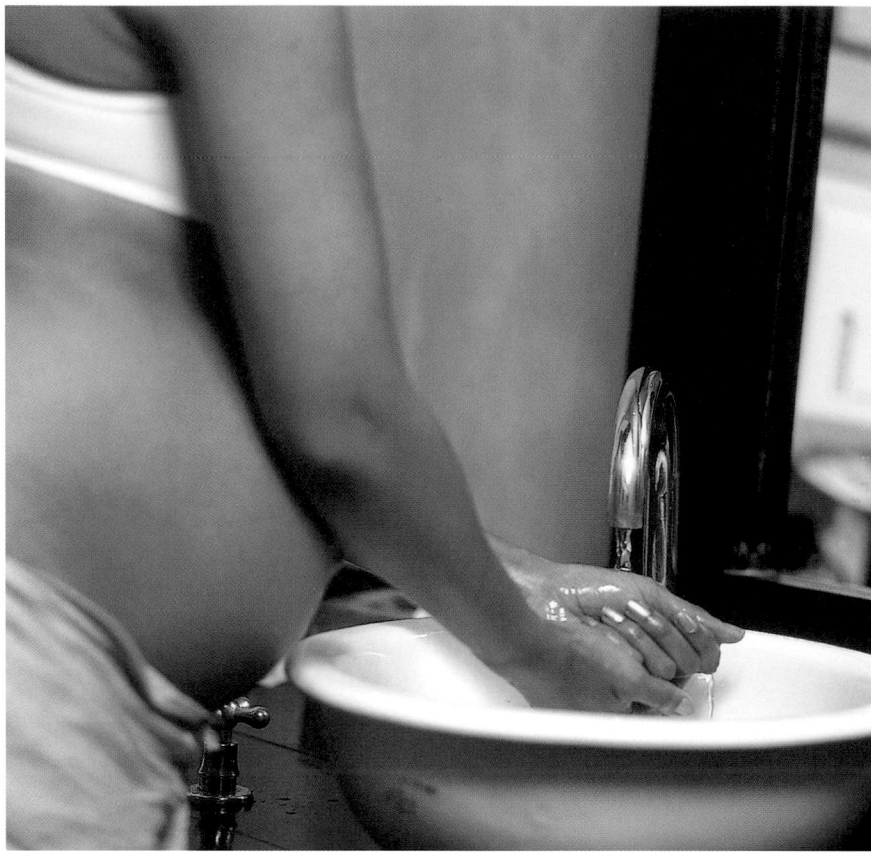

- avoiding soft cheeses (Brie and Camembert), and unpasteurized dairy products
- avoiding pre-mixed coleslaw, and paté.

Toxoplasmosis

Most people who are infected with *Toxoplasma gondii* do not show any symptoms. Toxoplasmosis can be transferred to the foetus, resulting in brain damage and blindness. If a woman is infected with the parasite before she becomes pregnant, the baby can still be infected. Always do the following to avoid poisoning:

- wash your hands, utensils and cutting boards after handling raw meat to prevent contamination of other foods
- do not drink unpasteurized milk
- cook meat all the way through

Above Wash your hands thoroughly after handling raw meat or working in the garden.

- avoid cleaning a cat's litter box
- wear household gloves when gardening.

Botulism

Botulism is a case of severe food poisoning, which is caused by the microscopic organism *Clostridium botulinum*. It produces a toxin that does not give off a bad odour or taste in food and is, unfortunately, not detectable by smell, or taste for that matter.

It breeds most commonly in food that has been improperly canned at home. To avoid food poisoning, do not eat foods from bulging cans or cans with bulging lids.

Substances in moderation

The following substances are normally fine, but during pregnancy they should be eaten in moderation otherwise they could affect the health of your unborn baby. These are by no means toxic but in large amounts can negatively affect the foetus.

Caffeine is a stimulant that crosses the placenta and affects your baby's heart rate and breathing. Although the research linking caffeine to pregnancy complications is inconclusive, the Food and Drug Administration (FDA) and the American College of Obstetricians and Gynaecologists recommend no more caffeine than that in two cups of coffee per day. There is also caffeine in tea, cola drinks and chocolate.

Vitamin A If eaten in large quantities, vitamin A can be teratogenic (*see* opposite page). Be very careful when taking supplements and do not overindulge in the following foods: liver, kidney, milk fat, fortified margarine and egg yolk.

Sugar, in moderation, adds to the palatability of your food. Sometimes, when aversions rule and you are not eating properly, a bit of sugar can help to meet the increased energy requirement that you have. However, sugar contains 'empty' calories and is not the best source of energy. Rather choose unrefined carbohydrates such as high-fibre cereals, wholewheat bread, and fruit and vegetables that are rich in vitamins, minerals and fibre.

Note: Since there are no specific safe recommendations regarding the use of artificial sweeteners in pregnancy, it is best to avoid them.

Fat You should limit the amount of fat that you consume. However, fats do contain important fat-soluble vitamins and essential fatty acids that are needed for the healthy development of your baby.

Instead, choose unsaturated fats and oils such as olive oil, sunflower oil, soft margarine, fish, olives and avocados, rather than saturated fats like red meat and full-cream dairy products.

General nutritional tips

- Eat a variety of foods.
- Eat plenty of high-fibre foods.
- Avoid eating fried foods: grill, steam, bake, poach or stir fry as much as possible.
- Eat as much raw fruit and vegetables as possible.
- Drink plenty of water: try to aim for eight glasses a day.
- Avoid alcohol!
- Avoid too much sugar and salt.
- Avoid too much fat.
- Avoid caffeine.
- Make sure that you have plenty of nutritious snacks available when hunger pangs strike.

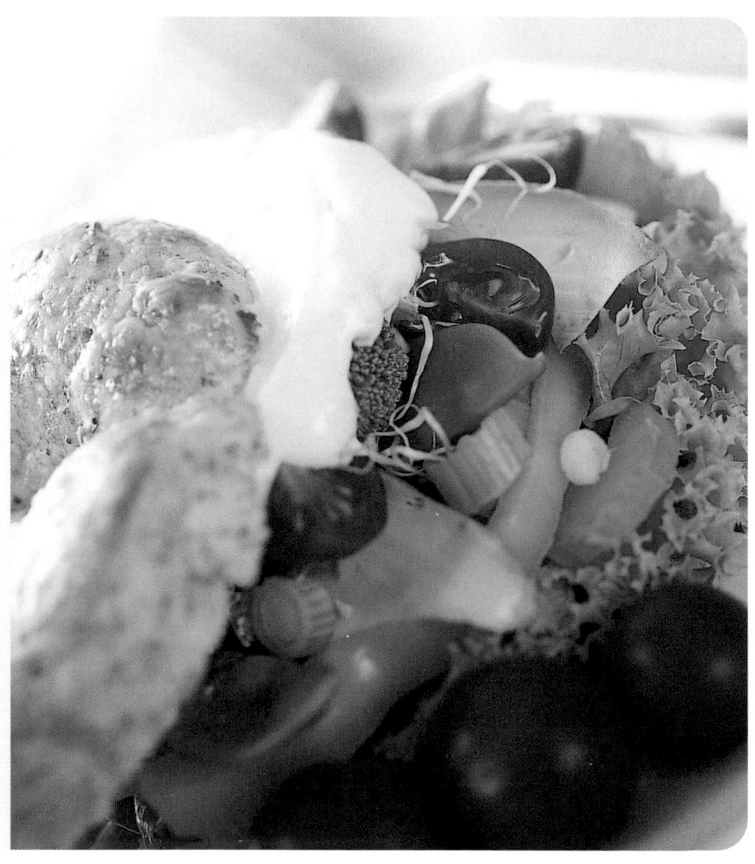

Right Make every meal count by eating healthy, nutritious foods that will contribute to your baby's health.

Cravings

Many pregnant women crave normal foods but in strange combinations. Cravings can indicate a nutrient deficiency – for example, a craving for strawberries may indicate a vitamin C deficiency. Changes in hormonal levels can also play a role.

Taste is very closely related to smell, using many of the same nerves and areas of the brain. The taste buds on the tongue are more vascular in pregnancy, which leads to taste changes during this time. The following changes that take place in your body might explain some of the reasons why you experience cravings:

- there are changes to your carbohydrate (or sugar) metabolism
- fat is usually stored in the body at a different rate than normal
- protein metabolism is different

- the thyroid hormone, responsible for metabolism, is related to the pregnancy hormone and also affects appetite
- the need for certain vitamins is increased during your pregnancy
- salt metabolism also changes, affecting thirst levels
- your taste threshold increases, making you want foods with a higher concentration of flavour.

Pregnancy is an emotional time and your eating habits are very strongly influenced by emotions. You may be feeling unsure of yourself and your changing body. Responsibilities at work may be getting the better of you because you are more tired, uncomfortable, forgetful and emotional. If you have other children at home, they may not understand why mom is not herself. All these factors can leave you feeling emotionally and physically drained, which can impact on your eating habits.

If you do experience moderate cravings or feel like eating something you would not normally eat, it is not a problem to indulge occasionally. If you have a severe craving for a specific food, make sure the rest of your diet is sufficient, and that this specific food is not harmful to you or your baby. Aversions normally come and go throughout your pregnancy.

Pica

Pica is the ingestion of non-food substances in response to a craving. Examples of unusual substances craved are: chalk, clay, soil, laundry detergent or starch, ice, baking powder, baking soda, cement, paint and ashes. The incidence of pica varies ethnically and regionally.

Pica probably will not be harmful if it consists of an occasional desire for ice cubes, but other substances may cause gastrointestinal problems. Dirt and clay may contain parasites and laundry products are likely to contain harsh chemicals and perfumes. The ingestion of these substances should be reported to your doctor immediately.

Another phenomenon, called 'olfactory craving', is when pregnant women smell selected substances in response to cravings. This may occur alone or together with pica.

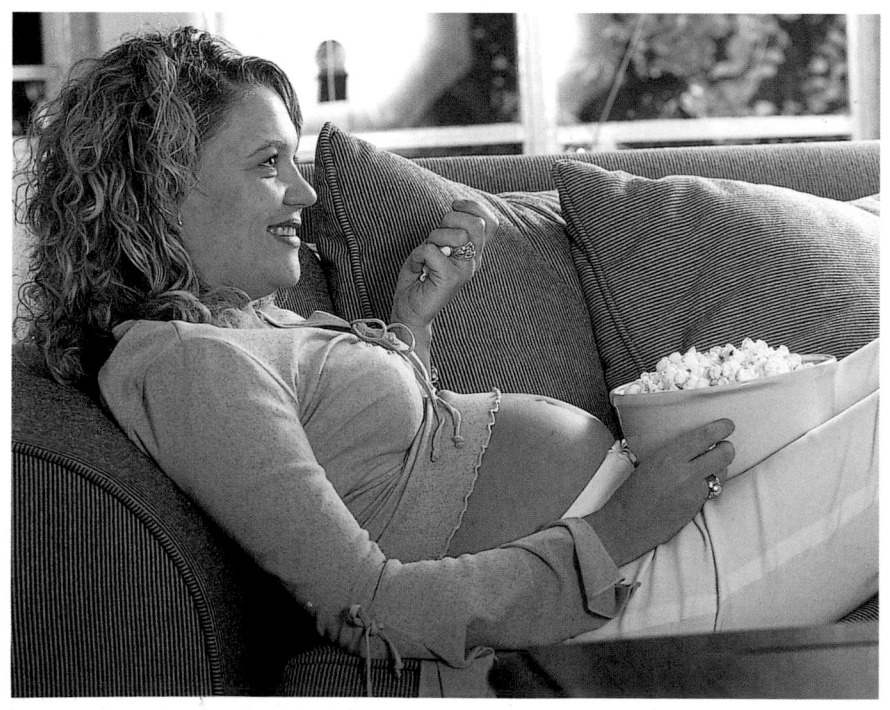

Left You might find that you crave foods that you normally would not eat; this is completely normal but try to avoid foods that have a high sugar, salt or fat content.

Harmful substances

Smoking

Pregnant women who smoke are nearly twice as likely to deliver low birth-weight babies (infants who weigh less than 2.5kg/ 5.5 lb) who are more likely to have health and developmental problems after birth. The decrease in birth weight is dose related; babies born to heavy smokers (more than 20 cigarettes per day) are more affected than babies born to light smokers. Smoking reduces the flow of oxygen and nutrients to the foetus. Nicotine impairs the absorption of calcium, vitamin C and other vitamins and minerals required by a developing foetus. Some researchers suggest that smoking may lead to lower caloric intake by the mother and her smaller weight gain may account for the lower birth weight of the baby. Smoking has also been associated with poor breast milk supply. Cutting down or switching to a low tar cigarette is not the answer either. Ideally, quitting is the only way to protect your baby, although cutting down is better than doing nothing.

Alcohol

Foetal Alcohol Syndrome (FAS) is a range of defects or abnormalities in the foetus while in the uterus, caused by alcohol in the mother's bloodstream. The gestational age of the baby at exposure is very important – the highest risk period is when your baby's organs are developing (between weeks four and 14). Alcoholism in the mother is usually

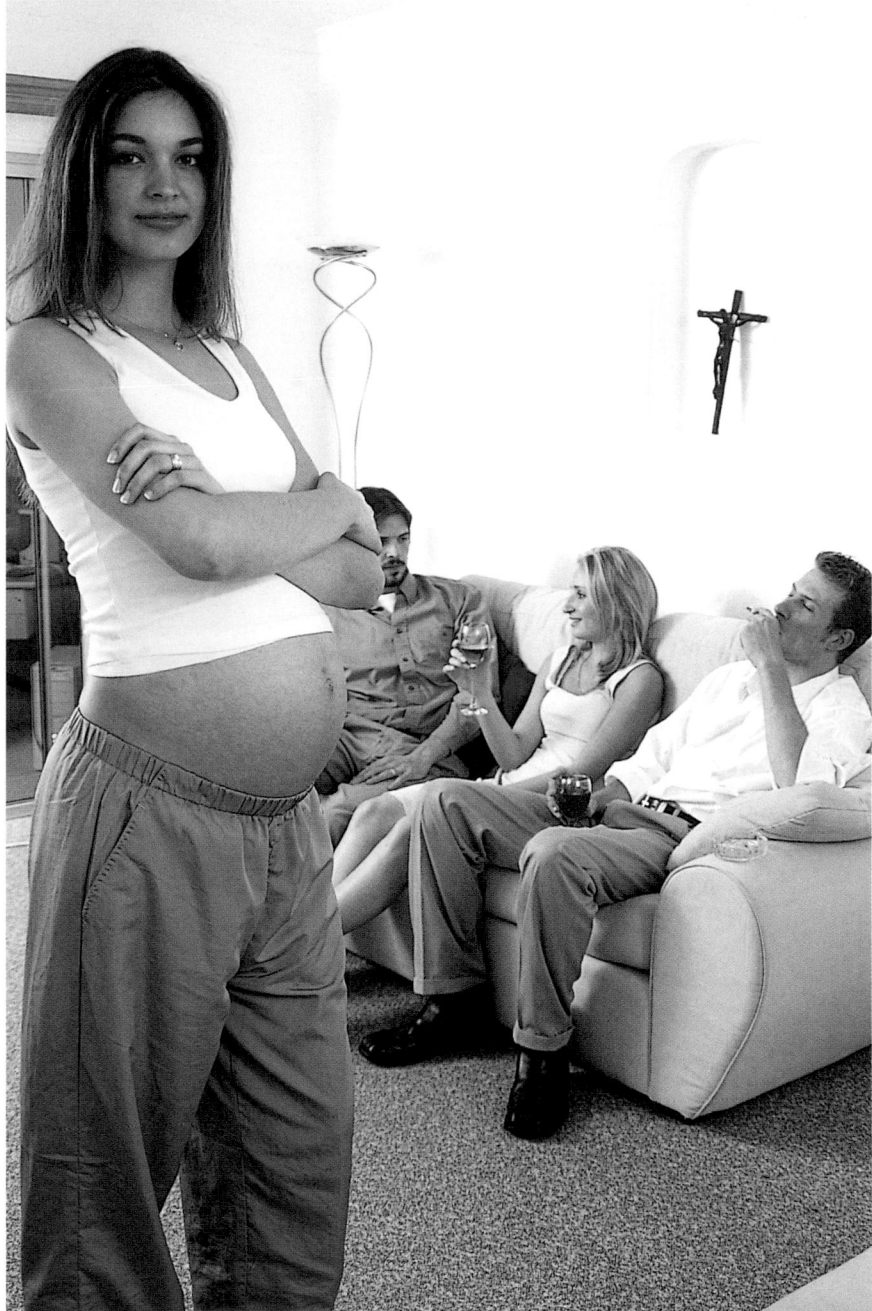

the cause, however, consuming large quantities of alcohol regularly, or binge drinking, will affect your baby. The alcohol will not only move via the placenta into the baby's bloodstream, but it can also reach higher levels in the baby than in the mother. Furthermore, the baby's immature kidneys

Above *Avoid alcohol and tobacco smoke as these substances are harmful to your baby.*

and liver cannot process and break down these chemicals so they can, potentially, reach a high level of toxicity in the baby.

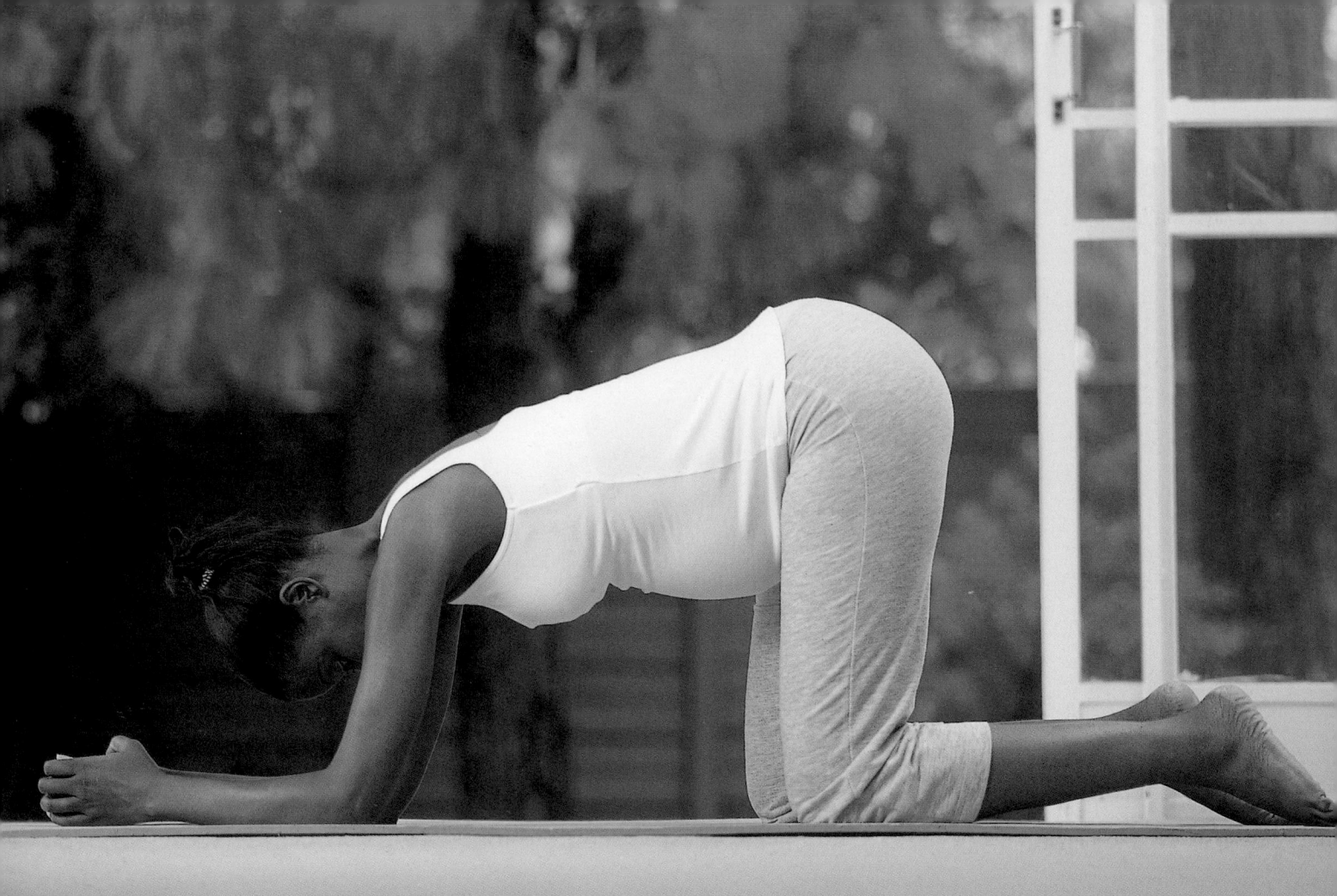

Exercise during pregnancy

Keeping active and preparing for labour and the challenges of motherhood are vital. Most pregnant women benefit enormously from doing regular exercise. Specialized classes are not always readily available but, with minor modifications to your lifestyle, you can still get fit and keep fit.

During pregnancy your body undergoes changes, which you have to accommodate. You are more vulnerable to injury during the latter part of pregnancy, so taking care of and respecting your body is all-important. You should make an effort to increase strength and stamina and keep energized, but maintaining a moderate exercise regime is the responsible thing to do.

LISTEN TO YOUR BODY'S SIGNALS AND DO NOT OVEREXERT YOURSELF

What you should know

When you exercise, different body systems are affected. Exercise changes hormonal activity, raises body temperature, activates muscles, changes mineral and fluid balance, speeds up metabolism and uses up stored energy. This is something the body likes; it feels good. How easily your body adapts to exercise depends on your age, weight, diet, health and level of fitness as well as the type, intensity and duration of the workout. Exercise causes you to use more oxygen, therefore you will take in more oxygen. The more you take in, the more you will burn stored fat. Your muscles and bones also become denser and stronger.

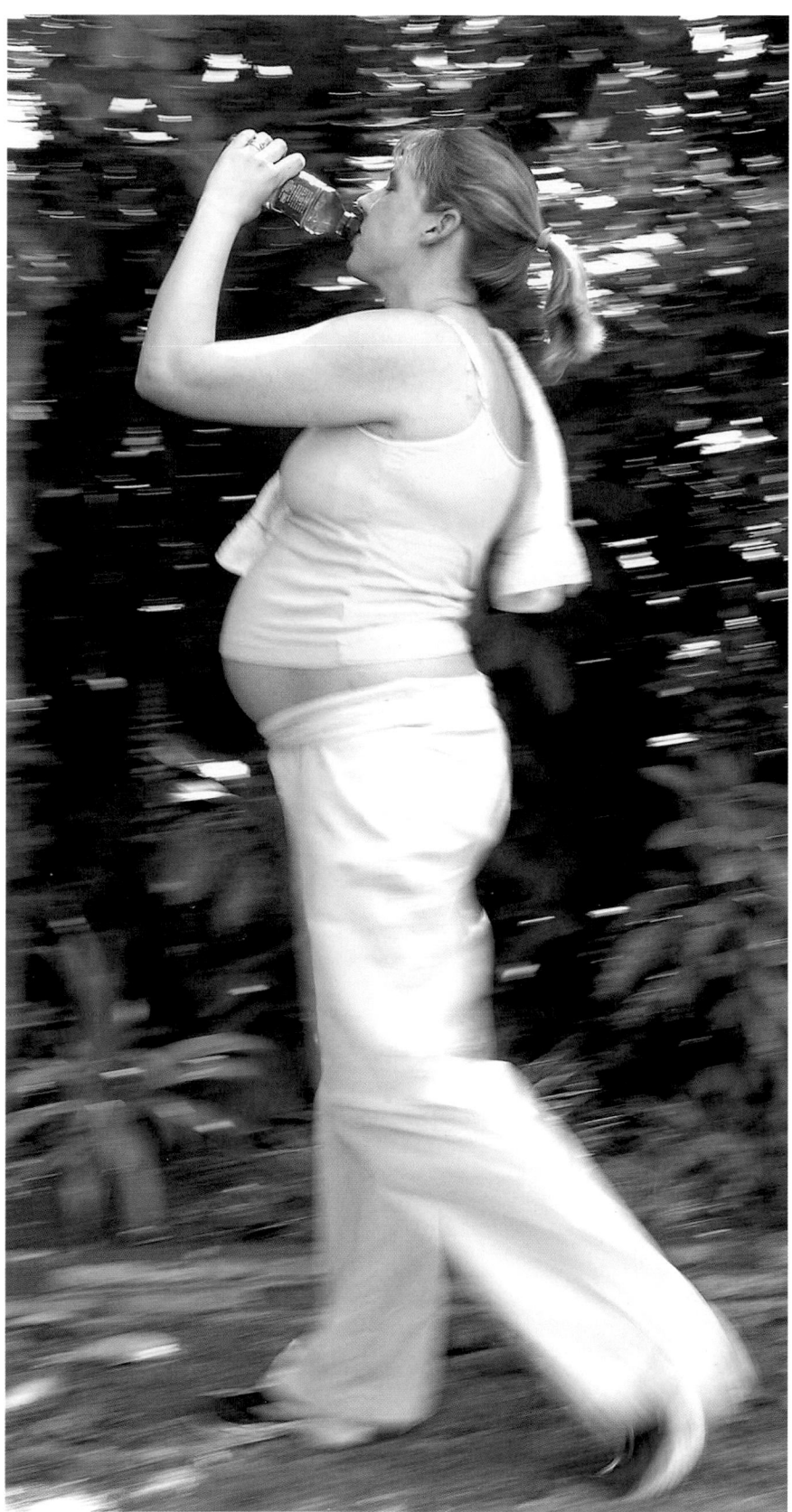

Right Remember to drink enough water to avoid dehydration when exercising.

Benefits of regular exercise

- Exercise improves blood circulation, which can reduce the severity of varicosities. Building muscular strength may help you reduce the discomfort of existing varicose veins (*see* p61).
- It can enhance muscular balance and strength. Learning good posture (*see* p84) and how to cope with postural shifts associated with pregnancy are essential to guard against muscle and joint soreness.
- Mild exercise may help reduce swelling and oedema (*see* p64) and return mobility to swollen joints.
- Exercise eases gastrointestinal discomfort and constipation.
- It may reduce muscle cramps.
- Exercise strengthens the abdominal muscles which provide stable support to the back and contribute to the efficiency of the second stage of labour (*see* p119).
- It helps you adopt alternative positions more easily if you prefer an active birth.
- Exercise that includes the physical practice of the birth positions and breathing techniques for birth are also beneficial for active labour.
- Postpartum (*see* pp146–148 and Glossary) recovery is swifter.

Above Start your exercise session with slow, gentle warm-up techniques so as to avoid muscle cramps and injuries.

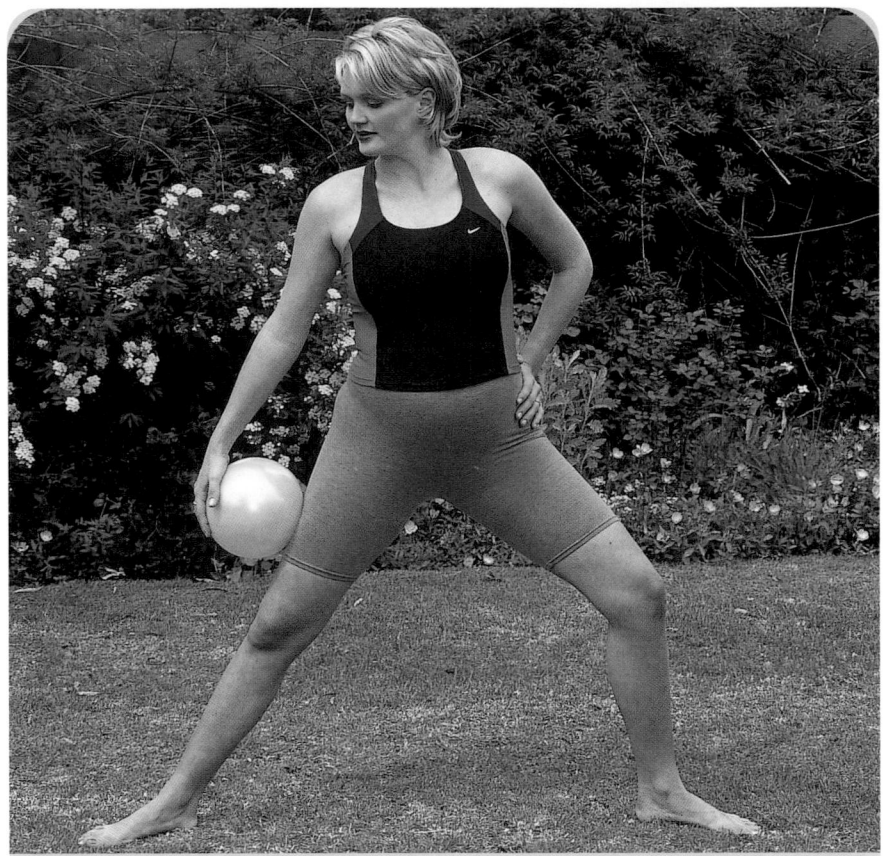

Helpful hints

- Be consistent with your workouts. Irregular workouts can do more harm than good. Work out at least three times a week, each session lasting a minimum of 20 minutes.
- Listen to your body and do not overexert yourself.
- Drink plenty of water before, during and after a workout.
- Warm up slowly before a workout and cool down afterwards.
- Rest and relax after exercise.
- Breathe easily as you exercise; you should not become breathless (slow down and drop your arms if this should happen).
- Tone down on the high-impact classes and attend classes that are slower paced.
- Always keep one foot on the ground at all times – this will prevent any strain and jarring to your joints and prevent pelvic floor discomfort.
- Avoid doing sit-ups or crunch-type exercises after the fourth month of pregnancy – modified exercises such as pelvic tilts or cat stretches are just as beneficial and effective if done correctly.

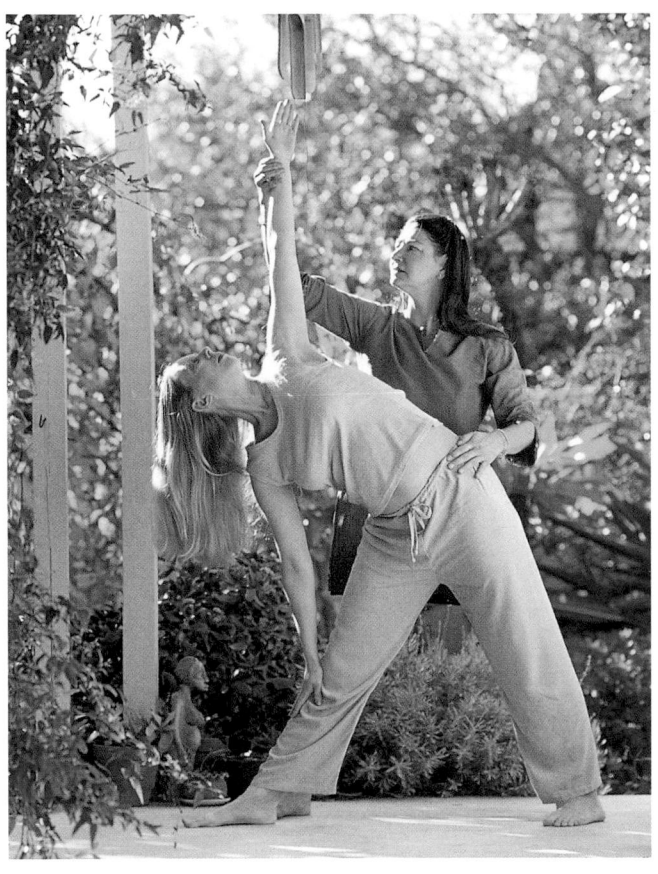
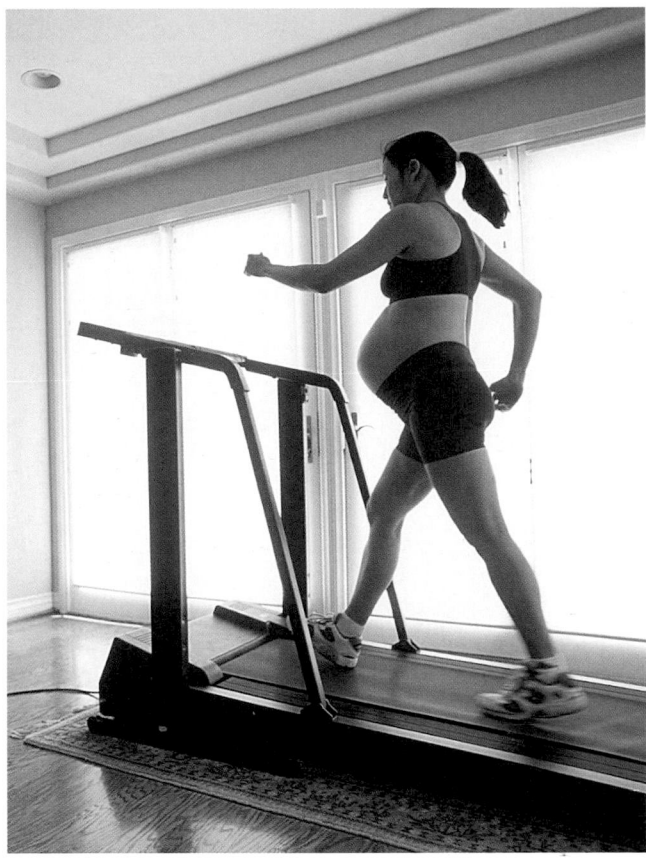

Suggested activities

Yoga

Many women find that yoga, with its gentle stretching and concentrated breathing techniques, is the perfect form of exercise and preparation for childbirth. It relieves tension, tones muscles and enhances flexibility.

During pregnancy, women should avoid strenuous upward or backward stretches or any bending seated positions that put pressure on the uterus. Forms of yoga that include vigorous abdominal contractions should be avoided. Mild forms of abdominal contractions such as the gentle taking in and pushing out of the stomach can be performed. Tell the instructor beforehand that you are pregnant.

Treadmill

The pregnant exerciser may continue to use a motorized treadmill but should monitor her pulse rate at all times, and in noting any discomfort, change her use of the treadmill accordingly. A walking or moderate jogging pace can be set up on an individual basis. Each session must include a warm-up and cool-down period. Keep the workout to 15-minute sets. Your balance is affected during pregnancy, and you should take extra care when getting on and off the treadmill.

Walking

If jogging has become uncomfortable, you should consider walking instead. Although the speed of walking may vary, the rhythm of both the walk and your breath should

Above left Yoga increases suppleness, making it the perfect preparation for childbirth.
Above right The advantage of a treadmill is that you can set a comfortable walking pace for yourself that you can maintain with ease.

remain consistent. You should transfer your weight from one foot to the other in an even pattern. Walking in gentle coordination with breathing allows your mind to clear and sharpen on your surroundings. Ensure that the area you choose to walk in is safe.

Getting in touch with nature is a wonderful way to get in touch with yourself. Hard, brisk walking while taking in the sights, sounds and smells of your environment will definitely make you feel good.

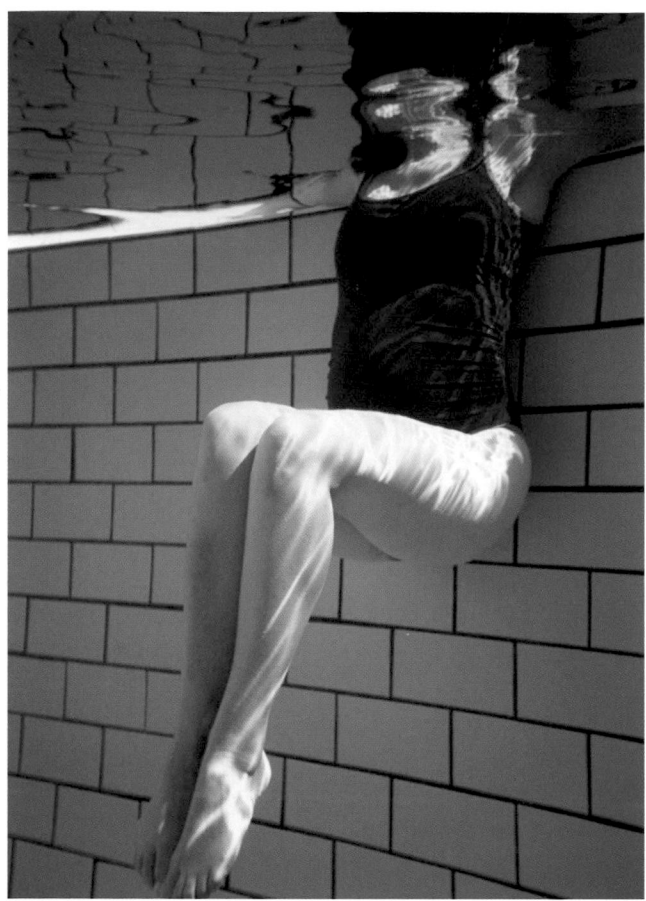
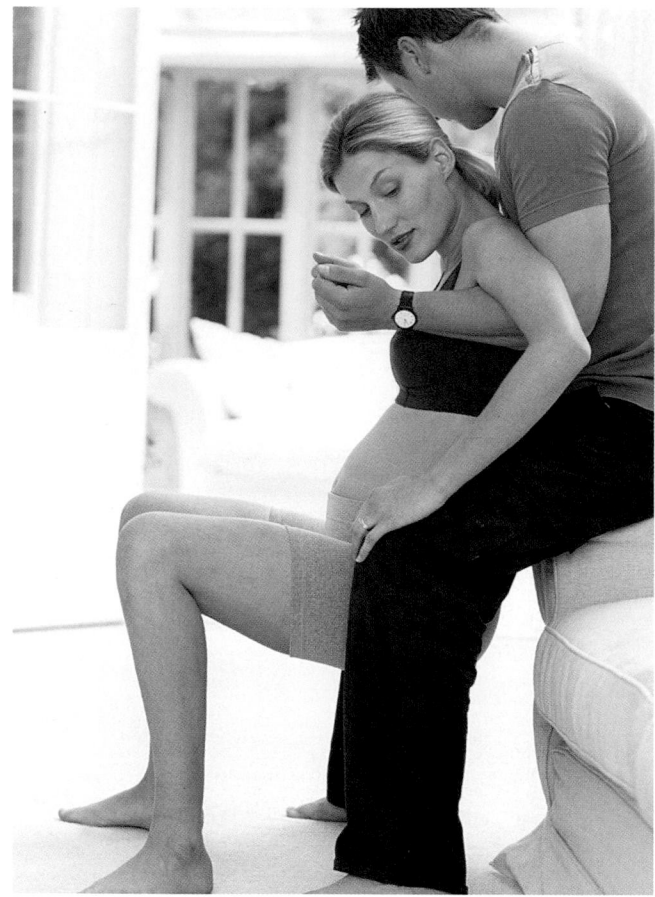

Above Exercising in water is excellent because the water provides resistance and supports your weight.

Above right Practise birth positions as part of your exercise routine; have your partner support and assist you with these.

Swimming

Swimming is a wonderful way to exercise and will strengthen and tone the whole body throughout pregnancy. In many ways it is an ideal way to exercise. Treading water is also excellent and provides a total body workout.

Swimming is an excellent way to train for the breathing of labour. Do not hold your breath for extended periods, as this could compromise oxygen supply to the baby. If a woman feels abdominal 'pulling', she should avoid the back crawl stroke. If her back hurts, she should try sidestroke. The breast-stroke is a gentle, adaptable stroke and easy to do. Diving should be avoided. If you are not feeling up to swimming, simply walk in the water – it is an excellent form of exercise because the water provides resistance. Research has shown that women who swim during pregnancy have increased abdominal strength and tone.

Stretching

Stretch and tone classes can be continued throughout pregnancy, with the mother making adaptations if any exercise or position causes even slight pain. Stretching exercise lengthens and strengthens your muscles and ligaments, and decreases your chances of injury and muscle soreness. When you stretch, take it only as far as you feel comfortable. Stretches should never be taken to the maximum point of resistance.

Strength training

The benefits of improved muscle tone and strength are endless. A strong body is a huge advantage in carrying the added weight of pregnancy. Your stability and balance are improved, as are your energy level and sense of wellbeing. Endorphins (see p114) are produced during any exercise session and they raise your pain threshold, which is

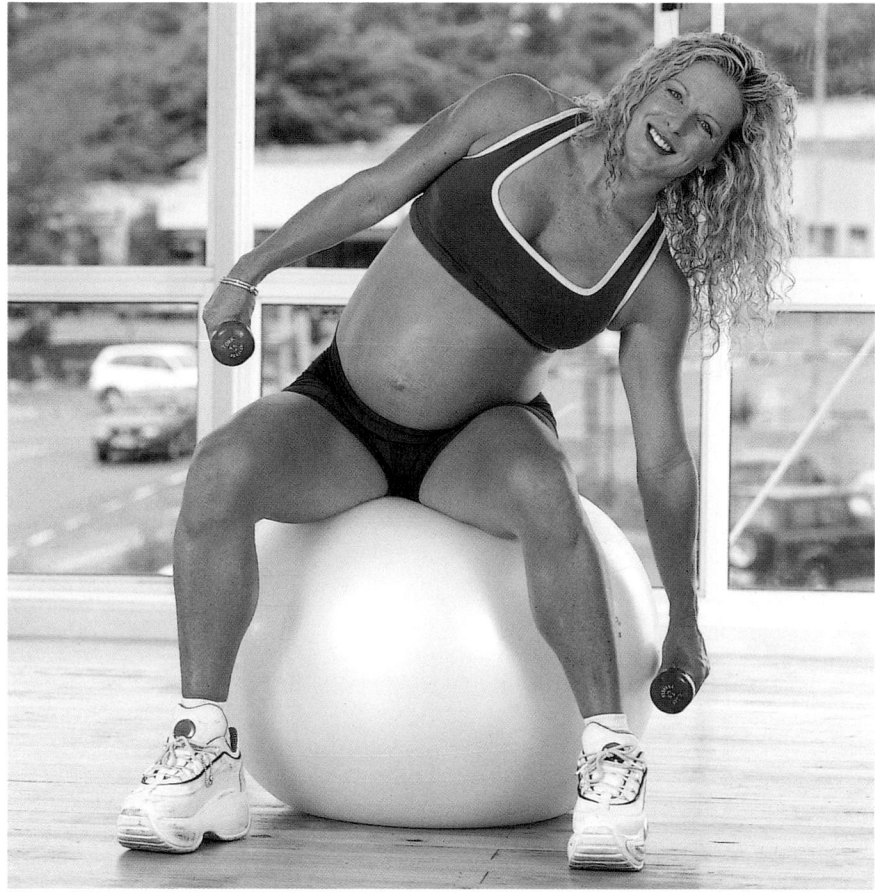

of enormous benefit to you and your baby in labour. Do not overwork or overstrain your muscles. Good body mechanics and breathing techniques are important. Work with light weights at a moderate intensity with high repetitions. Correct breathing is the key: inhale on the easy part of the exercise and exhale on the exertion.

Pilates

Pilates helps develop balance, control, strength, flexibility, alignment and posture. Under qualified instruction and modified movements, a pregnant woman can start pilates in order to develop trunk strength and stability. Remember to advise the instructor of your pregnancy if it is not obvious.

Ball classes

The exercise ball is a useful and fun training aid, especially great for pregnant exercisers. There are many techniques that can only be done on the ball – get used to sitting on it before becoming too adventurous. The ball is excellent for balance, a safe abdominal workout as well as for exercising the pelvic floor. It has many uses in the postpartum period and toddlers love it! Be sure to get instructions on use before using it alone.

You can use it throughout pregnancy and it is excellent in dealing with backache. The ball has been a therapeutic 'tool' for many years and only recently has it been used for recreational purposes as well as to get fit. It is used to improve flexibility, postural

Above left When sitting on the exercise ball, you are working the stabilizer muscles in the torso to keep you upright.

control, coordination skills and balance; it is also ideal for a full-body workout, relaxation or fun games. The ball can be used in conjunction with other training aids such as hand weights, bands and other smaller balls.

Alexander technique

The Alexander technique is a form of sensory re-education that teaches people how to change detrimental body habits that cause strain and stress commonly exhibited as backache, headaches and other physical disorders. It will give you insight into the importance of correct movement and posture, not only for pregnancy and labour but for life in general. It must only be done under the instruction of a qualified person, and is safe to do throughout pregnancy.

Posture

Good posture, especially during pregnancy, is all-important. If you maintain good posture at all times, it helps to prevent one of the most common problems in pregnancy – chronic backache!

There are a few things you can do to avoid poor posture: do not stand for too long, make sure your handbag is not heavy and wear the strap of your handbag across your chest, and when carrying parcels, balance the load equally in both hands.

Left *The illustrations show the difference between good and bad posture.*

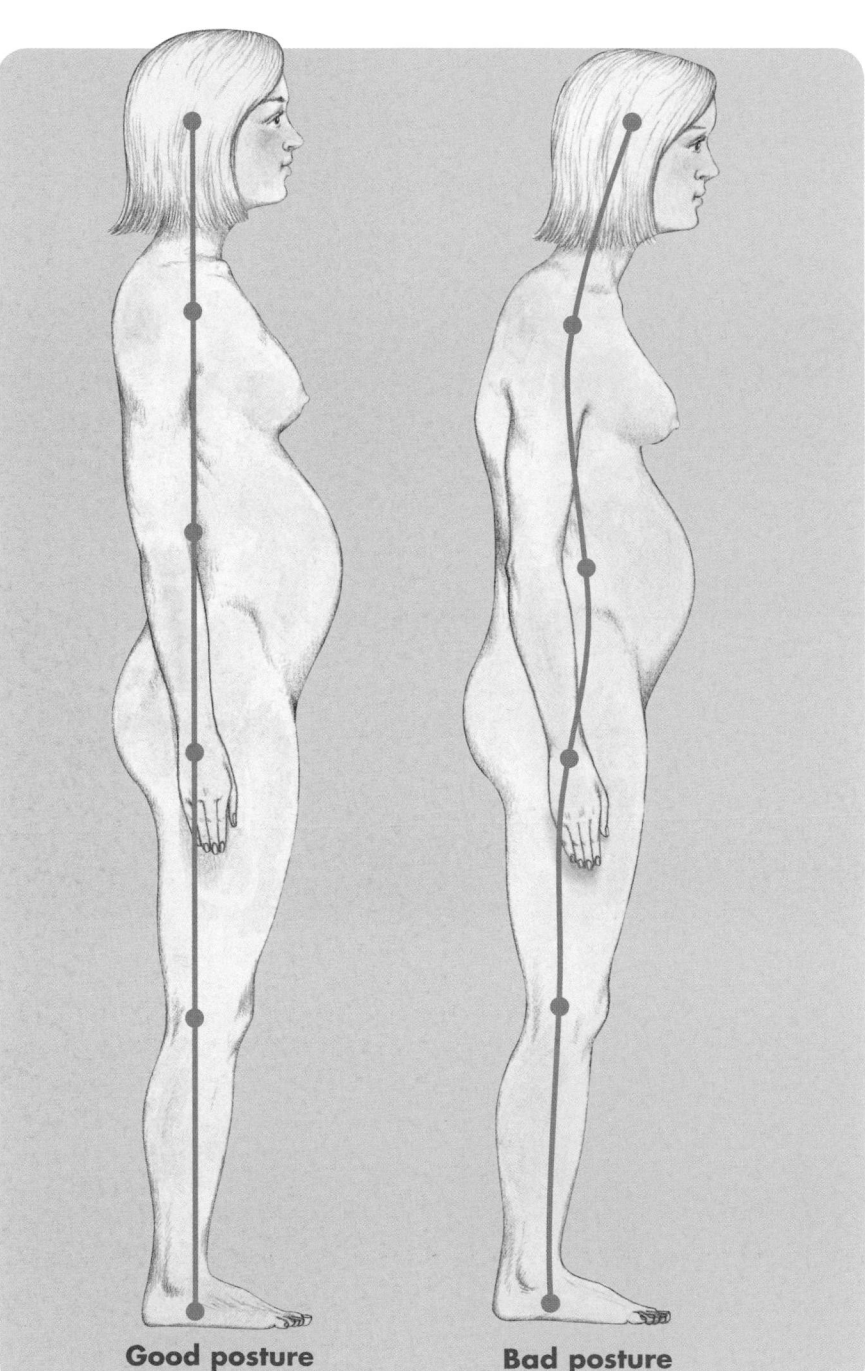

Good posture   **Bad posture**

When to avoid exercise

Pregnant women with the following conditions should not exercise, except with the approval of their caregiver and under the strict supervision of a qualified instructor:
- hypertension
- anaemia or other blood disorders
- thyroid disease
- diabetes
- history of early labour
- history of foetal growth retardation
- history of bleeding during present pregnancy
- breech presentation in the last trimester
- seizures
- irregular heartbeat
- excessive obesity
- excessively underweight
- have a history of an extremely sedentary lifestyle
- physical problems involving the spine, limbs or other body parts.

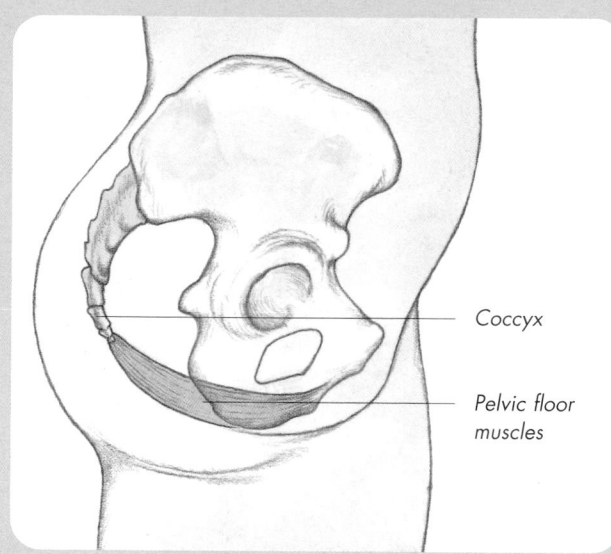

Coccyx

Pelvic floor
muscles

Kegel (pelvic floor) exercise

One of the most important groups of muscles that come under great strain during pregnancy and childbirth are the pelvic floor muscles. Give these top priority as far as preparation is concerned.

The pelvic floor is the base of the abdominal/pelvic cavity. It consists of layers of crisscrossing muscles that stretch like a hammock from the pubic bone in the front to the coccyx at the back. It is a sling of muscle inside the bottom of the pelvis (between your legs) that helps to hold the bladder, uterus and bowel in place, and to close the bladder outlet and back passage.

The most important muscle is the figure-of-eight muscle that circles the urethra and vagina in the front and the anal sphincter at the back. Like any other muscle in the body, the more you use and exercise the pelvic floor, the stronger it will be. Pelvic floor exercises strengthen the muscles so that they provide support and improve bladder control and prevent leaking of urine. The changes that take place in your body during pregnancy – more fluid retention, increased blood volume and the growth of the baby and the uterus – add to the weight your pelvic floor has to bear. During labour it will stretch even further as the contractions nudge the baby down toward the vaginal exit. The muscles will stretch around the baby's head and may even be cut or tear slightly.

Learning the exercise

These exercises are designed to strengthen and give you voluntary control over a specific muscle of the pelvic floor called the pubococcygeus (PC) muscle. This is the support muscle for the genitals in both men and women.

1. Sit comfortably with your knees slightly apart. Now imagine that you are trying to stop yourself passing wind from the bowel. To do this you must squeeze the muscle around the back passage. Try squeezing and lifting the muscle as if you really do have wind. Your buttocks and legs should not move at all. You should be aware of the skin around the back passage tightening and being pulled up and away from your support. Hold tightened for at least five seconds if you can and then relax.

Repeat at least five times (slow pull-ups). Now pull the muscles up quickly and tightly, and then relax immediately. Repeat at least five times (fast pull-ups).

2. Now imagine that you are passing urine. Imagine that you are trying to stop your urine midstream. You will be using the same group of muscles that you used before, but do not be surprised if you find this more difficult than exercise one. As with the first exercise, repeat this at least five times.

3. Do these two exercises – five slow and five fast at least 10 times a day.

You may have noticed that when you pull up and tighten your pelvic floor, your abdominal muscles also get involved. This is a good sign that you are doing the exercise correctly, since these two sets of muscles often work together.

Once you have identified where your pelvic floor muscles are, tighten them all together now: then one, two three and pull up. Try not to tighten any other muscles, and do not hold your breath. You might find this difficult at first.

These are invisible exercises and you can do them anywhere at any time. As you 'pull up', the entire sling of muscles across your pelvic floor lifts upward. This is called the 'pelvic smile' because it is the shape your muscles are now making inside you.

Abdominal muscle strength

Pushing out your baby will be a strenuous activity that requires great strength and knowledge of your body. This exercise helps to develop the necessary muscles in order to use them in the most efficient way.

By working your abdominal muscles safely during pregnancy you will not only regain your lean look sooner after birth, but also enjoy a more comfortable pregnancy because backache and poor breathing are less likely. During the second, expulsive stage of labour, having strong 'stomach' muscles may alleviate the need for intervention (in the form of forceps) during pushing. Getting to know and understand your abdominals is the key in using them effectively during pregnancy, labour and after birth.

The muscles of the abdomen are layered longitudinally, horizontally and diagonally. They stretch tremendously during pregnancy to accommodate the growing uterus. Weak abdominal muscles allow the pelvis to rotate forward, aggravating the curve in the lumbar portion of the spine. It is important to exercise the muscles to strengthen them; do not strain them, however.

Abdominal exercises have to be modified during the second and third trimester of pregnancy, and checks for separation of the recti muscles, known as diastasis recti, should be done. This occurs when the recti muscle separates painlessly to accommodate the expanding uterus. It is no cause for alarm, just the body protecting itself from over-stretching. It is important that you avoid crunch-type abdominal exercises (sit-ups) if this has happened to you.

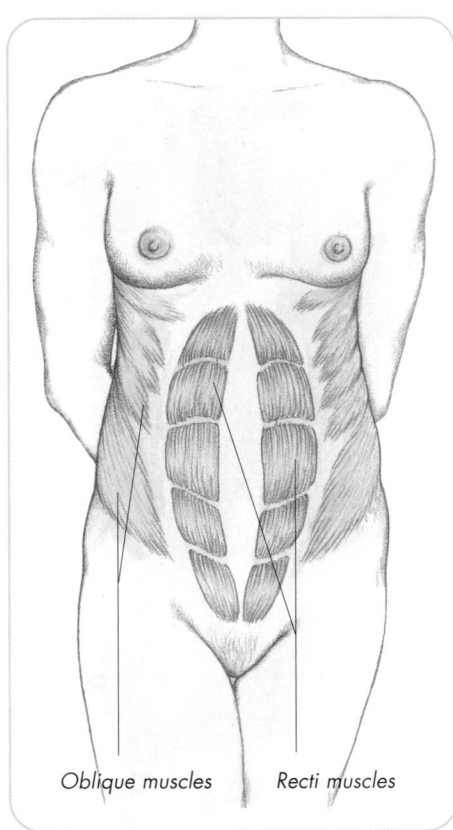

Oblique muscles   Recti muscles

Above During mid to late pregnancy, the recti muscles will start to separate.

Right Safely work your abdominal muscles as much as possible in preparation for labour.

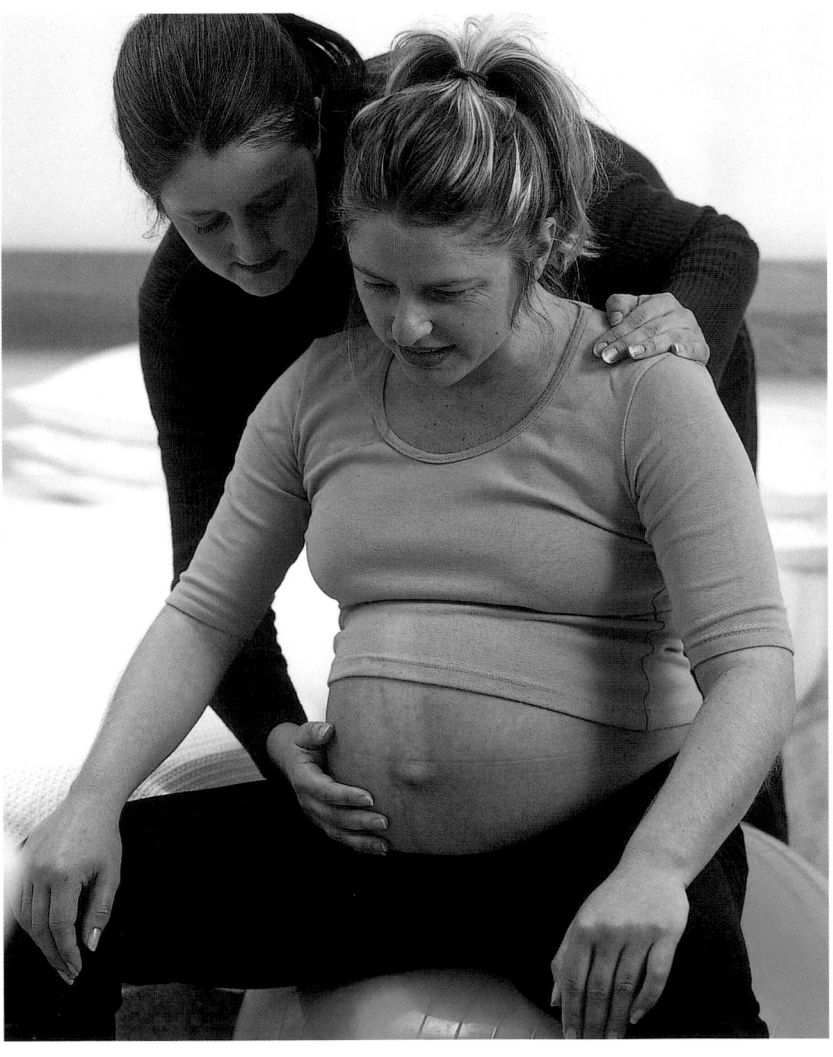

The American College of Obstetricians and Gynaecologists' guidelines for exercise in pregnancy (ACOG)

1. Regular exercise (three to five times a week) is preferable to occasional activity.

2. Swimming, stationary cycling and brisk walking are highly recommended.

3. Exercise sessions should be preceded by a five-minute period of muscle warm-up, for example, slow walking or stationary cycling at low resistance.

4. Exercise should be done on a safe surface, such as a wooden floor or tightly carpeted area to reduce the risk of injury.

5. Moderate to intense aerobic activity should be limited to 15–20 minutes. Lower intensity activities may be conducted continuously over a longer period, but should not exceed 45 minutes.

6. Heart rate should be measured at times of peak activity and should not exceed 140 bpm. One way to determine this is to perform the 'talk test': if the pregnant woman is unable to converse normally while exercising, she is over-exerting herself.

7. Care should be taken to rise from the floor gradually so as to avoid an abrupt drop in blood pressure, and to continue some form of activity involving the legs for a brief period.

8. Exercise sessions should be followed by a brief cool-down period of gradually declining activity that includes gentle stationary stretching. Stretches should not be taken to the maximum resistance.

9. A pregnant woman should consume enough calories to meet the needs of her pregnancy (300 extra calories a day) as well as her exercise programme. Weight loss should not be a goal of exercising during pregnancy.

10. Exercises that require jumping, jarring motions or rapid changes in direction should be avoided.

11. After the fourth month of pregnancy, exercises done lying flat on the back should be avoided. This position could allow the mother's expanding uterus to compress the vein that carries blood to the heart, which could interfere with blood flow to the uterus.

12. Strenuous exercise should not be performed in hot, humid weather or during illness accompanied by fever.

13. A pregnant woman's temperature should not exceed 37°C (99°F) while exercising. She should drink plenty of water before, during and after exercise to prevent dehydration and hyperthermia and take a break if more water is needed or if she is tired.

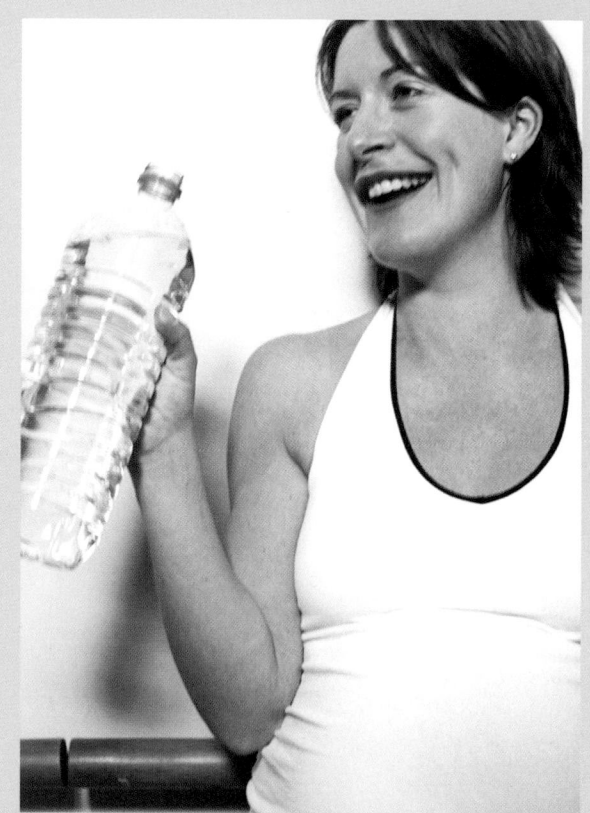

Above *Drink plenty of water after your exercise session to keep your body temperature normal.*

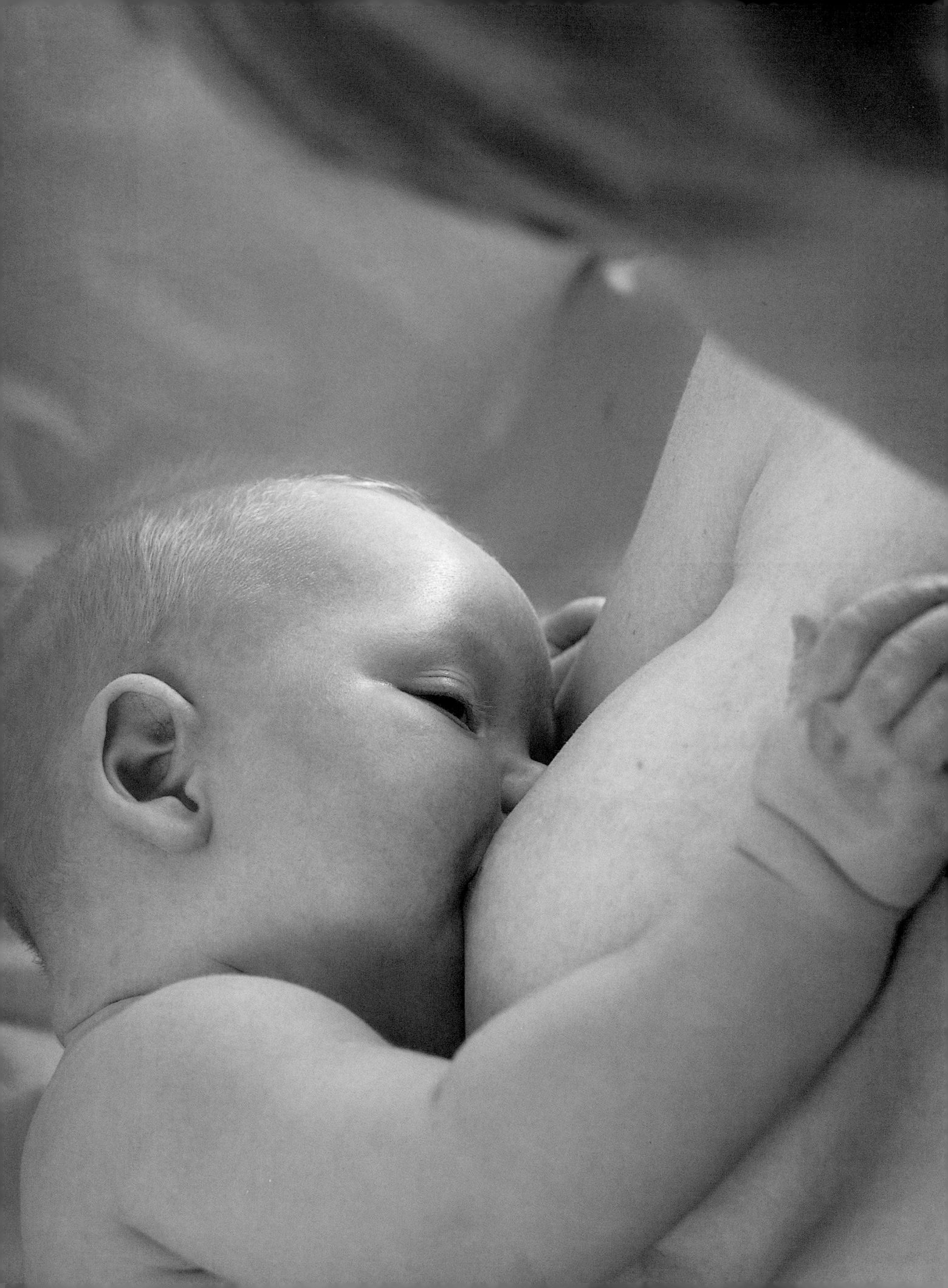

Part II
Childbirth

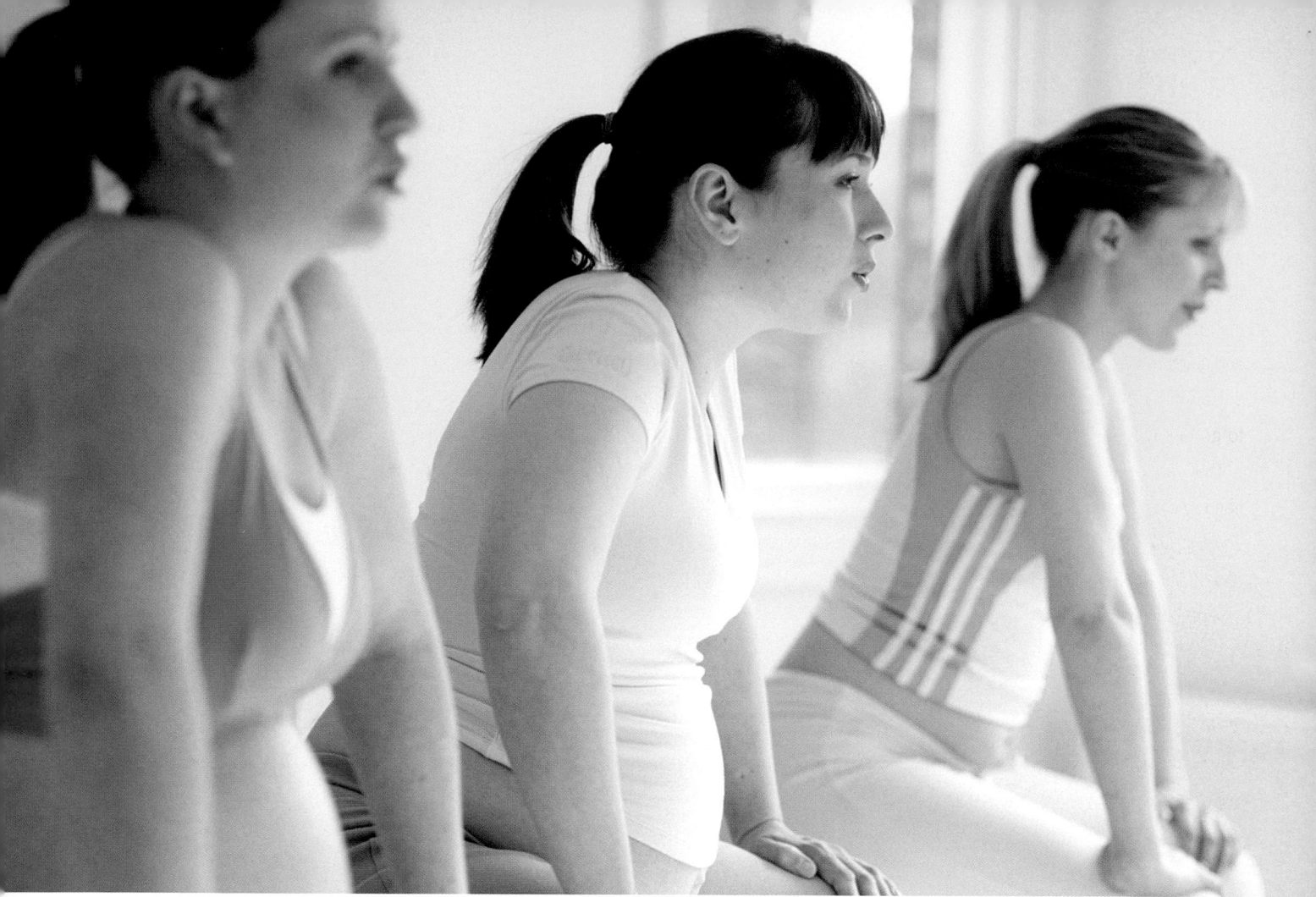

Preparing for childbirth

Giving birth is one of the most creative, challenging and life-altering events you will ever go through. Preparing for your baby and gaining knowledge of the birth process is not only essential, it is the most responsible thing you can do. Books and magazines provide vital information but if you are able, attend childbirth education classes; they will not only 'fill in the gaps' but you and your partner will meet other couples who are about to go through the same experience.

GIVING BIRTH IS A CREATIVE, CHALLENGING AND LIFE-ALTERING EVENT

Childbirth education classes should ideally be aimed at couples, as many partners want to be part of the process of bringing the new life into the world. Women and men need to understand what labour, birth and early parenting are all about. This is a potentially stressful time for any couple to go through.

This chapter deals with subjects that you need to explore in preparation for childbirth. You will learn coping skills and techniques and understand where the pain of labour comes from and how to deal with it.

Below Taking time out to relax and focus on correct breathing will be beneficial in preparing you for labour and early parenting.

Breathing techniques

You can practise breathing techniques anywhere at any time, as long as you are in a comfortable position. Sit, stand or lie down, then try the techniques given below.

Breathing awareness

Being aware of your breathing can help you to relax, reduce pain and create a mental distraction during difficult contractions. Try the following exercise with or without a partner.

1. Choose a comfortable position. Once you are breathing at a comfortable pace and level, keep breathing at that depth for a minute or two. Try out different paces to find out what is comfortable for you.

2. Place one hand (or your partner's hand) slightly above your navel and one hand on your chest near the top of your breast. Notice how your breath rises and falls under your hands. If you are breathing mostly into the chest area, try to breathe deeper into the stomach. It may be easier to allow the breath to come in and out of your mouth although breathing through the nose may be more comfortable for you.

3. Allow your jaw to drop open slightly and release any sounds or sighs on the outgoing breath. As you breathe, think about the air flowing into and out of your body. Note the coolness of the incoming breath and the warmth of the outgoing breath. Some women imagine the inward breath as a light colour and the outward breath as a dark one.

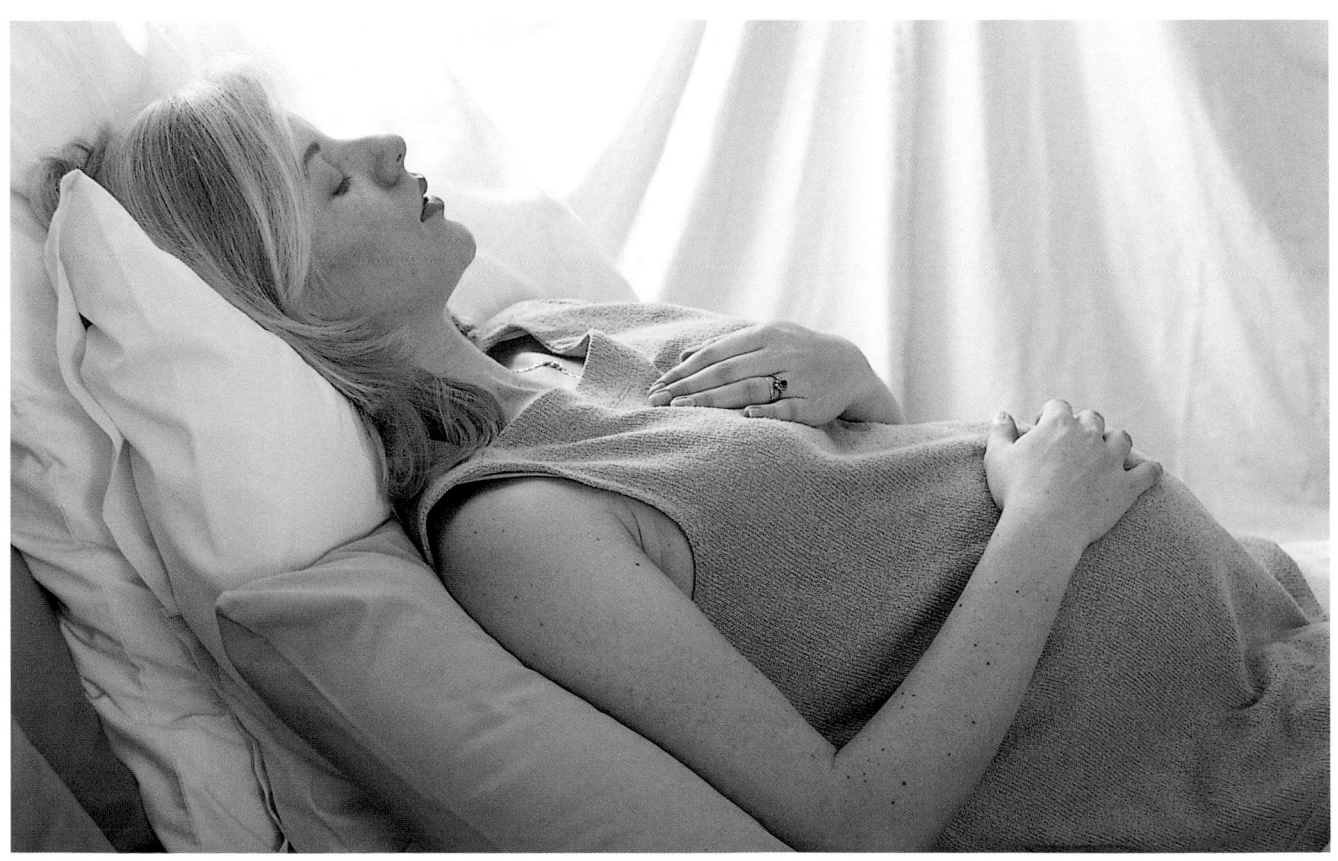

Deep breathing

Most people tend to use the muscles of the neck and shoulders when they breathe instead of the deeper, stronger abdominal muscles. When you breathe lower into the stomach, you will find that you are able to take deeper breaths than if you were breathing from the chest area. Some women breathe very slowly and naturally; others find a less full breath more comfortable. Do not force a particular pattern of breathing that may feel unnatural; rather find your own pattern of breathing that helps you to relax and feel comfortable. It is important to be aware of your breathing and how it changes during labour. Pregnancy is the perfect time to practise and develop your breathing awareness. Apart from preparing you for labour, it can also help to ease insomnia, poor circulation, breathlessness and many other discomforts.

Breathing in labour

A heightened awareness of breathing gives you the ability to respond spontaneously to the challenge of labour and feel more relaxed and comfortable. Your breathing changes throughout labour – the more active your labour, the more active your breathing will be. Try to keep your breathing even and easy, although it may become more difficult as the intensity of labour increases – try to not let your breathing become too fast. Taking a slow, comfortable breath at the beginning of each contraction will help you to focus and centre yourself, and alert your partner to the contraction. Try to breathe slowly throughout the contraction. As the

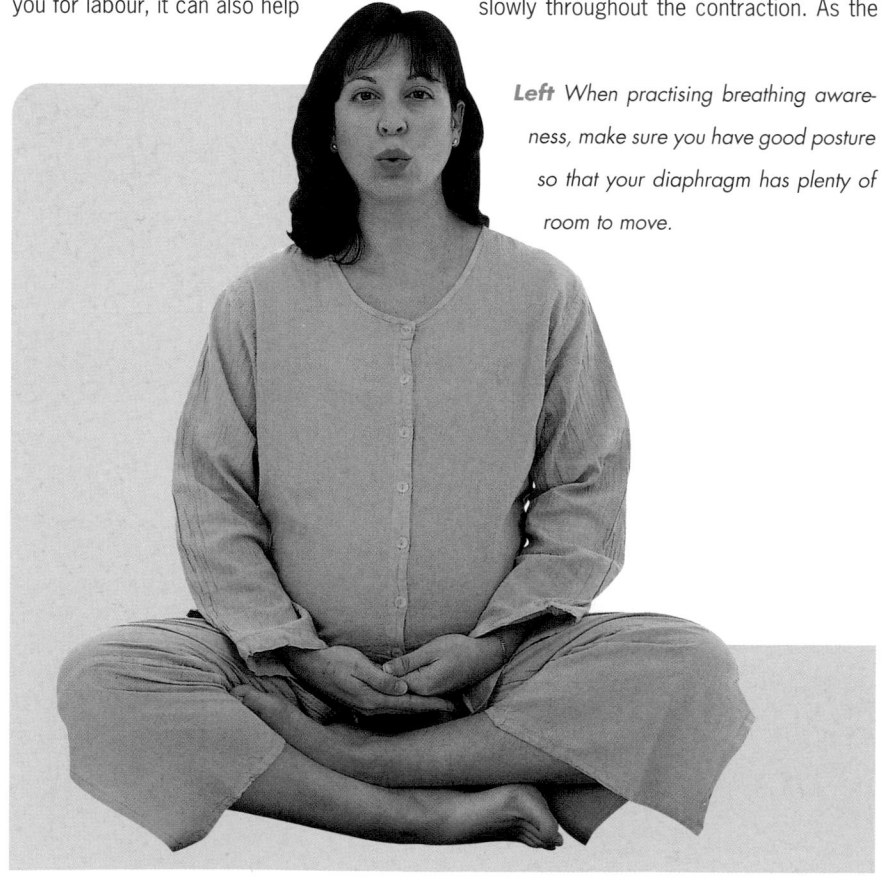

Left When practising breathing awareness, make sure you have good posture so that your diaphragm has plenty of room to move.

pain intensifies, you may tend to breathe faster and shallower but concentrating on breathing in a slow, controlled manner will help prevent panic, anxiety and breathlessness. Once the contraction is over, take a relaxing breath as if you were sighing to signal that the contraction is over and let go of any tension that may have built up. Keep breathing in a relaxed and free fashion between contractions; this will help you conserve energy and you will not feel like you are fighting labour continuously.

Once you have become a mother, your breathing and relaxation skills will keep you calm in the many stressful situations associated with early motherhood.

Relaxation

Breathing techniques and awareness will not work if you do not know how to release and express your feelings. Women who approach labour with fear and anxiety tend to have more difficult labours. Anxiety causes you to meet every contraction with tension and, as the pain increases, so does the tension. Unfortunately, anxiety can heighten your perception of pain, use up all your energy and inhibit your body from working effectively.

One of the greatest 'tools' with which to cope in labour is the ability to relax or to 'let go of your tension'. Relaxation involves mind as well as body. It is associated with the reduction of tension in muscles and the protective response that alleviates the fight or flight response, and decreases the heart rate, metabolism and breathing rate to bring the body into balance.

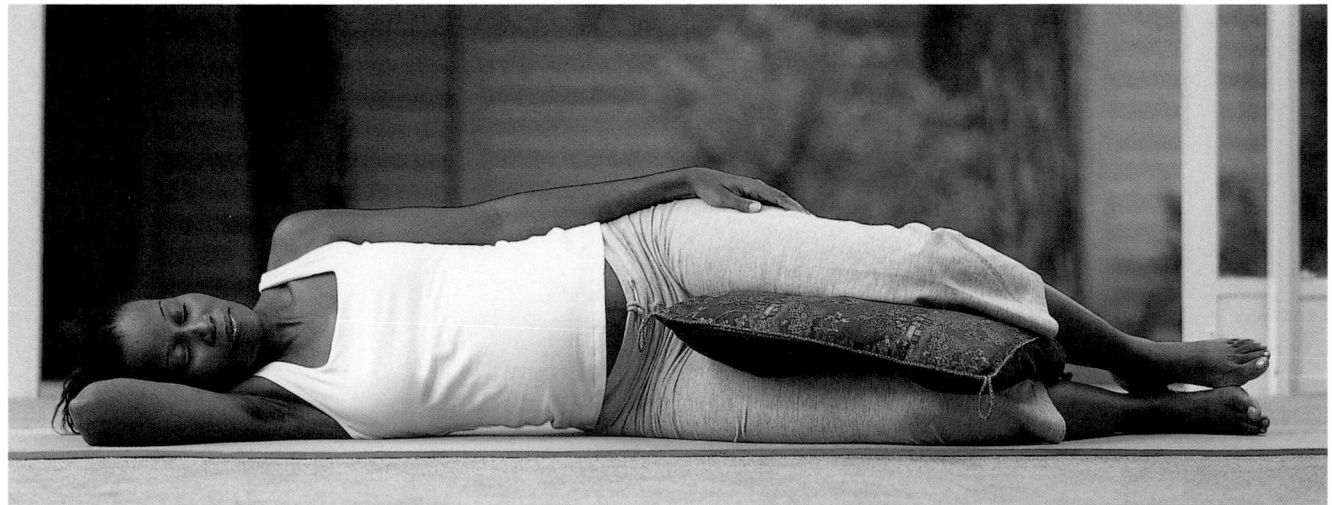

Above When you first start using visualization techniques, find a position that is most comfortable for you, and use pillows for extra support.

Relaxation techniques are taught in childbirth education classes but these require individual effort and diligent practice on a daily basis.

Tension and labour

If tension is allowed to become excessive in labour, it can hinder progress. Fear and anxiety cause a release of adrenaline, which prepares the body for rescue. Oxytocin, the hormone that stimulates the uterus to contract, is inhibited by the release of adrenaline resulting in labour being slowed down. Tension results in even more resistance from the uterus, causing a tug-of-war effect that slows labour and increases pain.

Understanding the source and the role of labour pain and knowing that it will end does much to alleviate the fear that so often accompanies birth.

How to release tension

Preparation is important – being comfortable, undisturbed and feeling secure will improve the quality of the experience. Wear comfortable, loose-fitting clothing; take off your shoes, watch and glasses. As you start to relax, your metabolism slows down and your body will start to cool. Keep something light and warm near, in case you start to feel chilly. Practise this exercise.

- Settle into a comfortable position, and close your eyes.
- Release tension from all your muscles, starting with the feet, ending with your face. Feel yourself becoming limp.
- Notice the depth and the rhythm of your breathing. Allow the breaths to take place quite naturally.
- Each time you exhale, recite the word 'one' under your breath. Repeat the word slowly every time you breathe out.
- If thoughts intrude, try to ignore them and continue repeating the word 'one'. Keep your attitude passive and allow relaxation to occur in its own time.

- Do this for as long as you are comfortable, maybe 10–20 minutes.
- Constantly 'scan' your body for any residual tension and mentally 'massage' that area, releasing the muscle with each outward breath.
- When you are ready to end your quiet time, continue to sit quietly for a few minutes with your eyes closed.

Visualization

Relaxation of the mind involves using mental imagery or visualization. This means having the ability to turn inner positive thoughts into pictures in order to bring about a desired situation. It stops the mind from wandering and reminding you just how uncomfortable you may be feeling. During pregnancy, as a result of the presence of the feel-good hormone endorphin, you are already becoming more distracted and full of daydreams, which goes hand-in-hand with positive affirmations and meditation. Visualization is most effective in preparation for childbirth than in any other field or situation.

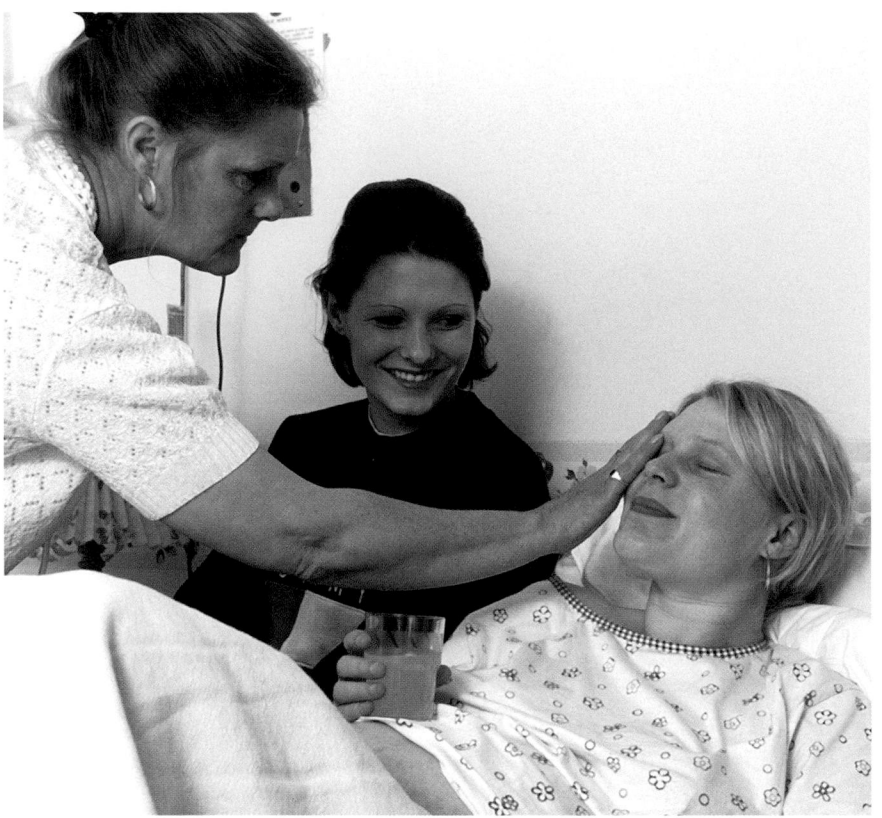

The pain of labour

Whether you want to attempt a drug-free labour or not, preparing for birth and learning how to cope with childbirth pain is vital. There are many reasons why labour hurts, and understanding the sources and mechanism of labour pain goes a long way to helping you manage it. Pain has both physiological and emotional components. It may be seen as a unique form of pain, which is not directly the consequence of injury. Although injury may be incurred during the process of labour, it is more likely to be as a result of intervention rather than a consequence of natural labour.

The pain of labour initiates hormonal responses that will benefit both mother and

Above Having loved ones to support and encourage you through the earlier stages of labour will help you deal with the pain.

baby. Research has shown that complete pain relief does not necessarily mean complete satisfaction. In fact, it is the presence of a caregiver – either a birth partner or a midwife – that reduces a woman's need for other forms of pain relief. You are at your most vulnerable and a good support system makes all the difference.

It is important to remember that pain in labour usually means progress, and at the end of the process there is a beautiful baby. Most of labour is pain-free, but we tend to talk about the pain-filled moments. When you hold your baby, you will soon forget about the pain.

Understanding labour pain

Describing the pain you will experience is complicated, as it does not bear any similarity to anything you have felt before, and each individual's perception is unique. Pain in labour has a predictable pattern, which is associated with the contractions of the uterus, and the location of the pain will change constantly along with duration, intensity and frequency.

Initially pain alerts a mother to seek a safe place to give birth. In the first stage of labour (*see* p116), the contractions build in intensity as the baby descends and the cervix opens. The pain at this stage is due mainly to the stretching and opening of the cervix. As a woman approaches the second (pushing) stage of labour (*see* p119) she may find it increasingly difficult to manage her pain and will often ask for pain relief.

Labour is painful because giving birth demands the cooperation of many parts of the body. The uterus and cervix have nerves that are sensitive to stretching, and the lack of oxygen causes the nerve endings to become very 'agitated'. Therefore, it is important to breathe in order to keep the working muscles oxygenated.

The strong uterine contractions often cause pain sensations that may radiate into the thighs and around the back.

The pelvic floor muscles and perineum also contain many nerve endings and pain receptors. When stimulated by contractions, they send messages via your spinal cord to your brain, which register as pain.

The weight of the baby on the uterus, lower back, sacrum and tailbone is also a cause for pain. This area of the body contains many nerves, and when pressure is applied, it can be painful – producing a sharp or dull backache. As the baby moves down the birth canal, there will be a lot of rectal pressure. Close to delivery the vagina and the vaginal opening stretch to capacity and this causes a burning, stretching-like sensation. The physical and emotional challenge of labour causes great fatigue so you feel more vulnerable to pain; a full bladder and dehydration can increase pain; fear, tension, incorrect positioning and lack of knowledge of the process may also magnify your perception of pain.

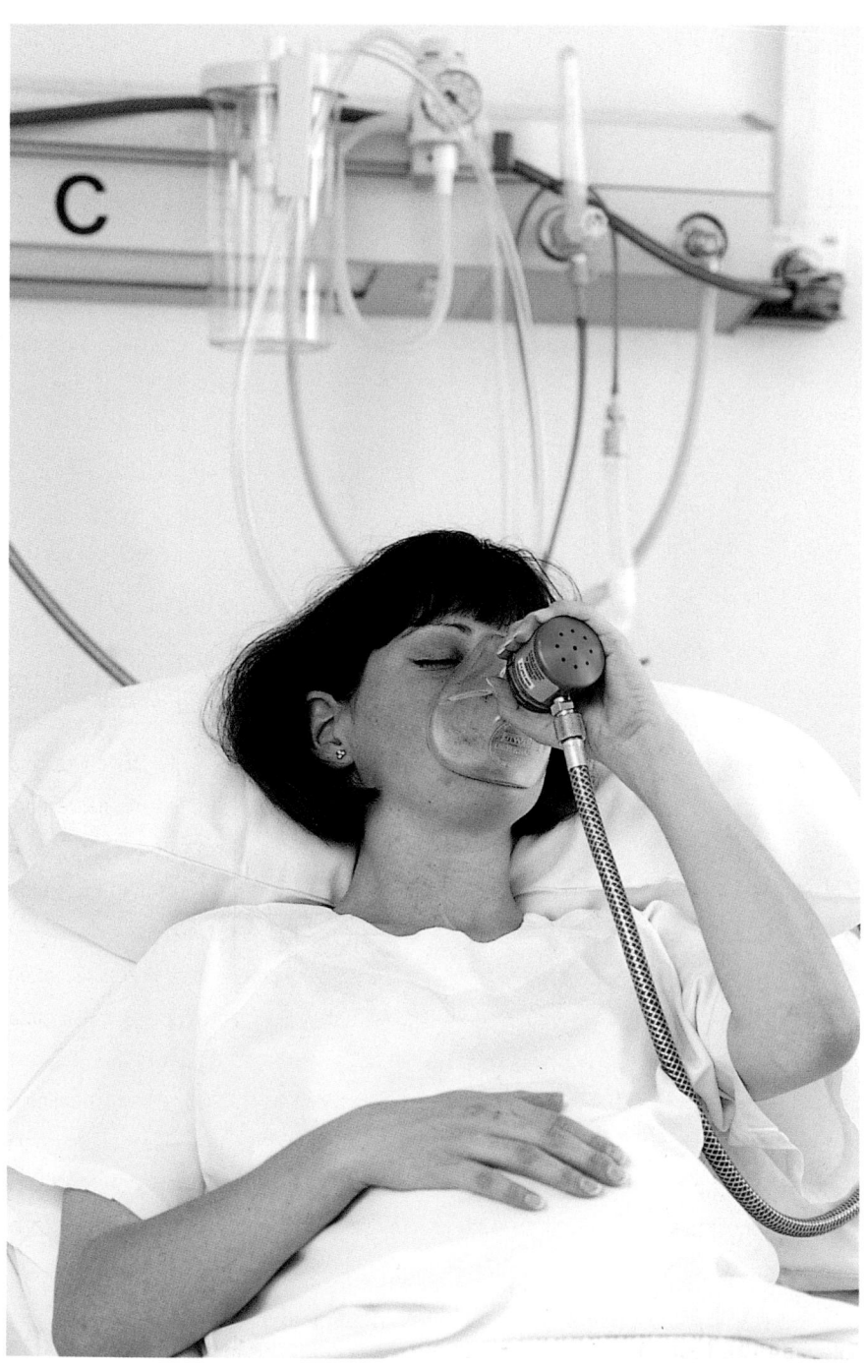

Coping skills

Stay calm Stress hormones cross the placental barrier, so find ways to remain calm and positive.

Draw up a birth plan Do not leave this to the last minute! Practise perineal massage and Kegel (pelvic floor) exercises often (*see* pp85 and 129). This will prepare the muscles for labour.

Get fit and strong Strengthening and toning the muscles will increase your ability to handle the hard work ahead. You will also be able to more easily adopt any position to help your labour along.

Gain knowledge Childbirth education classes will help you to understand the birth process, which will decrease your fear and increase your confidence.

Relaxation and visualization techniques The ability to release tension at will and turn inner positive thoughts into pictures is not only a labour tool but also a life skill.

Left You may be given entonox – a mixture of equal amounts of oxygen and nitrous oxide – to help take the edge off the pain, and you control the amount you take in.

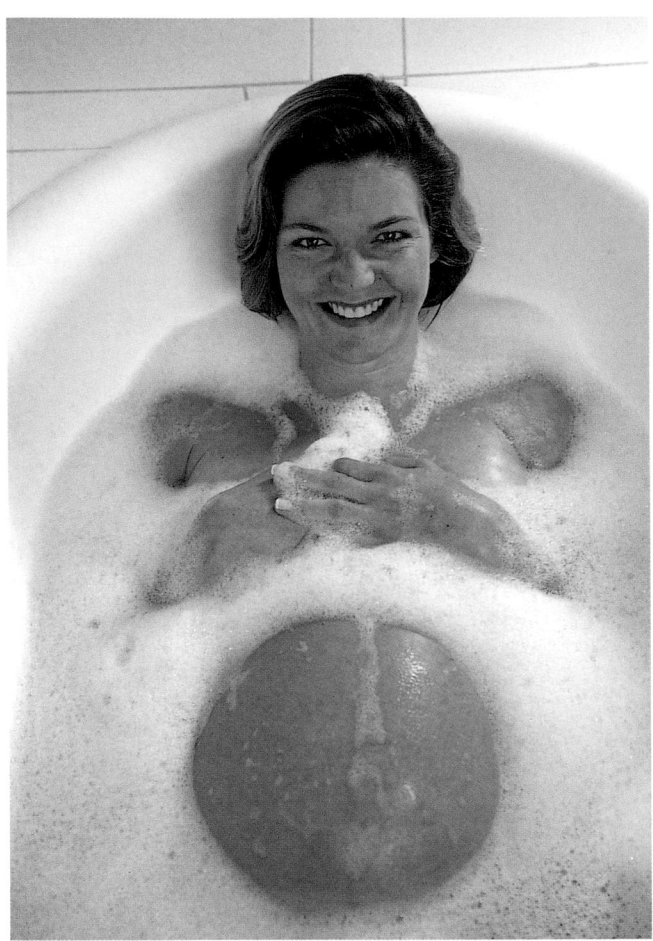
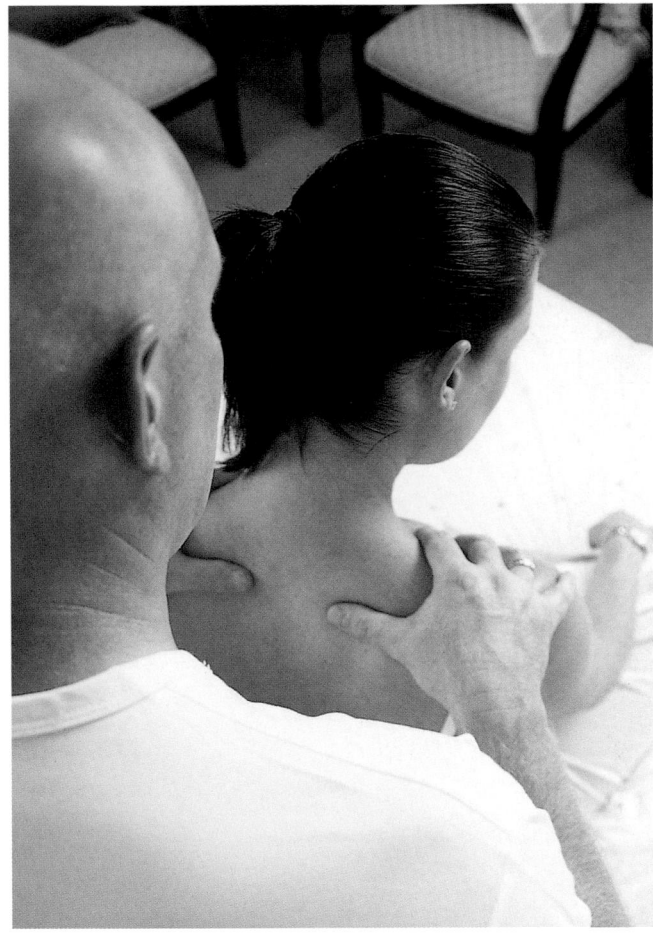

Breathe with purpose and intention Breathing well will ensure that you oxygenate your baby and the uterus, as well as help you deal with the contractions more effectively. Practise breathing techniques (*see* pp91–92).

Positive thinking and positive people will get you through labour and stressful nights with a new baby. Practise positive affirmations during pregnancy and gather supportive people around you. Your state of mind influences your labour more than you realize!

Use gravity Change positions constantly during labour. Movement dissipates pain and will change your perception. Stay as upright as possible and use the force of gravity to bring your baby down and open up your pelvis.

Make a noise Do not try to behave like a woman who is not in labour. Moaning and groaning helps with the release of endorphins, which will benefit the baby as well.

Empty your bladder often A full bladder is extremely uncomfortable during labour. It can also hold up the labour process and increase your level of pain.

Get into water Water has amazing pain-relieving powers. Water can be used at

Above left Warm water has amazing pain-relieving properties.
Above right Massage helps with the release of endorphins – the body's natural painkillers.

home or in hospital. A powerful showerhead directed onto your back can ease backache. If you do not have access to a birthing pool, use your own bath – the deeper the water in the bath the better.

Remember the baby has a part to play too – an active baby helps herself get into the world. Nudge your baby every now and then and remember that she is using her

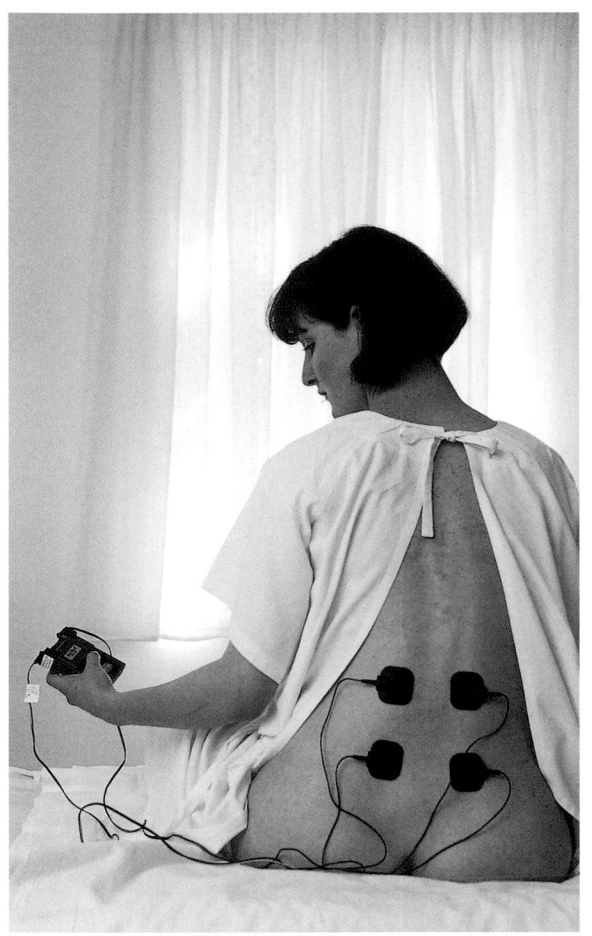
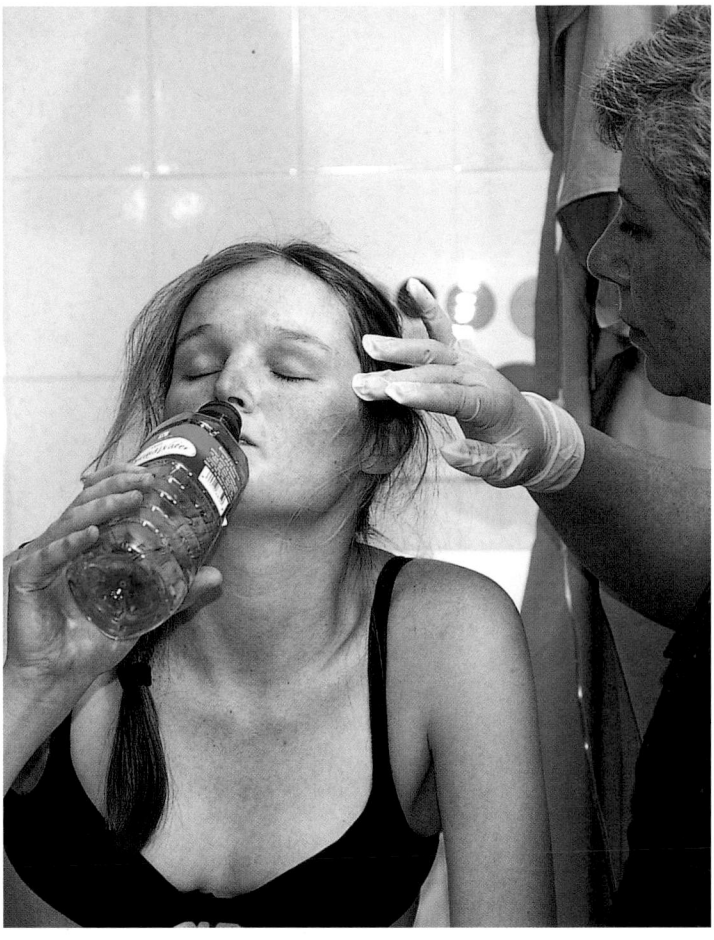

body to work her way into the world. Whatever you do affects her, so breathe, move, sing and relax. Again, these release the body's natural painkillers.

Listen to soft music Music is a 'universal language' and has many pain-relieving properties. Choose a variety of music beforehand and listen actively – use earphones to ensure you do not disturb others.

Touch and massage The power of touch should never be underestimated. Although many women love being touched in labour, some do not! The way you will want to be touched during the different phases of labour will change from soft and sensitive to hard, firm pressure on certain parts of the body, which will change the way you perceive pain.

Emotional support Having you family and and close friends encouraging and praising you goes a long way in helping you get through the hardest contractions of labour.

Environment If a woman feels safe in her environment, she is more likely to find it easier to relax. Stay at home for as long as possible, where you can wear your own clothes, listen to your own music and do whatever you like to keep comfortable. Once in hospital or your birthing facility, continue

Above left Trans Cutaneous Electrical Stimulation (TENS) interrupts the pain message to the brain, altering your perception of pain.
Above right Keeping well hydrated during labour will help lessen pain and discomfort.

to listen to music, use your oils and keep as private as possible. Many facilities today try to make a mother feel as if she is in a place that is comfortable and familiar. A harsh and noisy environment is not conducive to an easier labour.

Use aromatherapy Aromatherapy oils can change the smell of a harsh labour room into a welcoming, soothing environment that reminds you of a more familiar place. Oils such as lavender and chamomile have a wonderfully soothing effect on the psyche and the body!

Use **alternative forms of pain relief** such as movement in the form of walking or rocking, or using the TENS machine, which sends electrical impulses to the brain, releasing your body's endorphins and changing your perception of pain. Acupressure and having your heels rubbed will also help ease pain.

Always keep well hydrated. Dehydration can make uterine contractions far more painful, so sip little bits of water or clear fluid all the way through labour.

Focal point Many women find it helpful to focus on something during a contraction. It may be a picture or a sentimental object. Eye contact or an altered breathing pattern may help.

Use homeopathy Find out from your childbirth educator or caregiver what homeopathic preparations can be used in labour.

Medication Pain-relieving drugs are useful to help with pain IF they are necessary and worth the risks involved. They have nothing to do with the idea of success or failure. Be sure to examine all your options long before your due date and share your fears and concerns with your labour partner.

Above right Lean against a chair for support when you are upright during labour.

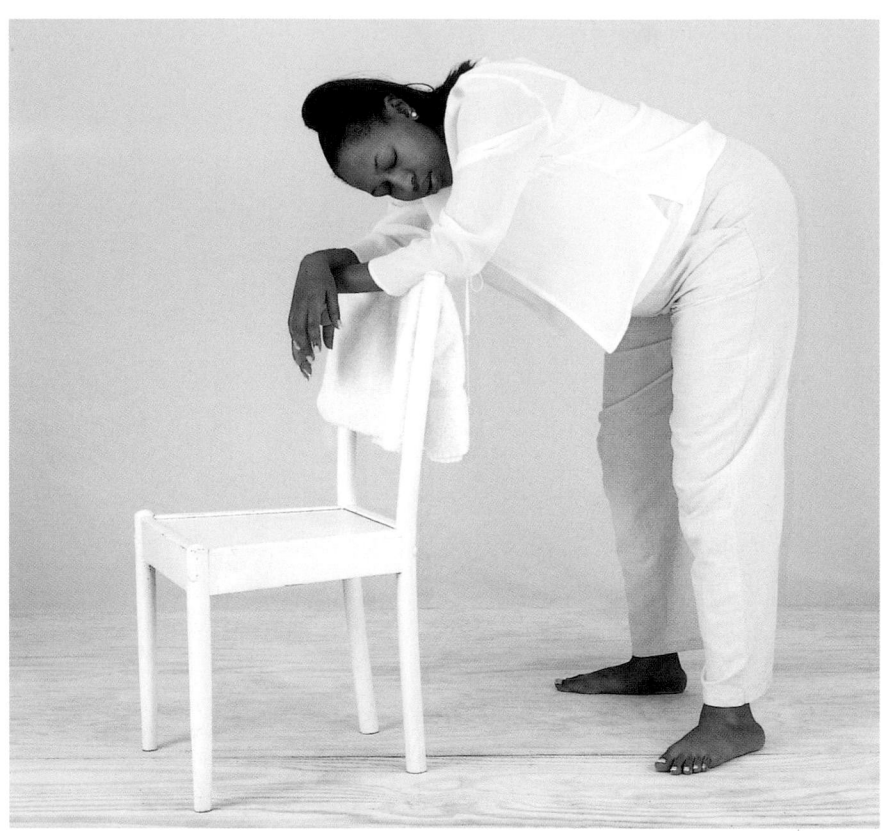

Positions for delivery

There are two reasons why you should adopt different positions during labour: it encourages the descent of the baby and it lessens pain because you are not lying on the major nerves, the blood vessels or the spine.

The more upright and mobile you are, the faster your labour will progress. Besides utilizing gravity, contractions in the upright position, especially the standing position, are usually stronger, longer and further apart and perceived to be less painful by most women. They also seem to be more effective because the baby descends, cervical pressure is increased evenly and usually less painfully than if you were semi-recumbent (semi-sitting).

Being mobile during your labour gives you a sense of being actively involved, in control, as well as keeping your mind focused. If you feel that you want to lie down at times during your labour, lie down on your side rather than on your back. Not being on your back also allows the coccyx to move back and out of the way.

The woman who lies in bed during her labour is at a distinct disadvantage. Physiologically, she loses most of the advantages of gravity. Being up and about and remaining mobile for as long as possible will keep up a good circulation as she takes charge of what happens to her body, her baby and her labour. Psychologically, if she is recumbent, she takes on a more passive role, leaving decisions for her wellbeing in the hands of others. She invites others to do things for her and to her, rather than remaining in control herself.

It is important to remember that resting is appropriate, especially if labour turns out to be a long one. You will need to alternate periods of activity with periods of rest. Listen to your body's signals and respond accordingly. Be aware of holding tension in any of your muscles – prolonged tension leads to fatigue, which leads to more pain. Use the relaxation techniques discussed earlier to release tension (*see* p93), and this

Below Adopting the 'all fours' position will help your baby get into a good position for birth. It is also an excellent position if a woman is experiencing back pain.
Below right Your partner can support you when adopting the squatting position.

will 'free' your breathing as well as your pain. Developing good body awareness during your pregnancy will enable you to get 'in touch' with and trust the signs and signals your body will send you.

Upright position

Remaining upright does not mean that you need to stand; leaning against a window sill, wall or your labour partner is a good way to deal with your contractions. You should not stand unsupported but have most of your weight against something. You may wish to have your support person walk around with you to help you relax and keep focused.

'All fours' position

Many women instinctively adopt the 'all fours' position, especially if they are feeling pain in the back. Use chairs, bean bags, balls or large continental pillows to make yourself more comfortable in this position. This will

take all the pressure off your back as your stomach hangs away from the nerves and blood vessels supplying the uterus.

Squatting position

In the squatting position, your pelvis is wide open, inviting your baby to move down and through. If this hurts your knees, rather sit on a low stool, knees wide apart or sit back to front on a chair, once again with your knees wide open in a supported squat position. A birth ball is a wonderful aid in getting the pelvis to open to maximum.

Sometimes even after you have done all you can to assist with the movement of the baby through the pelvis, and you have used all the non-medicated forms of pain relief available, you may end up having a Caesarean section or asking for medication. This is OK! What does count is that you have done all you can, which often gives you a sense of satisfaction and comfort if your labour turns out to be different to the way you expected.

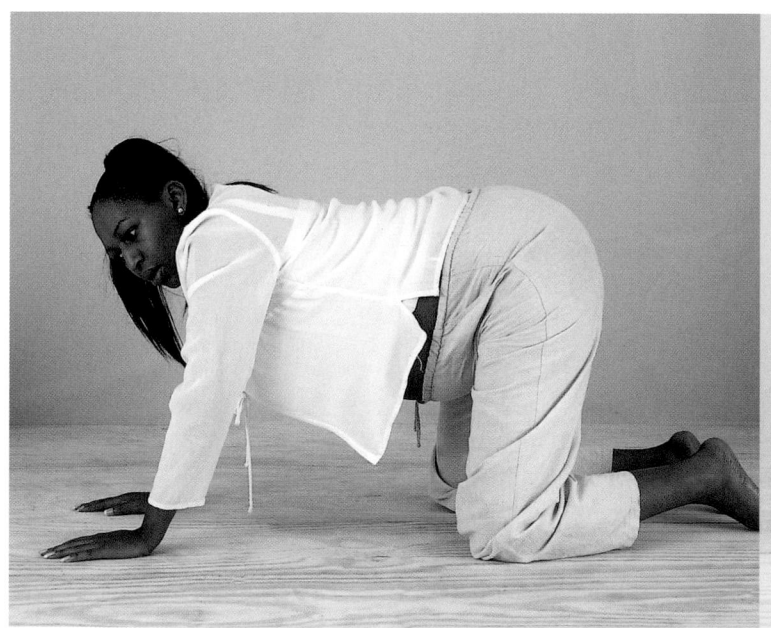
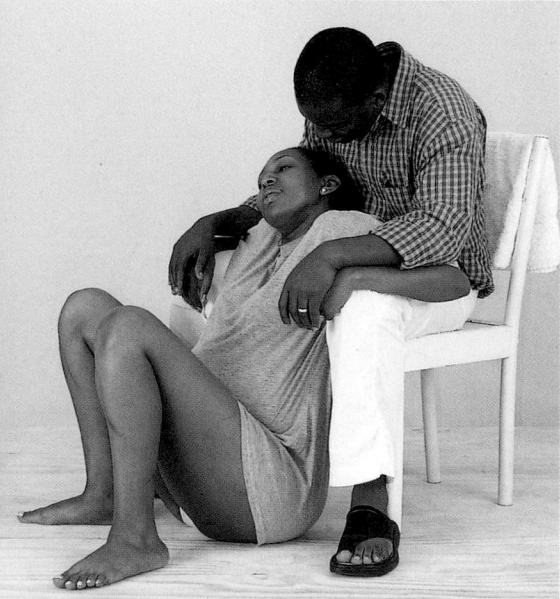

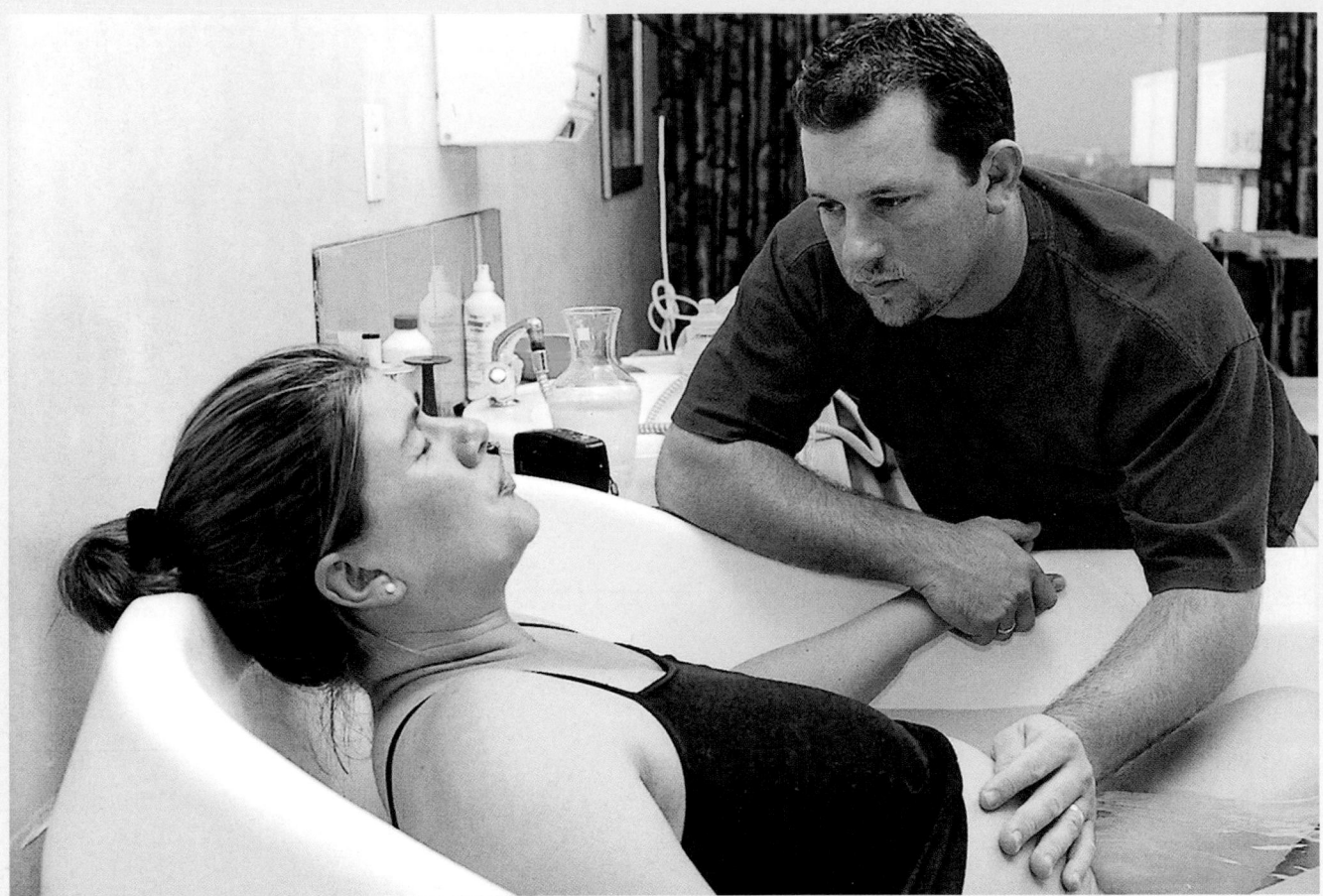

Dedicated to dads

Labour support

In most cases, the father will be with the mother for most of her labour and birth, and will be her advocate, her guide and her biggest supporter. Many fathers-to-be have shared their concern about not knowing how to be a good labour supporter. Watching a loved one in pain can be a very frightening and disheartening experience. These feelings can be magnified, if you feel that there is very little you can do to help ease her pain and discomfort. You may feel detached with very little involvement. Everything seems to be happening to her and around her. They are unsure of what to do, where to stand, what to say and what not to say, when to ask questions and, most of all, how to assist this person they love deeply and how to help her manage her pain. It is important for you as the father or partner to have a few tricks up your sleeve, so that you too can feel a worthy part of the experience. She will need a variety of things from you – some are plain common sense and some will require some skill. You can be actively engaged in helping her feel comfortable and safe. You can protect her dignity and her privacy. You can ask questions on her

Above A woman in labour finds much strength in having her partner very close by during labour. Whisper words of encouragement and praise constantly.

behalf and offer words of encouragement, praise and empathy. Acknowledge her power, her wisdom and her courage. You will need to reinforce techniques learned in class and remind her to relax, breathe and visualize the baby moving down and out.

Do not make her feel weak and vulnerable by telling her you think she should opt for pain relief before she is ready to ask for it. She will tell you when she is ready. Respect her wishes and work with her in every way.

Must do

Have a positive attitude Be confident in your ability and in hers. Develop a positive attitude about birth. Birthing pain is not a sign that something is wrong; it is a sign that something is happening and if she 'listens' to the messages, her pain will tell her what to do, how to do it and when to do it. Birth pain is 'constructive' pain but it is also a force to be reckoned with, and pain management can include both natural and medicated remedies. Accepting the positive nature of this pain can enable both of you to be more receptive to it.

Become educated Attending childbirth education classes with her will help you gain a clear understanding of what causes labour pain, which in turn will alleviate your fears and help you gain clarity as to why certain positions help the pain and others hinder the progress of labour. As a woman moves through the stages of labour, she will display certain behaviours. Through education you will understand these behaviours, and you will be reassured (as will she) that this is normal and to be expected.

Say the right thing Help your partner find and use her confidence by uttering words of encouragement. Tell her how strong she is, remind her what is at the end of labour and acknowledge that this is indeed the hardest thing she has ever done, and also tell her that you are very proud and amazed at what she is doing.

If she ends up having a birth outcome that is unexpected (i.e an assisted/forceps birth or a Caesarean birth), she will need to fall back on what she has achieved as she comes to terms with the shift of her goals.

Take your role seriously She really does need you! You are more important than you know. Be familiar with the suggestions and tips you gain from reading and childbirth classes. Get feedback from her. Discuss options long before the due date; in this way you will learn what she likes and dislikes, and will come to understand what her hopes are for her unique birth experience.

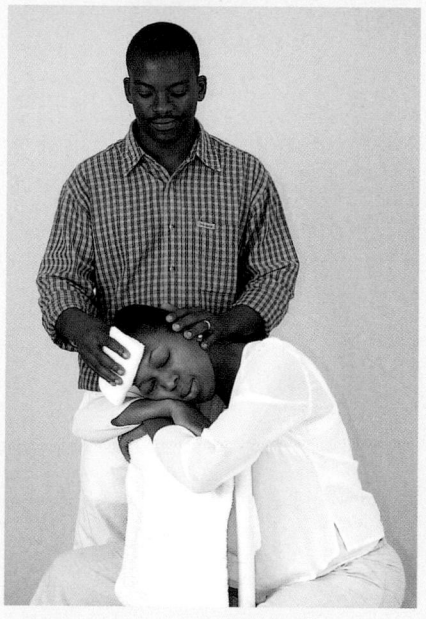

Above Make sure that you keep the mother relaxed and focused on her breathing. If she is feeling hot, dab a cool cloth on her forehead.

Learn about positioning techniques for comfort, breathing patterns, touch and massage FOR LABOUR, and how to prevent hyperventilation. You may be surprised to find that there are some massage strokes that she will not enjoy during labour.

Be open and flexible Acupressure is a wonderful skill to use in labour and she will be grateful that you know where and when to apply pressure and why. Use visualization and relaxation techniques to calm her down and keep her distracted. Keep her as upright and as mobile as you can for as long as possible. Ask questions on her behalf and do not leave her unattended – ever!

Must not do

- Do not breathe and blow in her face, this can be distracting for her. (If you think your breath might smell strongly, take some fresh breath mints with you.)
- Do not command or demand anything, and do not try to control her experience – trust her to know what she wants, when she wants it.
- Try not to get too involved in technology.
- Never leave her alone.
- Do not touch her in a way that you think she will enjoy. Do not be offended if she does not want you to touch her in a certain way.
- Never diminish her sense of pain and discomfort – we all feel pain differently.

Childbirth is a normal, healthy life event for most women. Of course there can be problems – perhaps minor, perhaps more serious. For most women, however, birth is a healthy challenge – one of many she will face as a mother. You should look forward to the time of your baby's birth with anticipation and celebration, not gloom, dread and fear. By supporting her, you can make all the difference!

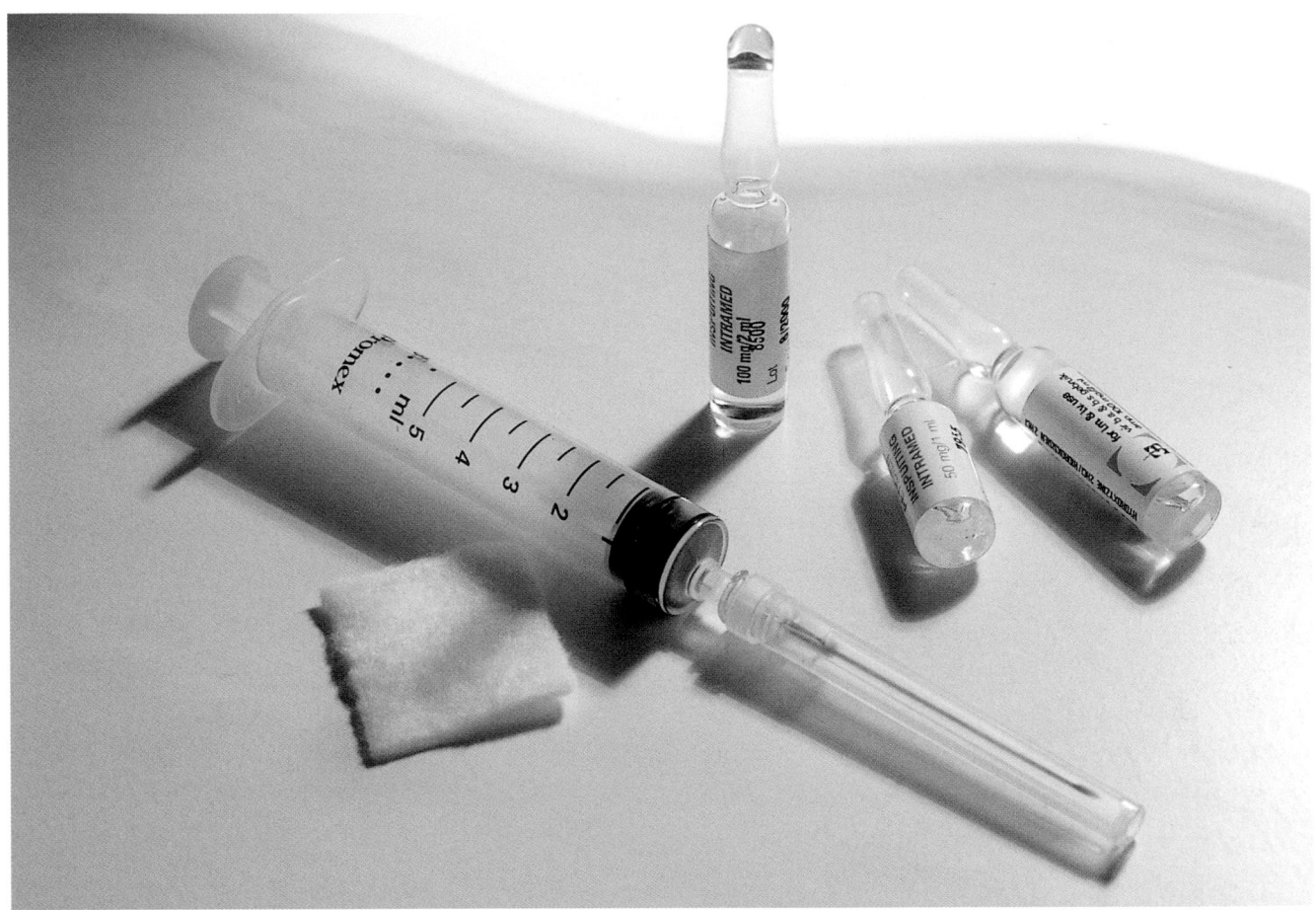

Anaesthetics

Anaesthetics are drugs that eliminate pain altogether, and can be administered regionally or generally. If given regionally, by injection, a loss of sensation will occur in a particular region of the body.

Benefits

- Anaesthetics provide complete pain relief in labour.
- They cause no maternal or foetal depression if administered correctly, and do not lead to complications.
- The danger of gastric contents being aspirated into the lungs, as in general anaesthesia, is virtually eliminated.

- If timed well, they will not slow down the progress of labour.
- With continuous infusion, anaesthesia can be extended for the duration of the delivery and can be modified if a Caesarean section becomes necessary.
- The mother is conscious during labour and delivery, and is involved on all levels as her child is born.

Risks

- Anaesthetics can only be administered by a highly trained person and, even with a skilled practitioner, a regional anaesthetic sometimes may not take full effect during the labour process.

Above If you do have an anaesthetic, you will feel absolutely no pain, but you should bear in mind that there are risks involved with these procedures.

- If given too soon, can slow down labour.
- They may restrict the movements of the mother during labour.
- Side effects, such as lowering blood pressure, can cause serious complications if not treated immediately.
- Contractions may slow down, resulting in a longer labour. The mother may need intervention in the form of synthetic oxytocin via a drip, to stimulate the contractions.

Pudendal nerve block

The anaesthetic is administered via the vagina into the pudendal nerve close to the second stage of labour. The timing of the administration is crucial to it being successful, as once the presenting part of the foetus is distending the perineum, it is too late. It takes effect quickly and lasts about one hour. It has been used for discomfort during the delivery or, in the case of an assisted delivery, where obstetrical instruments are used. The block will extend into the period when an episiotomy (*see* p128), if performed, will be repaired.

Local infiltration

This is an injection of local anaesthetic into the perineal tissue. It is performed during the second or third stage of labour, mainly for an episiotomy to be performed and then for the period after, when the incision is repaired or when lacerations or tears are sutured. The technique is a simple one and the success rate is almost 100 per cent. The injection can be given at any time, even when the foetal head is distending the perineum.

Saddle block

Saddle block is a low spinal anaesthetic. The mother must sit upright so that the solution gravitates downward. The anaes-

Right The procedure of having an epidural administered is virtually painless. You may be asked to sit up and lean forward or lie down on your side during the process.

thetic takes effect in about five minutes and the length of time the mother sits up will determine the level of anaesthesia. The perineal muscles become relaxed, and there is loss of sensation in the inner thighs and lower abdomen. It is usually administered in the second stage of labour, when the use of low forceps is anticipated, which may result in a drop in the mother's blood pressure.

Epidural block

The spinal epidural block has become increasingly popular for labouring women throughout the world and is considered the ultimate form of analgesia for women in labour. Unlike most of the other types of regional anaesthesia, an epidural can be given at any time during the first stage of labour and can extend into the second, third and fourth stages. If administered at the

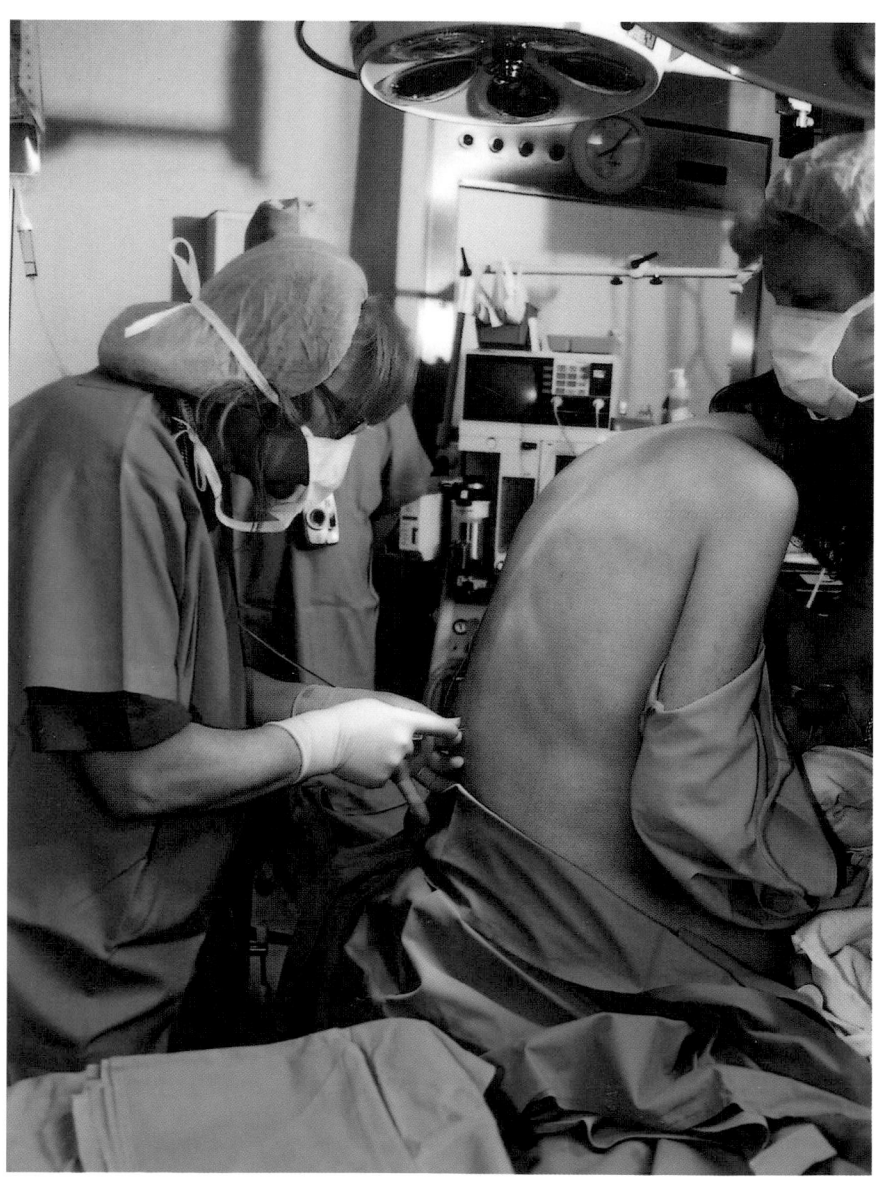

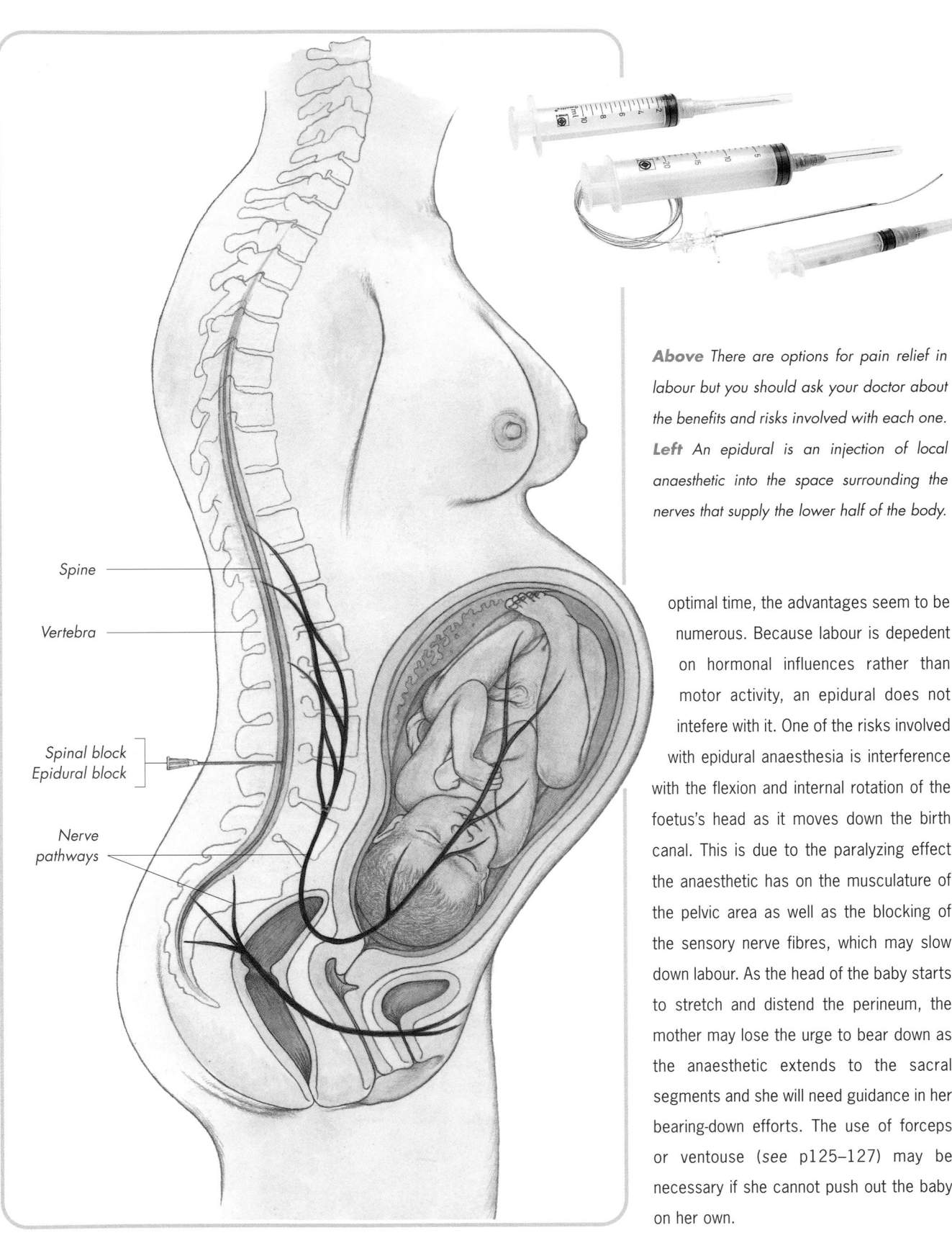

Spine

Vertebra

Spinal block
Epidural block

Nerve
pathways

***Above** There are options for pain relief in labour but you should ask your doctor about the benefits and risks involved with each one. **Left** An epidural is an injection of local anaesthetic into the space surrounding the nerves that supply the lower half of the body.*

optimal time, the advantages seem to be numerous. Because labour is depedent on hormonal influences rather than motor activity, an epidural does not intefere with it. One of the risks involved with epidural anaesthesia is interference with the flexion and internal rotation of the foetus's head as it moves down the birth canal. This is due to the paralyzing effect the anaesthetic has on the musculature of the pelvic area as well as the blocking of the sensory nerve fibres, which may slow down labour. As the head of the baby starts to stretch and distend the perineum, the mother may lose the urge to bear down as the anaesthetic extends to the sacral segments and she will need guidance in her bearing-down efforts. The use of forceps or ventouse (*see* p125–127) may be necessary if she cannot push out the baby on her own.

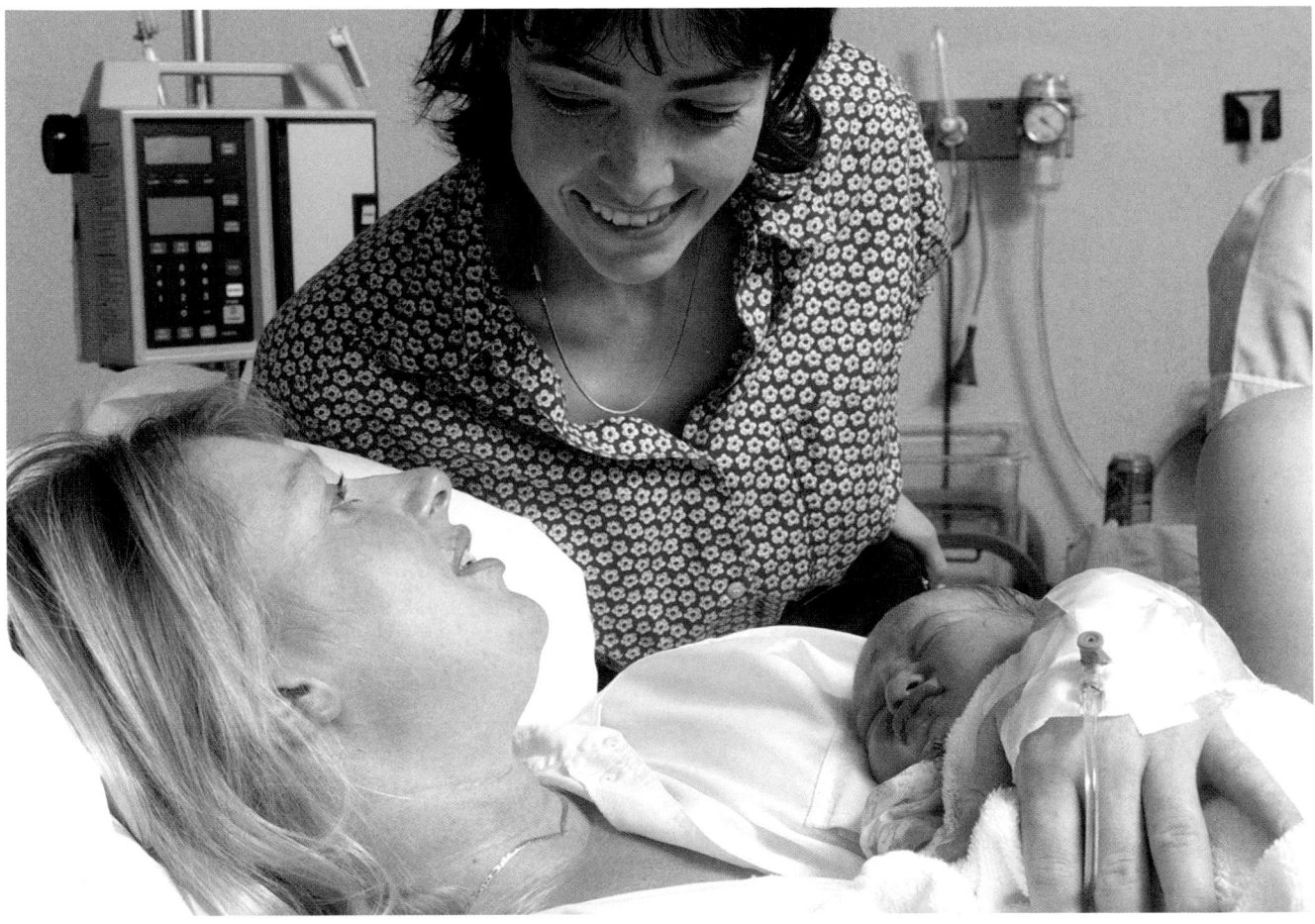

An epidural can be administered as a single dose block, which is effective in the latter stages of labour when delivery is not far off, or it can be given as a continuous infusion, providing anaesthesia for the greater part of the first stage of labour. The needle is inserted into the epidural space (extradural) and does not enter the spinal canal. The mother may lie on her side in the 'rainbow bend' position, or may sit in an upright position, with her head down – this usually depends on the personal preference of the anaesthetist. The mother will start to feel relief from pain within five minutes, and total effect within 30 minutes. Once the initial block is established it can be maintained by a constant infusion of the anaesthetic via the catheter left *in situ* in the mother's back, or by the intermittent injection of the drug when the mother starts to feel discomfort. The best time to administer this type of analgesia is when labour has progressed to the active phase and the cervix is 5–6cm (2–3in) dilated. An epidural may slow down labour, and other forms of intervention may be considered (i.e forceps or ventouse; see p125-127). Sometimes allowing the epidural to wear off before pushing begins can help to overcome this problem. Epidural anaesthesia does not work in a small percentage of women and may not take full effect in some others.

Above *The effects of an epidural can last into the third stage of labour and you can be cleaned and stitched, if necessary, while holding and bonding with your baby.*

An epidural is not advised if:

- you have a blood clotting disorder that significantly delays the clotting times of your blood
- you have open lesions on your back
- you have had surgery or trauma to your back, which makes it difficult for the anaesthetist to safely access the epidural space.

Mobile epidural

Recently, some obstetric units have been able to offer mobile epidurals. The advantage is that some movement is possible in labour, thus assisting their baby's journey into the pelvis. With the mobile epidural no catheter is required, but possibly the greatest advantage is that the woman still experiences the urge to push during the second stage of labour. The procedure for the administration of the epidural is the same. The difference lies in the mix of drugs.

Benefits

- A pain-free labour. It is the only form of total pain relief available for almost the entire labour and it brings about relaxation.
- Effectively decreases the mother's and her family's distress.
- Can be maintained for as long as is necessary during and after labour.
- The level of anaesthesia is controlled by the volume and concentration of the drug and, to a lesser degree, by the posture of the mother.
- If well timed, the mother can still feel the urge to bear down, which may result in spontaneous delivery.
- The mother is cooperative and alert.
- It is valuable in the trials of labour, and is a suitable form of anaesthetic should a Caesarean section become necessary. (The epidural would be modified.)
- Little effect on the foetus other than slight lowering of the heart rate.

Risks

- The strength of uterine contractions may be masked to a point where uterine rupture may occur. This is more likely to happen with the use of oxytocic drugs (*see* Glossary).
- In approximately 10 per cent of women, hypotension (low blood pressure) may occur. Doctors are aware of this and steps will be taken to prevent it or offer treatment to reverse the hypotensive effects of the epidural.
- No matter how skilled the practitioner, the dura mater (*see* Glossary) may become punctured, causing headaches.
- Some mothers have experienced backache with this procedure.
- Infection at the site of injection is rare, but the risk does exist.
- If administered before the active phase of labour, the epidural may affect uterine contractions. Labour may then have to be stimulated with the use of oxytocic drugs.
- If not optimally timed, and with large doses, the mother may lose sensation in her lower body and the urge to bear down. This may lead to the use of forceps or ventouse in the second stage.

Your self-help tool kit

It is a good idea to pack a bag of things that you are likely to use during your labour at least three weeks in advance of your due date. A few well-chosen personal items are all you need.

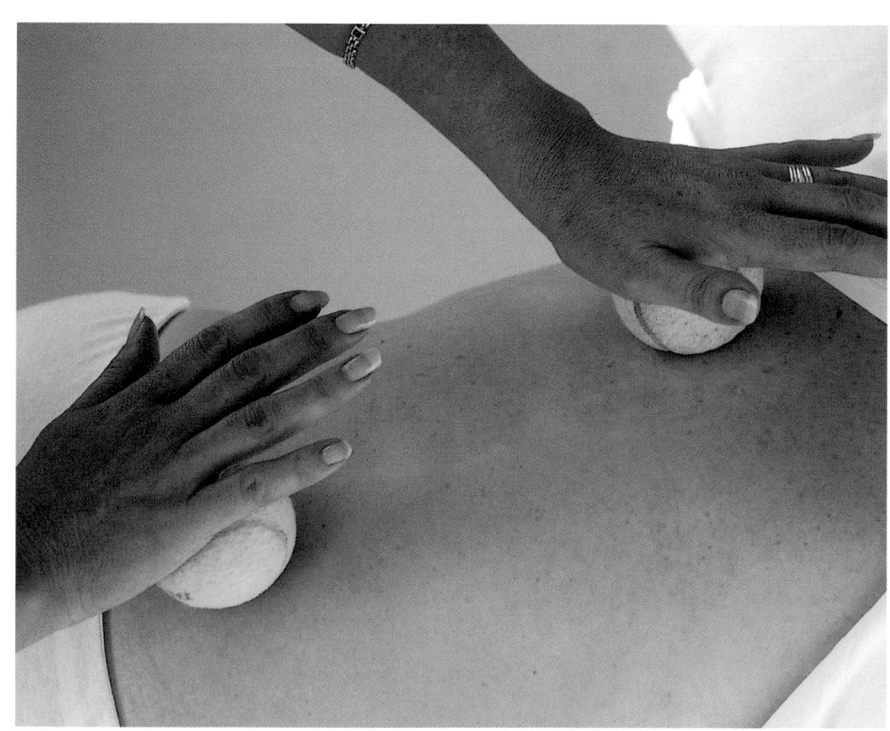

Below *Tennis balls can be used as effective massage aids to relieve backache.*

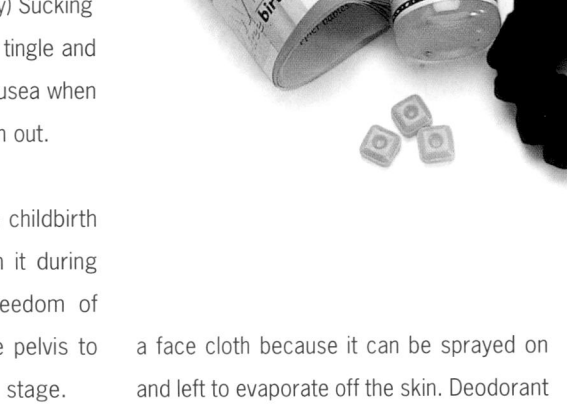

Lip balm Your lips may become dry and chapped due to heavy breathing.

Ice chips (only possible on the day) Sucking on ice chips will make your mouth tingle and quench a slight thirst or reduce nausea when labour is becoming long and drawn out.

Birth balls A new addition to the childbirth arena is the birth ball. Sitting on it during labour allows you a different freedom of movement and it encourages the pelvis to open to maximum during the first stage.

Cool or warm cloth (whichever makes you feel better) – to wipe down the face, neck, shoulders and chest when you start to feel hot and sweaty.

Massage balls or tennis balls There are many aids that one can use for massage during labour; these include tennis balls, rollers and reflex balls. Hands, knees and elbows are the best tools, of course, and firm yet gentle touching can be very reassuring.

Oil useful for massage.

Deodorant and rosewater spray Rosewater spray may be a better alternative to a face cloth because it can be sprayed on and left to evaporate off the skin. Deodorant spray also goes a long way to 'freshen' up damp skin.

Popsicles and boiled sucking sweets that contain sugar will help you keep up your energy levels. Remove during contractions and store in a cup of ice chips.

Fruit juice Natural fruit juice (diluted) will help keep you from becoming dehydrated, and is a change from drinking water.

Personal toiletries A toothbrush and toothpaste, mouthwash and moisturizer.

Hair accessories To keep hair away from your face.

Warm compresses Warmth can be very soothing to sore ligaments and painful joints. Hot-water bottles can be used, but the popular buckwheat huggers are safer – it is great for labours which are especially painful in the back.

Ice packs Buckwheat huggers can be placed in the ice chest of a refrigerator and used to cool a hot body or to numb a sore back – it is safer to use than ice. Never place ice directly against the skin.

T-shirt and socks A comfortable T-shirt and warm socks for cold feet.

Camera For taking pictures of the birth and your newborn.

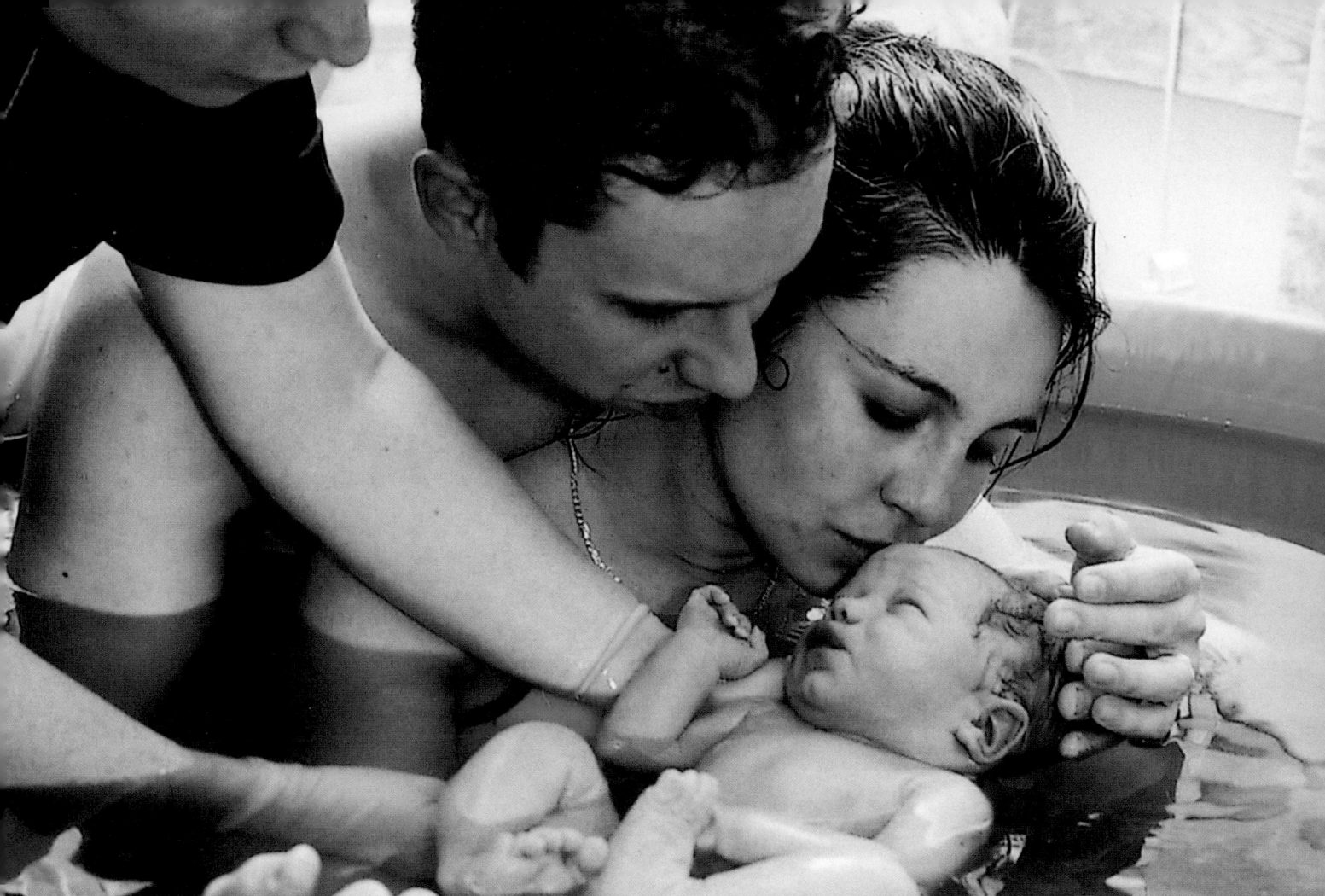

Giving Birth

Today's woman has many options and, as with any other important decision, finding out everything you can is vital before making a final choice about the way you will bring your baby into the world. Memories of this event will stay with you for the rest of your life and influence the way you feel about yourself as a woman and as a mother. Take time to explore your options before making final decisions and remember that we are all different and will experience this life-changing event in our own way.

EXPLORE YOUR OPTIONS BEFORE MAKING FINAL DECISIONS ABOUT YOUR BABY'S BIRTH

Active Birth

An 'active birth' means that you are actively involved in what is happening to your body during labour and delivery. It involves freedom of movement as you use your body in any way to make labour more tolerable. Positioning and movement play a big part in active labour and women who choose a water birth, home birth or birth in an alternative birthing centre are more likely to experience active birth.

Advantages

- Gravity helps the baby to move down onto the cervix and therefore assists with 'opening up' the body.
- The increased pressure of the abdominal wall and the diaphragm on the uterus maintains a 'resting phase' pressure between contractions.
- Owing to the fact that you are not lying on your back and not compressing the major blood vessels that lie behind the uterus, the foetus will be better oxygenated and the condition of the newborn is likely to be better.
- Changing positions helps to increase the strength and effectiveness of contractions, thus speeding up labour.
- You will not be treated like a patient – you are encouraged to participate and listen to and act upon your body's signals.

Right Staying upright and keeping mobile for as long as possible may assist in speeding up your labour. Your partner can assist by letting you lean on him for support.

- Psychologically, you will feel that you are contributing in a meaningful way to your birthing process.

Disadvantages of lying down

- Lying on your back is the one position that compresses the major blood vessels that lie behind the uterus, which may cause foetal distress and increase pain.

- Lying down does not permit mobility of the pelvic bones to the same extent; it also does not take advantage of the pelvic ligaments.
- The direction of the uterus's efforts conflicts with the direction of descent of the foetal head.
- Energy and effort is wasted.
- You will act and feel like a patient, and your caregivers will treat you like one.

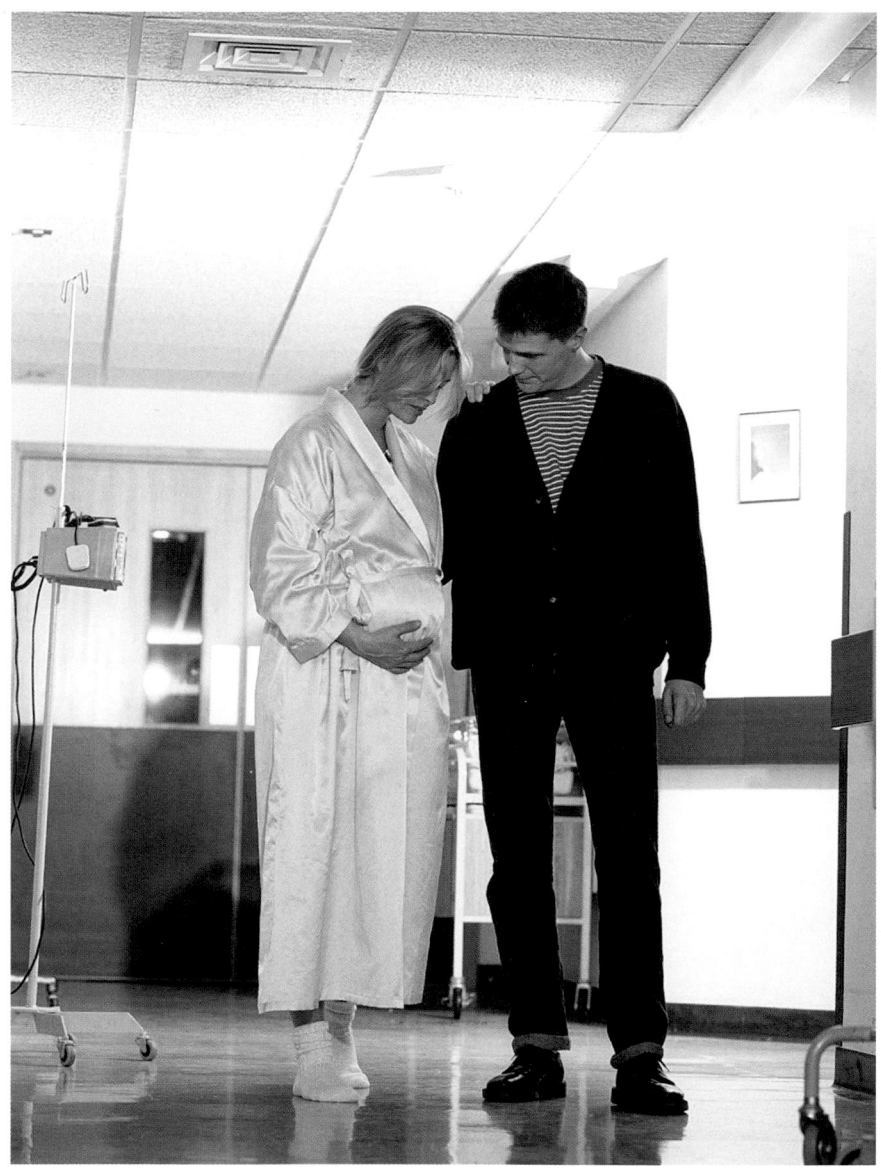

Home Birth

Women who have had a previous uncomplicated delivery may opt for a birth in the comfort and familiarity of their home. You are more likely to be actively involved in the labour and a midwife will assist you with the backup of a doctor. You will have to make sure that all you need is available on hand when you go into labour. Bear in mind that over 90 per cent of healthy pregnant women, receiving good antenatal care, will give birth spontaneously. However, if things do not run smoothly, you might need to be transferred to hospital.

Water Birth

Water birth is the vaginal birth of a baby directly into water. It may be in a hospital setting or at home in a special or normal bath. Remember that water birth is not a method of delivering but rather a tool to assist in the natural process of birth. Benefits include: freedom of movement, effective pain relief, natural acceleration of labour, lowering of blood pressure, less perineal trauma, less intervention and a gentler entry into the world for the baby. Much of this is borne out by available research. You will be actively involved in the labour and birthing process.

Water birth is not a good idea if:

- the baby is small for dates (see Glossary) or premature – in this case, you will need the safety net that modern technology can provide
- you are expecting twins – there is an increased chance of complications (although you may not experience complications at all)
- you have pre-eclampsia
- your caregiver anticipates birth complications. If your baby becomes distressed at any time during your labour or if the water are stained a green colour, this may indicate that the baby is not tolerating labour well. A constant, watchful eye in the form of a foetal heart monitor may become necessary for a while
- any unexplained blood loss occurs – it is cause for concern
- the mother has active genital herpes
- the mother has AIDS
- the baby is in a breech position
- there are any serious medical conditions present.

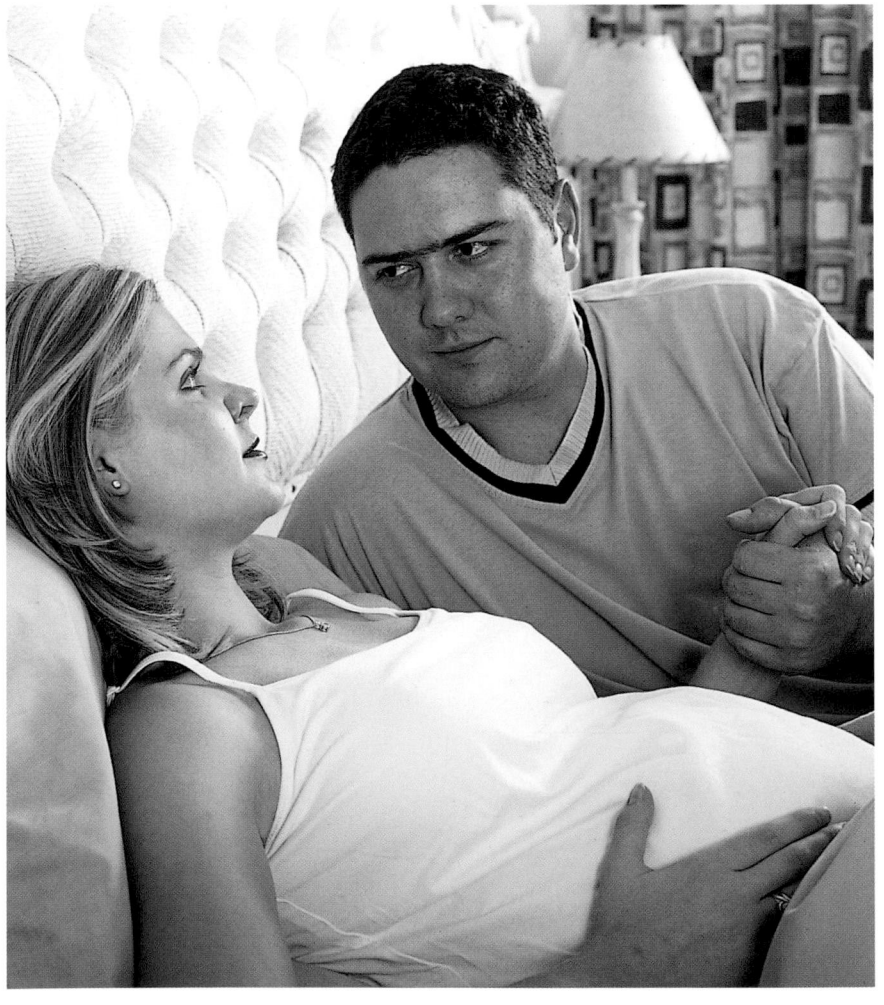

Left Having your baby at home may help you feel more relaxed and comfortable because of the familiar surroundings.

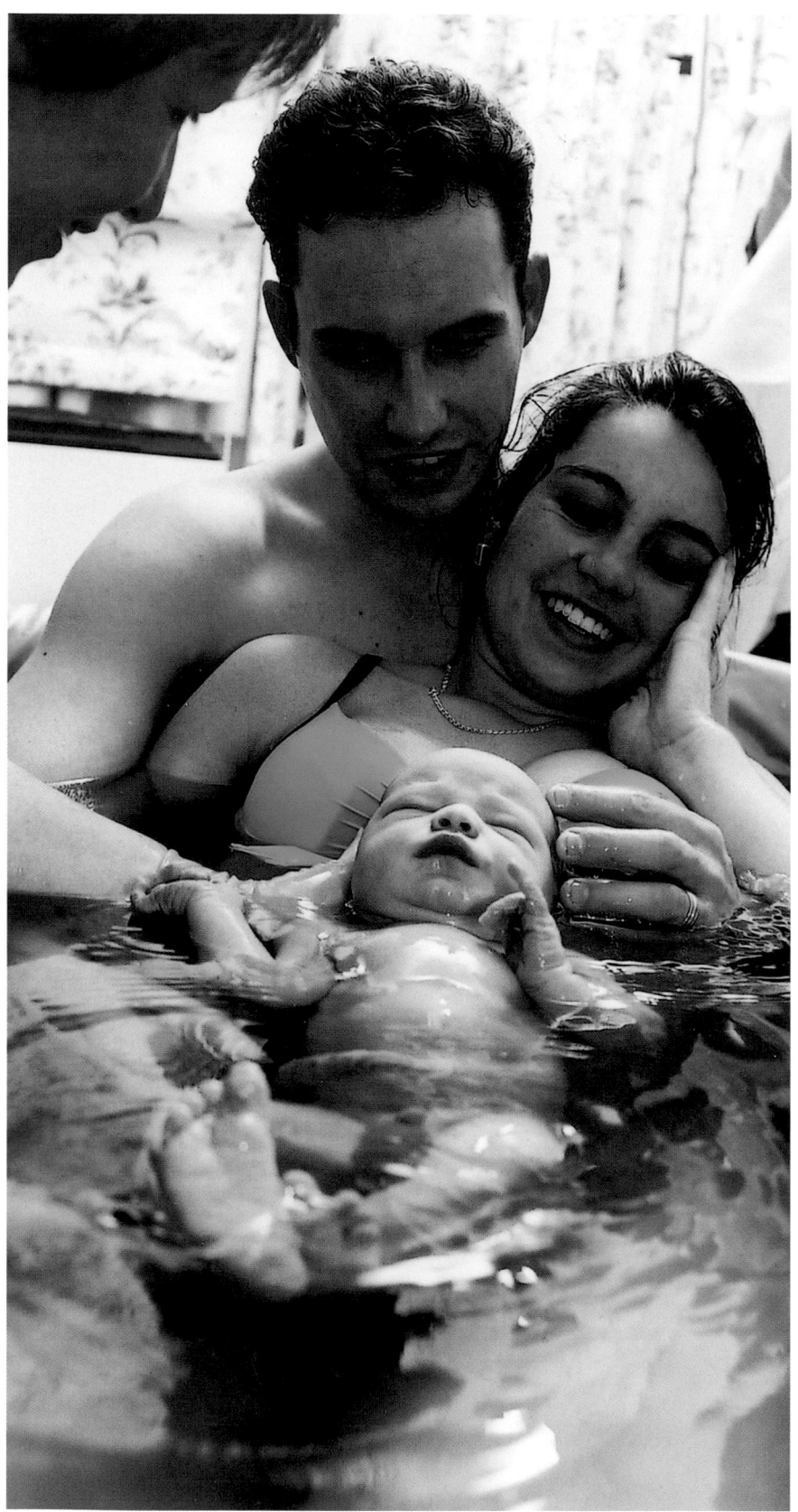

Vaginal birth after Caesarean (VBAC)

Vaginal birth after Caesarean (VBAC) means exactly that – a mother succeeds in her attempts to have her baby born vaginally after having her first child born by Caesarean section. Although VBAC has been common in Europe and other continents for many years, it was seldom considered in other parts of the world.

In the past, doctors were cautious about encouraging a vaginal birth after a woman had had a Caesarean because they knew little about it. However, they are now responding to the requests made by many women wanting to explore the possibility of a vaginal birth. If you are investigating the possibility of a VBAC, it is helpful to know why you had a Caesarean the first time.

Many of the former contra-indications for VBAC are being revised. Medical attitudes, training and experience, and the practice style of doctors, as well as the acceptance of new research and ideas will greatly influence your caregiver's willingness to allow a VBAC.

If the reason for the first Caesarean still exists, it is doubtful that you will be a candidate for a vaginal birth. These reasons could include diabetes, chronic high blood pressure, serious pelvic abnormalities or active genital herpes around the time of your due date.

Left *There are many advantages to labouring and birthing in water – one being a gentler birth process for your baby.*

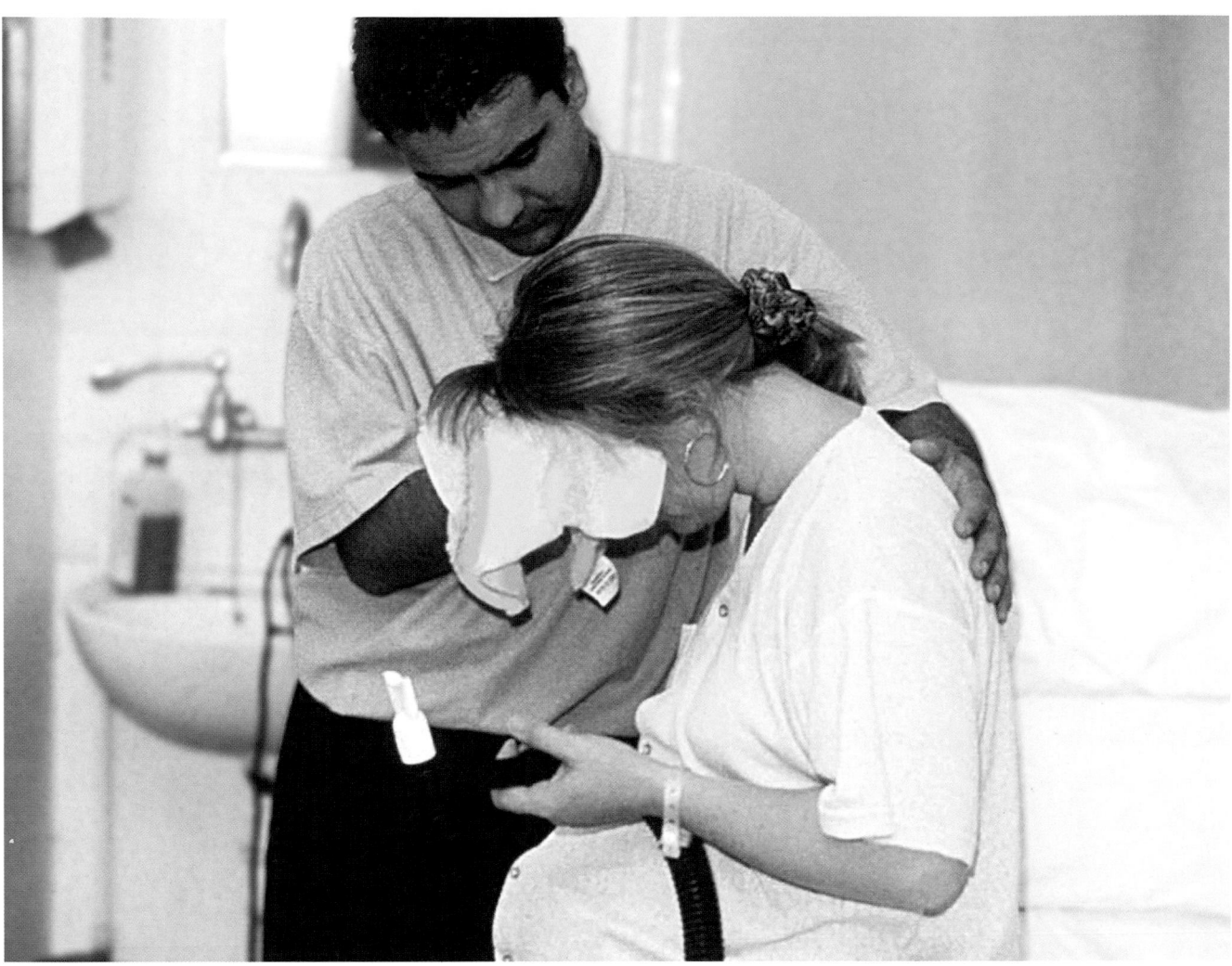

Labour

Labour is a process that every woman will experience in her own unique way. For some women the signs are very distinct; other women ease into labour with less easily defined contractions that start and stop over a period of time. Even so, there are definite stages with recognizable signs that will direct you through it. These signs are often referred to as pre-labour phenomena. There are clusters of signs that can occur over a few weeks, a few days, and even over a few hours. If you are unsure about whether or not it is the real thing, do not hesitate to contact the labour ward of the hospital where you plan to deliver or the midwife who will be delivering your baby. The following signs indicate that your body is preparing for labour:

- **Lightening** This is the term used to describe the change in your baby's position as it starts to dip its head into the pelvis. While you will find it easier to breathe, your bladder takes strain as the weight of the uterus rests on it. This causes you to visit the toilet more often.
- **Weight loss** You may lose a small amount of weight as your body gets rid of excess fluid, due to hormonal changes.
- **Burst of energy** It is common to get a sudden nesting urge. Conserve your energy for what is to come.
- More frequent **Braxton-Hicks** contractions. They may be so intense that you may want to go to the hospital, only to be told that you are having false labour.

Above Labour may be harder or easier than you think – be flexible and open-minded when entering this powerful experience.

Classic signs

Show
The mucus seal that has closed off your cervix from the vagina for the entire pregnancy dislodges itself; it may even have a streak of blood in it. It may occur over a few hours or for one to two weeks. It is not a definite sign of labour but watch out for something else to happen.

Contractions
These will get stronger, longer and closer together. Under the influence of the hormone oxytocin, the uterine muscle will start to contract (cause still unknown). These contractions will cause the top of the uterus to become thicker while the cervix becomes thinner and shorter.

Breaking of waters
The waters may rupture before or during labour, and some babies have been born 'in the bag'. There can be a break in the bag at a low point, resulting in a gush of fluid or the break can be higher, so there is more a trickle of fluid. The amniotic fluid has a sweetish smell and is straw-coloured.

Left You should be on your way to the hospital by the time you are having three to four contractions in 10 minutes!

True labour
In true labour, the contractions may be irregular at first but become more regular, longer, stronger, and closer together as labour progresses. Walking makes them stronger but, unfortunately, lying down will not make them go away. The contractions are usually felt in the back and radiate to the front. On internal exam, the cervix has thinned and it starts to open. A warm bath will not make contractions go away.

False labour
In false labour, the contractions felt are short and irregular. They do not get longer, stronger and closer together, and walking has no effect on the strength of the contractions. If you lie down, the contractions may disappear. False labour pain is usually felt in the front and groin area. On internal exam, the cervix does not thin out or open up.

The birthing hormones
There are three hormones that are that are actively involved in the birth process. Understanding how they work and how they benefit both mother and baby will help you work with them during labour.

Oxytocin
This hormone enables you to maintain effective contractions of the uterus up to the birth of your baby and placenta. The release of oxytocin peaks after birth, in order to allow the placenta separate easily and safely without significant bleeding. At this time, oxytocin loads the breasts with colostrum, warms the mother's skin and makes her more receptive

to receiving her baby. In order to maintain high levels of oxytocin, the mother has to have privacy and no demands must be made on her, except to focus on her baby. if the flow of oxytocin is left undisturbed, it will motivate breast-feeding. A term for this important stage of childbirth is 'bonding'.

Catecholamines (adrenaline and noradrenaline)

These hormones act on nerve endings of the nervous system and can cause symptoms such as agitation and restless body movements, rapid breathing, dilated pupils, shivering, raised blood pressure and rapid pulse. In labour, if you are feeling afraid and unsupported or even uncomfortable in a strange environment, your body will assume that you are in danger and release adrenaline to assist you. The level of oxytocin falls in direct proportion to the rising levels of adrenaline in the system, and contractions can slow or even stop if you are in early labour. The circular muscles in the cervix cease to dilate, resulting in a tug-of-war effect and increased pain is felt with little progress.

It is vital that you feel safe and private during your labour to prevent high levels of adrenaline in your system. Once the transitional stage of labour is complete, there will be a 'rest and be thankful' phase before the pushing stage, which will allow you to take a break, get a 'second wind' and renew your energy. The uterus gets ready to expel the baby. At this stage there is a peak release of all hormones, including the emergency hormone, adrenaline. When birth is left undisturbed, this is the time when your behaviour will change in response to the adrenaline rush. It is important to note at this stage that the level of oxytocin is so high that adrenaline will not cause a negative influence. From being withdrawn and focused inward, you will now be alert and full of energy. Some women have a very short episode of fear, which is a sure sign of adrenaline release.

Endorphins

These natural substances are similar to opiates in structure and appear when the body is stressed beyond its normal limits. They are the body's natural painkillers. When a labour is allowed to progress naturally, contractions will naturally get longer and stronger. Owing to the effects of this hormone, the mother has no perception of time and space. As the labour progresses, the endorphin levels rise to contend with increasing pain and fatigue. During the transitional phase of labour, the uterus changes its action from opening the cervix to pushing the baby out. At this stage, the contractions are long and strong and unrelenting. Endorphin production is then at its maximum, allowing you to manage your pain and also allowing you to 'switch off' and focus inwardly. This is often referred to as a 'altered state'.

The following table will give you some idea of what to expect from the different stages of labour and how to deal with them.

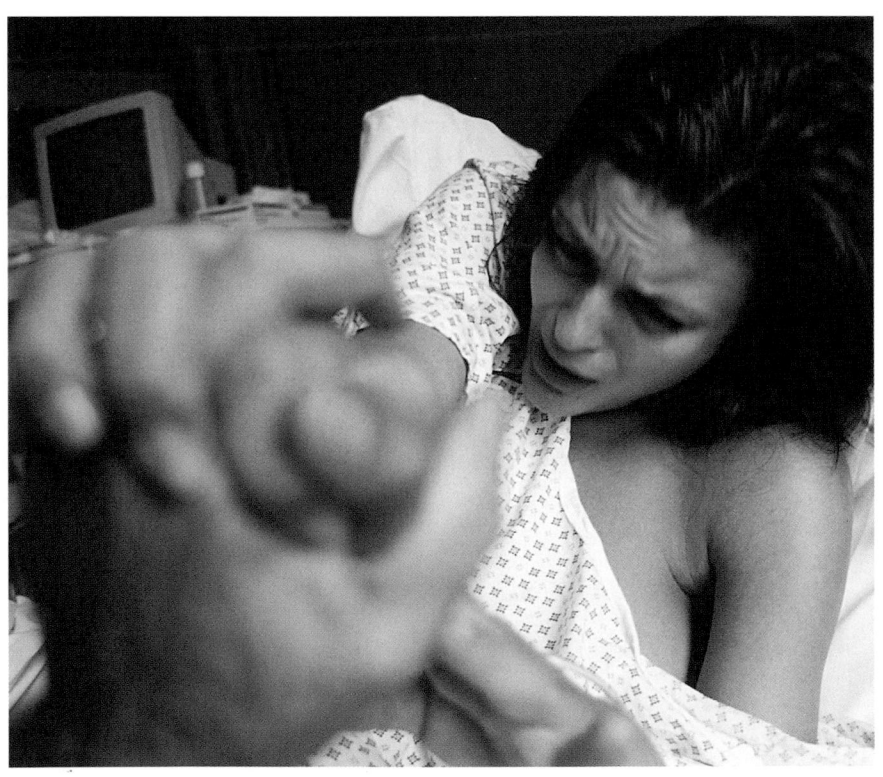

Above After the transitional phase of labour, there is a peak release of all the birthing hormones and you will feel a surge of energy as you enter the 'pushing' stage of labour.

Pre-labour clues

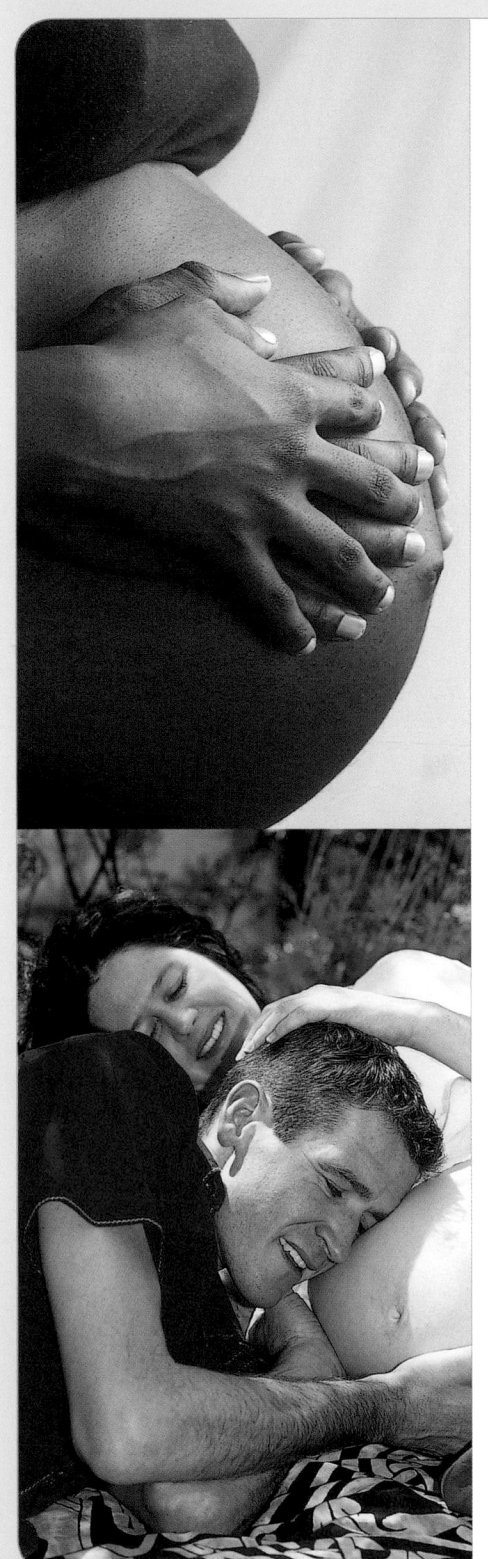

What happens inside

The cervix will begin to soften and thin slightly. Contractions are short, mild and irregular, and may be felt as a little backache or as 'period pain' low down on the abdomen.

Other signs

- Increased vaginal discharge
- Sudden weight loss
- Nagging backache.

Emotions

You may sense that something is different but often deny that it may be the start of labour. You may feel a nesting instinct kick in and start to clean, paint or wash baby clothes or you may find that you become more lethargic and sedentary, wanting to rest more. You may recognize subtle body changes.

Self help

Do not start anything strenuous. Pace yourself and rest as much as you can. Eat small 'snacky' high-energy fruit and carbohydrates. Drink enough water. When resting, focus on relaxing and breathing deeply as you start to tune in to your body.

Partner power

Partners can help by keeping the mother-to-be relaxed. Encourage her to slow down and help with any unfinished chores. Get the telephone list ready. Make sure the hospital bag is packed, the car has enough fuel and you know the quickest route to the hospital. Do not rush and do not panic.

Left Enjoy the quiet time before true labour starts in earnest. Take this time to reflect on what is about to happen.

Stage one – early labour

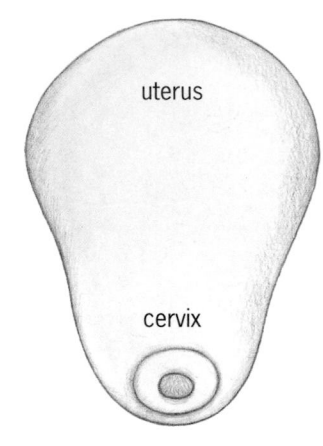

uterus

cervix

2cm (0.8in) dilation

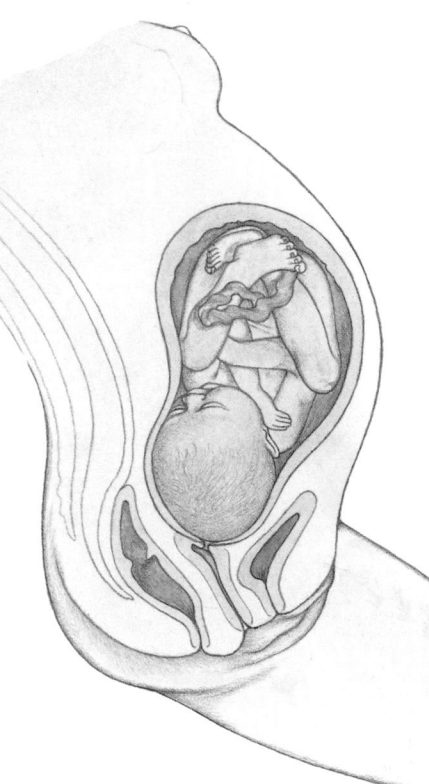

Above *The first stage of labour is all about the thinning out (effacement) and the start of dilation of the cervix.*

What happens inside

The cervix continues to thin out (efface) and starts to dilate. Contractions are five to 20 minutes apart, lasting 20–50 seconds. They are usually not painful but they do get your attention. Vaginal discharge increases and you may have a mucus show tinged with a bit of blood.

Other signs

Your bag of waters may break now (or it may happen later). Lower back pain may persist or increase with contractions.

Emotions

You may experience mixed feelings. You are excited that labour has started in earnest, but also apprehensive. You may feel anticipation, restlessness and nervousness; you may want to walk around, make eye contact, and just have a companion who will keep you distracted. You may want to leave for hospital or you may want to be in the comfort and familiarity of your home.

Self help

Eat lightly and sip clear fluids. Rest, sit in a rocking chair or take a slow walk. Distract yourself between contractions by reading, talking to someone, listening to music or making telephone calls.

Partner power

Stay clam and keep close to her. Help her to practise breathing while the contractions are still mild. Time the contractions to know when to go to the hospital. Massage her if she is willing. If she has backache, apply firm pressure or hot or cold compresses to her lower back. Make sure you are 'fed and watered' to keep up your own strength.

Stage one – active labour

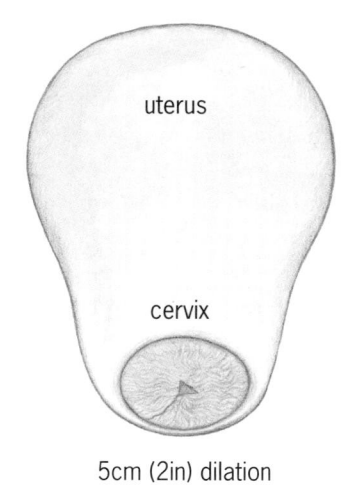

uterus

cervix

5cm (2in) dilation

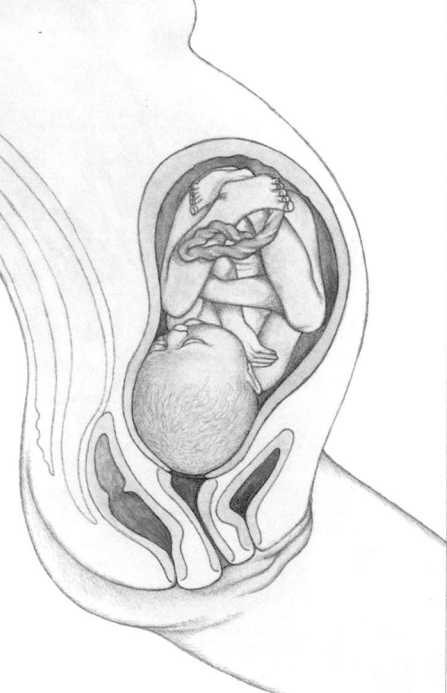

Above *During the active phase of the first stage of labour, you are already past the halfway mark.*

What happens inside

The cervix s completing thinning out and continues to dilate. Contractions are stronger, longer, and closer together (three to five minutes apart), lasting 50–60 seconds.

Other signs

Vaginal discharge is more profuse. The bag of waters may break now. Your labour may experience a plateau: contractions continue but dilation may cease or pause for a while.

Emotions

You will be alert and concentrating during contractions, and sleepy and tired between them. Your endorphin levels are very high. You may feel frustrated that labour has slowed, but try to relax – your body is taking a breather before the next step. Avoid conversation; rest quietly between contractions and become passive. Find your own position – placing your head on the arms of you birth companion's for non-disruptive support may help.

Self help

Change positions frequently to help your baby get into a good position and keep as upright as possible, using gravity to get your baby to move down into the pelvis. Empty your bladder hourly and rest between contractions. Use the visualization techniques you learned in childbirth class. Breathe in a way that keeps you focused. Remember that the uterus needs lots of oxygen to work efficiently and your pain will become less if you breathe with awareness.

Partner power

Provide whatever comfort techniques she needs. She needs you to help her make decisions and encourage her through these tough contractions. Remind her to change positions and help her to do it. Help her overcome her plateau by holding her and helping her to relax as much as possible. Praise all her efforts and expect her behaviour to change at this point. Do not panic – what you see is all within the nature of birth.

Transition – advanced labour

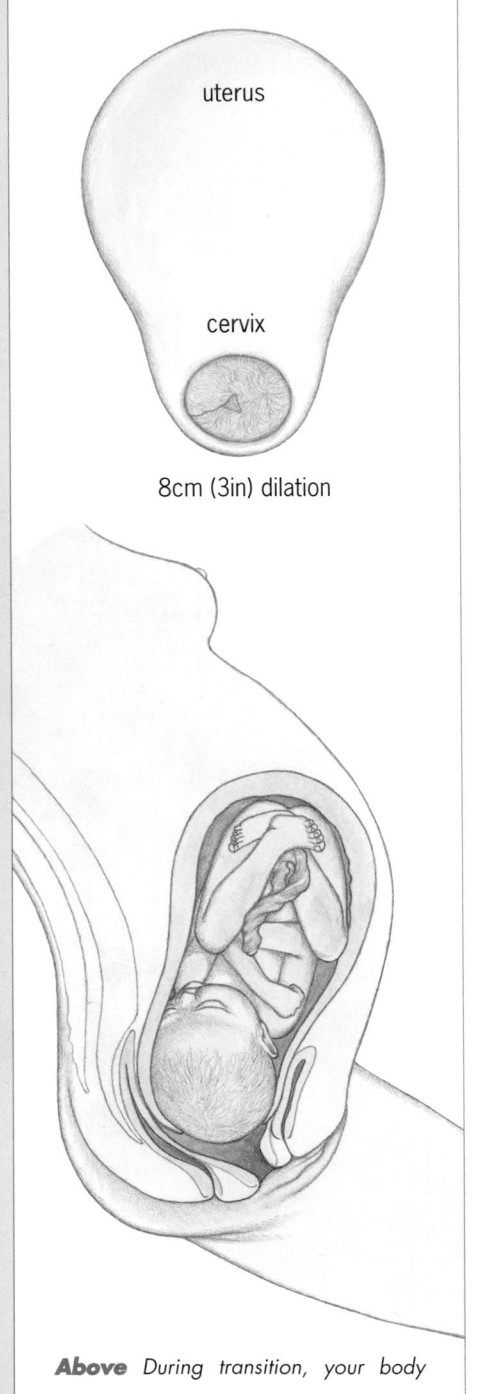

uterus

cervix

8cm (3in) dilation

Above *During transition, your body 'changes gears' as you move from first stage into the second stage.*

What happens inside

The cervix is almost fully dilated. Contractions are close now (two to four minutes apart), lasting 50–90 seconds. You will sense a change in the feel of contractions as their function changes from pulling open the cervix to pushing down to get the baby out. Oxytocin (the hormone that causes contractions) levels are very high.

Other signs

You may start to feel the urge to push (this does not happen to every woman). You will feel pressure and fullness in the vagina, rectum and groin area. It is common to shiver and feel nauseous due to high adrenaline and endorphin levels.

Emotions

Sudden changes take place: adrenaline gives you a 'second wind' and enhances your concentration. It also makes you aggressive to others and protective toward the baby. Some women become grouchy and confused, and extremely discouraged. At this stage, it is normal for a woman to express fear of dying. You may feel out of control and unable to cope. Remember: this is the darkest time before the dawning of the second stage.

Self help

Deal with one contraction at a time! Each contraction is one closer to seeing your baby. Relax as much as possible between contractions to conserve your energy for pushing. Pant or blow if you feel the urge to push before it is time.

Partner power

Remind her that she is almost there! Take care of her discomforts: give her ice chips to suck; she will be hot and sweaty, so place cool compresses on the back of her neck and tell her to slow down her breathing. Place your hands gently on the parts that are shaking. Work through each contraction as it begins and try to make eye contact with her. Direct her breathing if you have to. She needs a lot of guidance and encouragement to get through these tough contractions.

Second stage – pushing and birth

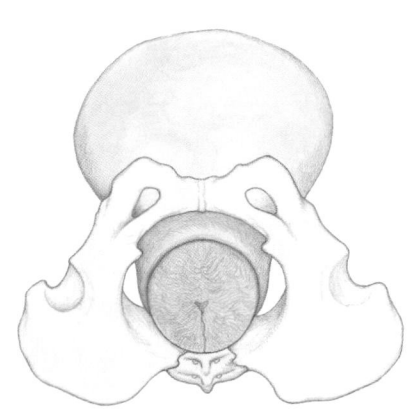

10cm (4in) dilation

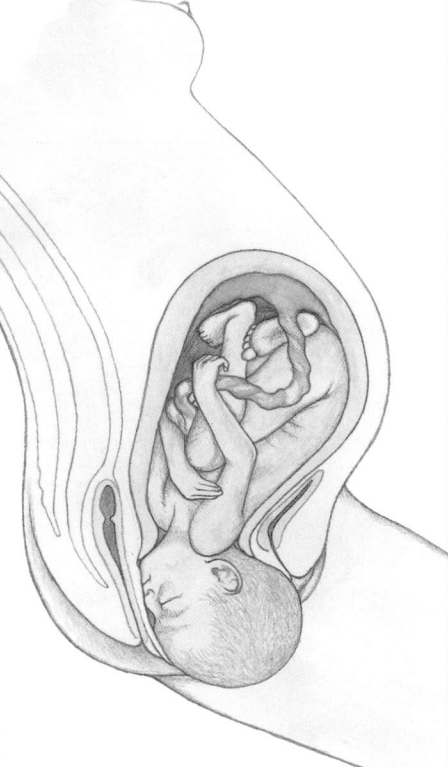

Above As your baby's head stretches the pelvic floor, you will start to feel the urge to push. If you have an epidural in place, you will experience more pressure than stretching in the vagina.

What happens inside

The character of the contractions changes and feels more manageable. They are two to five minutes apart, lasting 50–60 seconds. Uterus pushes down with each contraction. The baby moves down the birth canal, and pressure and burning is felt in the perineum as the head stretches the vagina.

Other signs

The uterus takes time to rest between first and second stages. This is normal and may take up to 30 minutes before beginning in earnest again. The contractions of second stage are often referred to as 'mother making' contractions.

Emotions

You become calmer as your second wind kicks in and a sense of purpose takes over. You experience intense concentration – you feel alert and eager as the birth of your baby approaches. You may feel tired and discouraged if pushing is taking a long time.

Self help

Only push with contractions; rest between them. Try short, sharp pushing techniques, rather than long periods of breath-holding that will tire you quickly. Get into a comfortable optimal position for pushing; the more upright the better.

Partner power

Support her body when she pushes. Now more than ever she needs your encouragement and praise. Help her relax between pushes and stroke areas of her body that are holding tension. Wipe her face and offer her sips of water or ice to suck between contractions. This is the hardest work of labour. Once the baby is born, you may want to cut the cord yourself. Speak to the doctor about this beforehand.

Third stage – placental expulsion and delivery

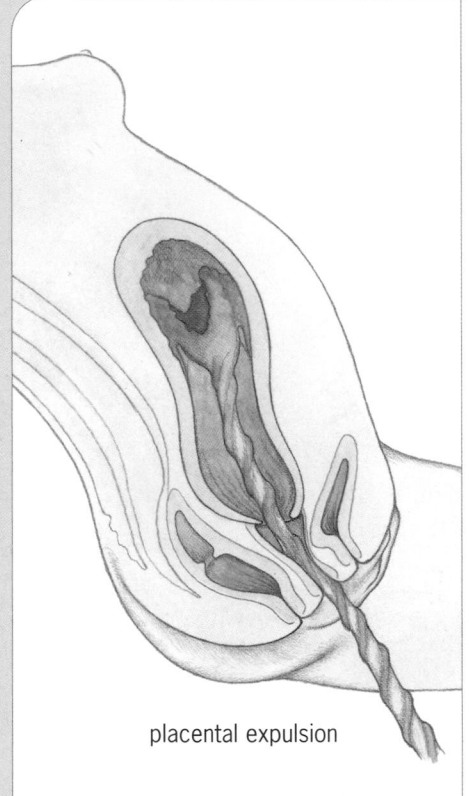

placental expulsion

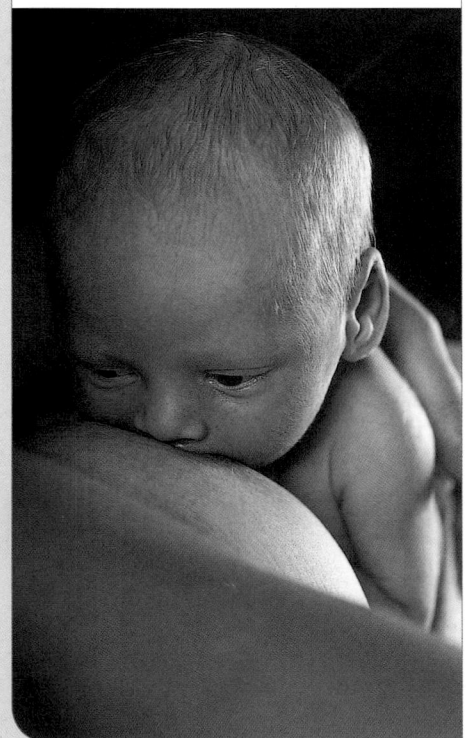

What happens

The uterus contracts to expel the placenta. The breasts become loaded with colostrum, ready to feed your baby and your skin temperature rises in order to keep your baby warm on your body.

Other signs

You may be asked to help with a few more little pushes to get the placenta out. You may feel cramping as the uterus contracts and it is common to shake or experience chills.

Emotions

You will feel relieved and happy, and eager to hold your precious baby. Do not be surprised by the utter exhaustion (physical and emotional) that you will feel. Endorphin levels and oxytocin levels are still very high. Place your baby skin-to-skin on your body.

Self help

Push as directed to assist with the expulsion of the placenta. Relax your legs and perineum if you need to be repaired due to a cut or tear. You should try to breast-feed your baby in order to help the contractions of the uterus. Breast-feeding causes oxytocin to be released, which causes the uterus to contract tightly and expel any unwanted leftover tissue.

Partner power

Praise her wonderful strength. Massage her shoulders. Tell her how proud you are of her. You may want to hold your baby.

Left Try to breast-feed your baby as soon as possible after birth. Remember, you have to arrange this with the doctor before you go into labour.

Stage four – the first hour after birth

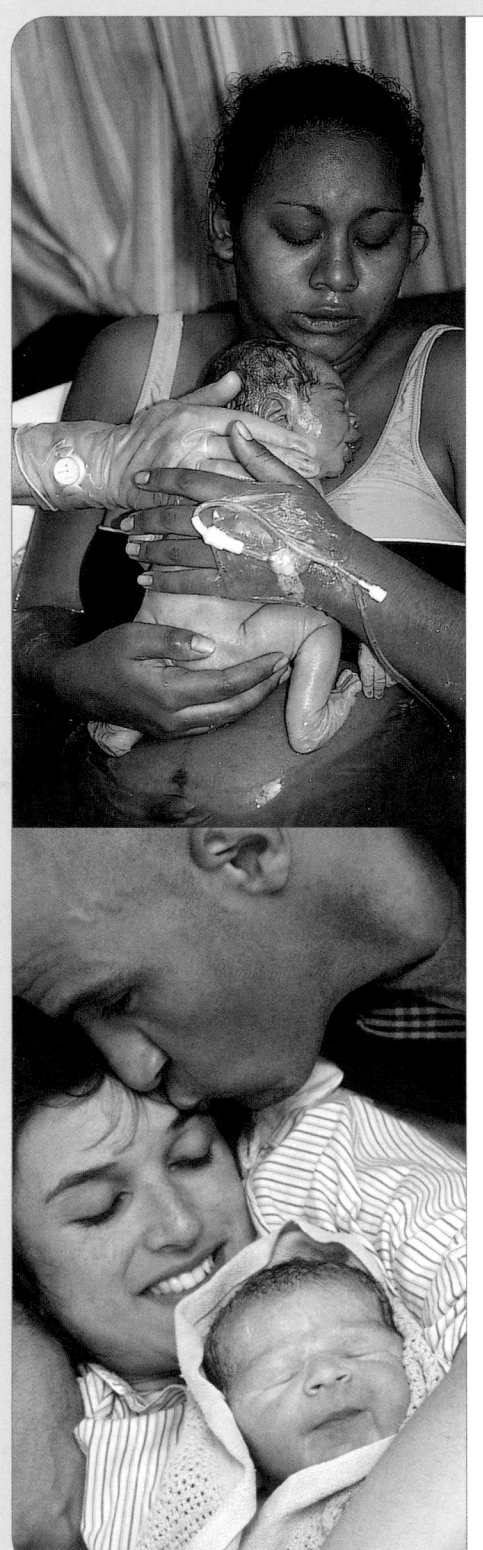

What happens inside

The uterus is resting now but you may feel mild contractions as it begins to shrink back to its normal size. Vaginal discharge is heavy and bloody.

Other signs

Contractions will resurface during breast-feeding. You may still experience chills and shivering. Your vagina will feel tender and uncomfortable.

Emotions

You are likely to feel many different emotions. You may feel elation, joy and extreme love for your baby. Perhaps disappointment and exhaustion if labour was longer and harder than you expected or did not go according to your expectations. If you feel very little after the event of labour, do not be concerned. Once you have had a chance to rest and recover, you will start to feel like your old self.

Self help

Rest, relax and take it easy. Focus on your baby and offer your baby the breast. Breathe through the uncomfortable examinations that you may need to endure. You may be offered a cup of tea and may be surprised to find that you are ravenous. Share this special time with your partner as your new family is born.

Partner power

Ask for a warm blanket to ease her chills. Remind her that shaking is normal. Obtain some food and drink for both of you (this is usually offered by the hospital). Hold your baby, relax and rest, and draw close to your partner at this special, momentous time.

Congratulations!

Left Skin-to-skin contact will warm up your baby immediately after birth and your baby will recognize you by your smell.

Your birth 'wish list'

No-one can predict exactly what your baby's birth will be like. A birth plan is a chance to let your caregivers know in advance what kind of birth you are hoping for. It is a way to ensure that there will be continuity of care even if you have different people looking after you. It is not always necessary to have a birth plan if you have communicated your wishes to your midwife or doctor with whom you have a good level of communication. The best kind of plan or guide is one that develops as your pregnancy does. As you learn more about what is happening to you, you will be asking more questions and may need to change some of your ideas. Ideally it is best to formulate a birth plan with the guidance of your midwife, consultant and partner because this can mean the difference between a good birth experience and one that may not meet all your expectations. It will also empower you at a time when you may feel as if you have no control over what is happening to your body.

Opposite Develop your birth plan as your pregnancy progresses. Be sure to make a copy for your caregiver and the hospital-ward staff, so that everyone knows what you are hoping for.

When compiling your wish list, be:

Reasonable in your requests. This is not a contract! The tone you strike and the way in which you make your request will help you get what you want. Think it through thoroughly and bear the following points in mind:

Brief

Never write more than two A4 pages.

Polite

Use the words 'prefer' and 'please'. It is in your own interests not to annoy the hospital staff before labour begins.

Flexible

It is important to remain flexible for your health and the baby's. Your individual labour and delivery may require last-minute adjustments. There is no such thing as a right or a wrong birth plan. You can change your mind if you wish to.

Clear

Know what you want but be clear about alternatives and be prepared to take them if you are medically advised.

Realistic

If labour turns out to be more complicated and painful than anticipated, you may have to think fast and re-evaluate your choices. You and your partner need to know and understand your options as well as the alternatives should things not go according to plan. Do not be disappointed if things work out differently to what you had hoped for. The most important thing to remember is that if you and the baby are well, you have achieved your most important goal.

Confident

Talk to your partner and discuss your feelings with him. Very often he will turn out to be the one who will do a lot of communicating on your behalf, and you will feel a lot more relaxed and confident knowing that there is someone who has your interests at heart. When you reach 34-36 weeks of pregnancy, share your birth plan with your caregiver, and establish their attitudes to your requests and preferences. You may wish to give a copy of your plan to be kept with your notes. Keep the other with you when you go into hospital.

Giving birth is not meant to be an endurance test or a test of strength. It is the natural process of bringing a child into the world safely and achieving the best possible experience that you can at the same time.

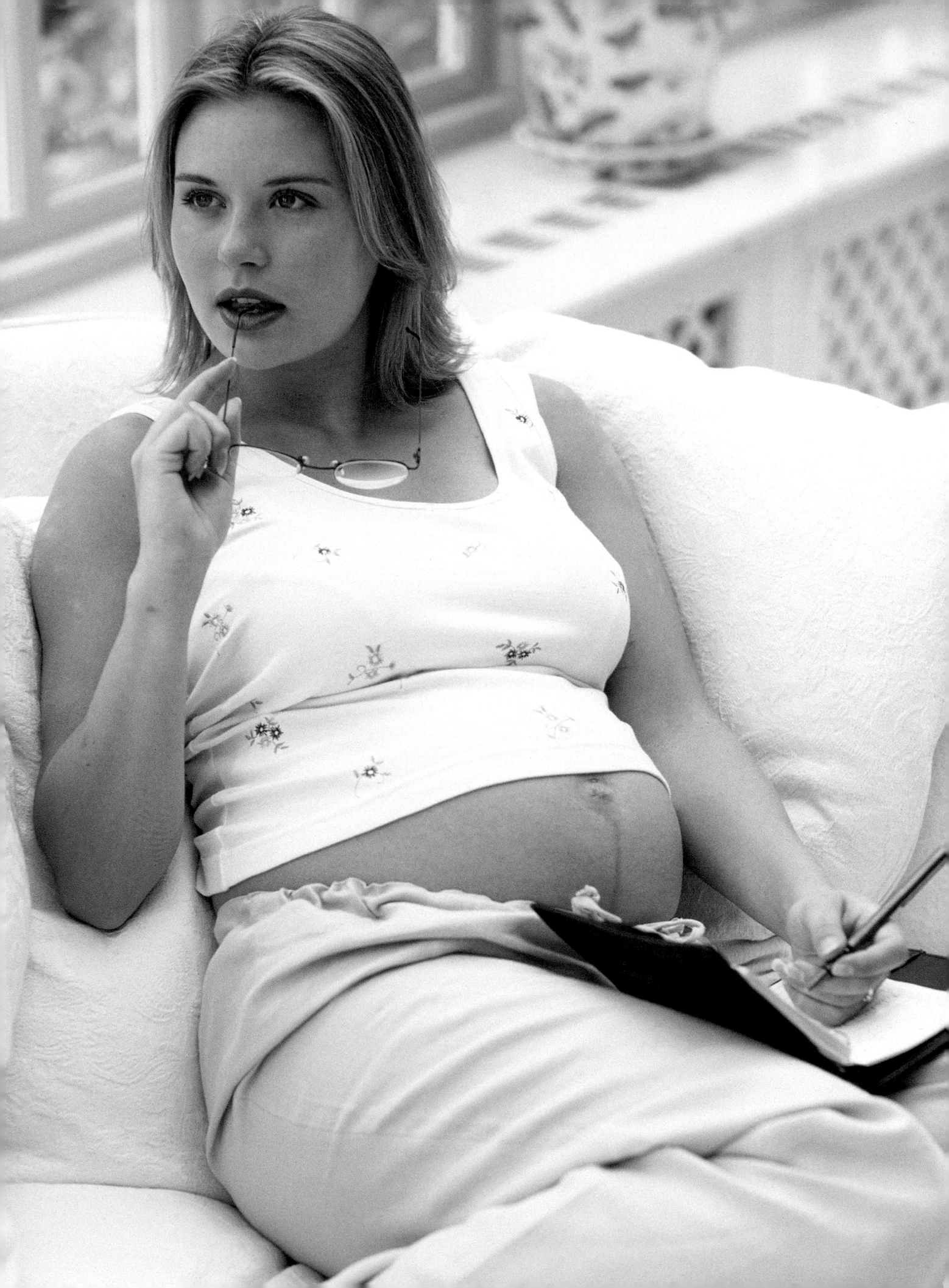

Medical intervention

In some instances, labour may start spontaneously but the contractions are not effective or are infrequent or irregular and labour does not progress. Augmentation of labour means that natural labour is accelerated and can be done in many of the ways described.

Induction

Induction is when your doctor starts labour artificially, causing uterine contractions. It can only be done in a hospital setting. Induction may be considered necessary when the mother's and/or baby's health is in question. Induction is considered a safe procedure but not necessarily a quick one.

There are a number of ways labour can be induced once the decision has been made. Before the induction is started, the mother will have a vaginal examination to assess the condition or 'ripeness' of her cervix. Induction is less likely to succeed if the cervix is not ready. If this is the case, your doctor will order medication in the form of pessaries or jelly that is inserted into the vagina to soften and prime the cervix.

Right Your midwife will keep a watchful eye on your progress and monitor your baby's heart rate constantly.

Syntocinon drip

A very effective and successful method of bringing on labour – if the cervix is ready or has been 'primed' – is by administering Syntocinon (synthetic oxytocin) via an intravenous drip over a few hours. A special infusion pump, set by your caregiver, regulates the rate and amount of the hormone that goes into your body.

Risks

As contractions become more frequent and intense, they may become difficult for the mother to cope with, as the pain level may rise out of proportion to the rate of dilation. This means that the mother tires quickly and may become very negative emotionally. This may also increase the need for other forms of intervention, such as electronic foetal heart monitoring.

Stripping the membranes

Your caregiver inserts a finger between the amniotic membranes and the cervix during an internal examination. This may be done in the rooms or in the labour ward. This frees the membranes from the lower part of the uterus

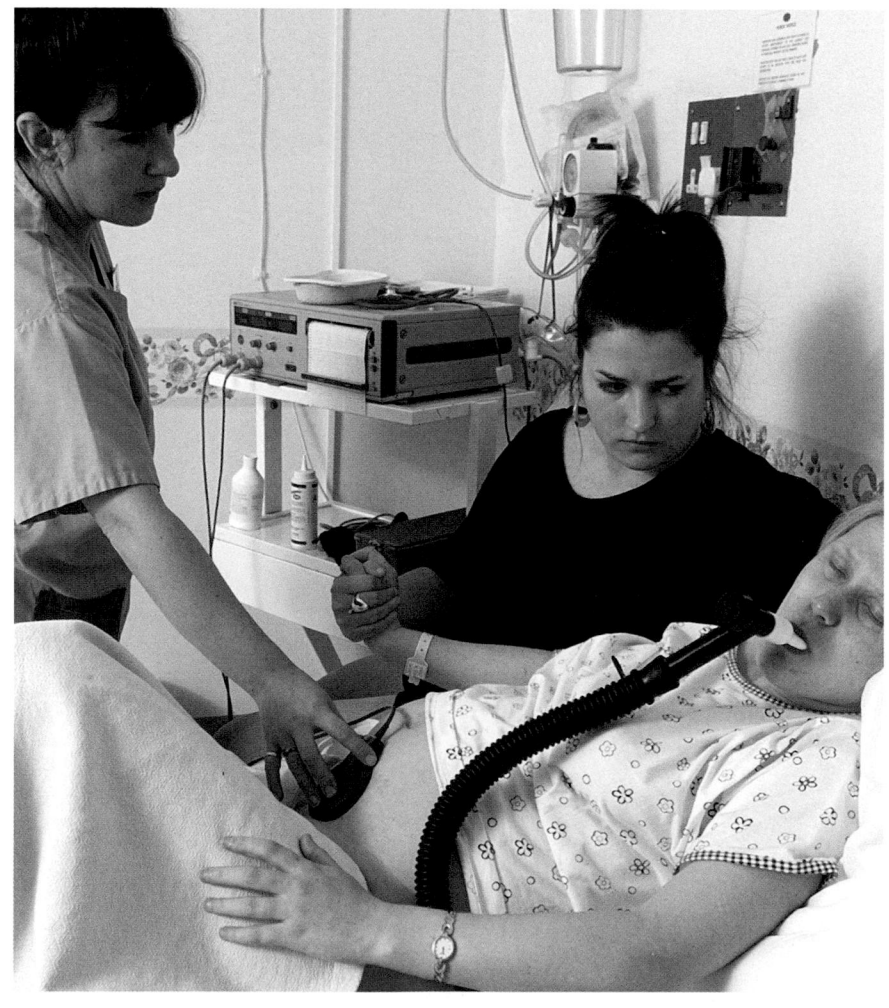

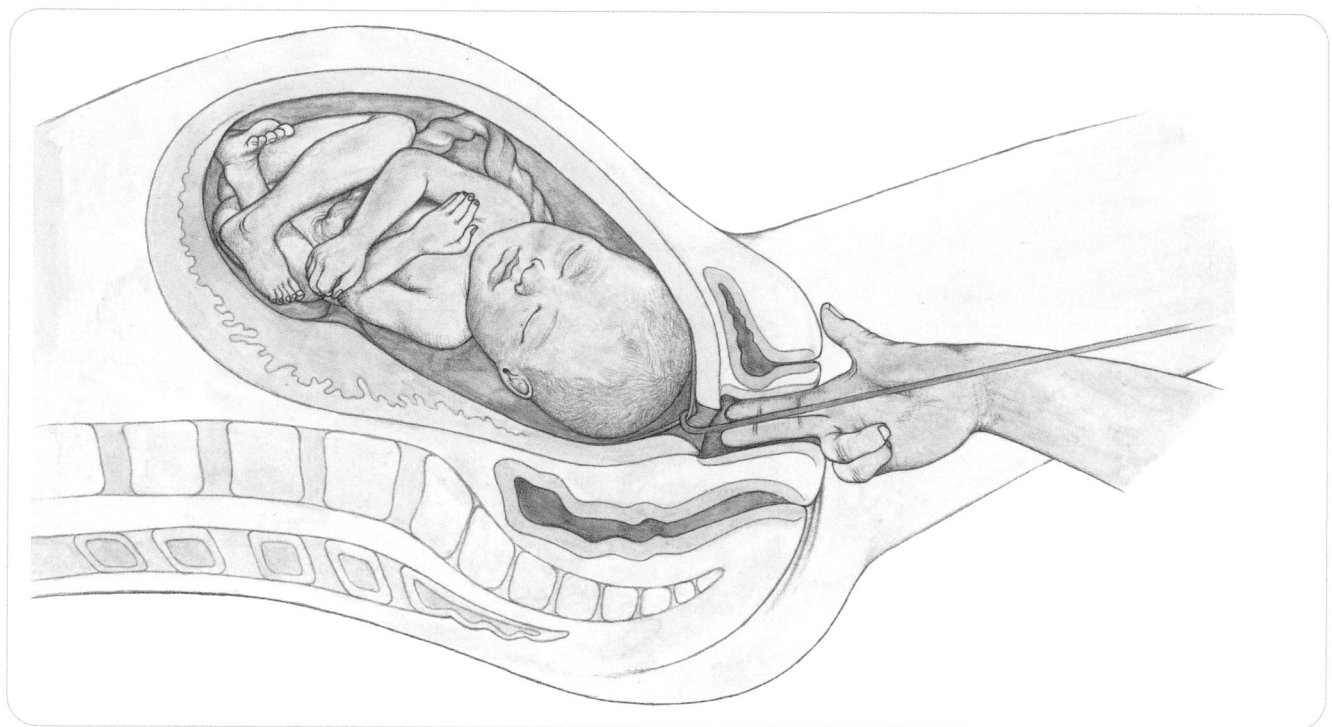

and stimulates the release of natural prostaglandins. This may or may not start labour and may cause the bag of waters to be broken before the time is right. This is a safe and effective way of starting labour close to or at term. Some women find this painful.

Assisted delivery

Sometimes the baby does not move into the vaginal opening in the second stage of labour. This could happen if the baby is very large or in a difficult position or the mother is tired and she cannot push. If the baby is not getting enough oxygen, your doctor might use forceps or ventouse to help the baby out. This is known as assisted delivery.

AROM (Breaking the waters)

This relatively painless procedure involves the puncturing of the amniotic sac, either before or during labour. A plastic instrument called an amniohook is used to make a tiny hole in the double membrane, thus allowing the amniotic fluid to leak out of the vagina in a controlled way. This is done with the mother lying on her back during an internal examination. It may be done in conjunction with a Syntocinon drip. It is important to remember that this is an irreversible decision. Once your waters are broken, you are committed to having this baby, usually within a 24-hour period. It is important that the baby's head is well down and firmly applied to the cervix and ideally the mother should be at least 2cm (0.8in) dilated.

Once your labour has been started, remember to apply all the other self-help measures, such as walking and maintaining an upright position, breathing and relaxation as well as adopting positions that will help your body open up.

Above Before your waters are broken, make sure you understand the reason behind this invasive procedure.

The forceps

Forceps are used if the baby is in distress and needs to be delivered quickly, or if the baby is in an awkward position. The mother may be tired and unable to assist in pushing. Forceps consist of two metal blades, rather like curved spoons, that lock together to form a protective cage around the baby's head. There are different types available, and the shape of the blades varies, as does the length of the handles. The type used depends on the reason for use and the user's preference. The forceps are separated and slipped in one at a time over the baby's head. The handles are then locked together and traction applied, during a

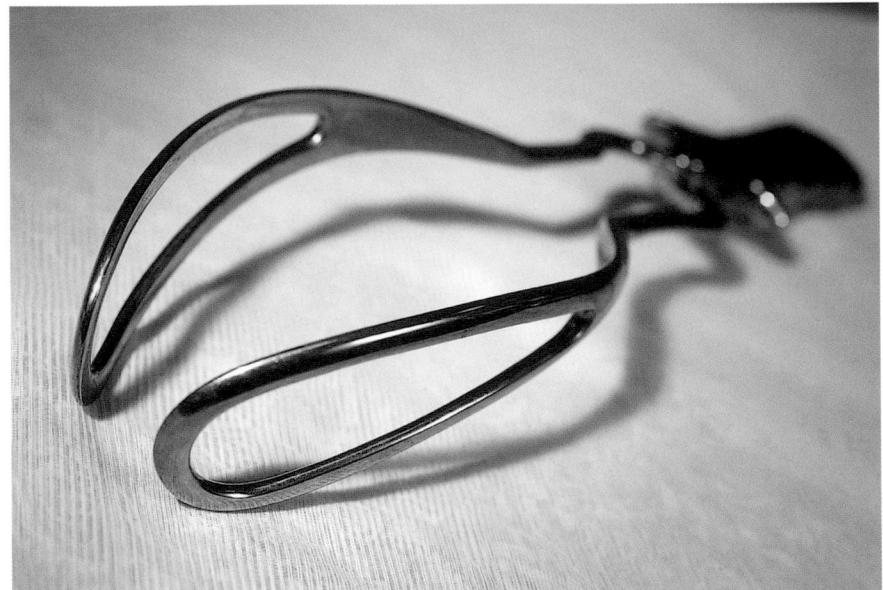

contraction, to deliver the baby. The baby is usually delivered after only a few pushes. An episiotomy is usually required when using forceps to aid delivery.

You will be required to push with each contraction and, at the same time, the doctor or midwife will apply traction using the forceps. Once the head is delivered the forceps are removed and the shoulders and the body delivered normally.

The ventouse (vacuum extraction)

A cap is attached to the baby's head, which is then connected to a suction machine. Once the cap is secure on the baby's head, the doctor will apply traction while you bear down with each contraction, until the baby's head is delivered. The cap is then removed and the rest of the body delivered.

Less anaesthesia is needed for ventouse, although a local anaesthetic will probably still be given to someone without an epidural. An episiotomy is not always required.

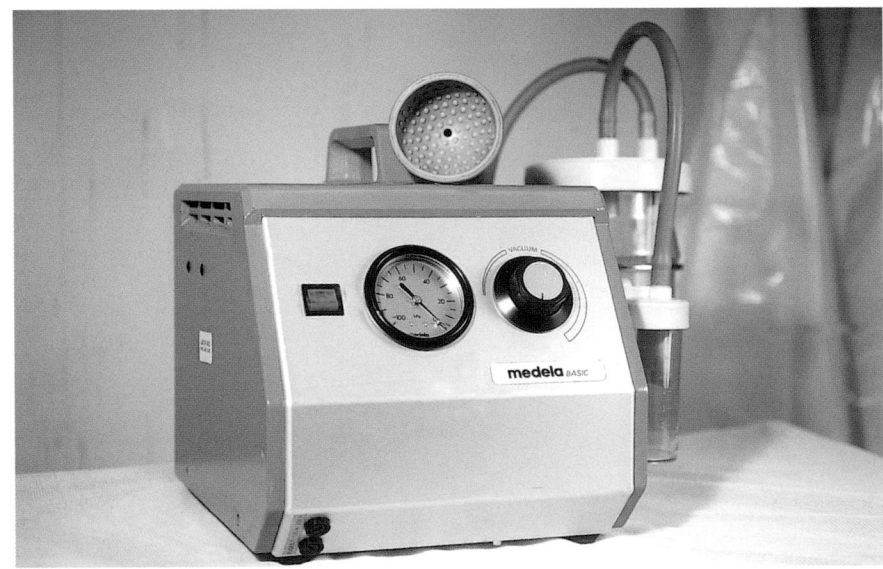

Effects on the baby

- Forceps leave marks on the baby's scalp or face, depending on where they were applied. These may be quite prominent at first but will fade after a couple of days.
- The suction cap of the vacuum extractor will leave a raised red area on the baby's scalp. This is also quite prominent initially, but will subside over the next week.

- There is a higher incidence of neonatal jaundice in babies delivered by ventouse.
- Babies delivered by ventouse tend to have a higher Apgar scoring than those delivered by forceps. The Apgar score (see p138) only reflects the baby's wellbeing up to 10 minutes after birth. No conclusive evidence is available on the long-term differences between babies delivered by forceps versus ventouse.

- If the baby has experienced a long labour or foetal distress, he may not initially latch onto the breast or feed well. Be patient and persevere.

Effects on the mother

You will have bruising to the perineum, which can be relieved with ice packs.

- Passing urine may be sore initially, as may opening your bowels.

- In the case of an episiotomy, having stitches may feel uncomfortable for the first few days.
- Take analgesia as prescribed; you may take regular salt baths if you wish, and the use of ice packs may also offer relief.

Electronic foetal monitoring (EFM)

A baby's condition and how it is tolerating labour is assessed regularly throughout labour and birth. Regular monitoring can be done with the use of a handheld Pinnards stethoscope, a sonic aid in the form of a Doppler or by EFM.

EFM involves two belts being fastened around the mother's abdomen, one with a pressure-sensitive device that picks up the foetal heartbeat and the second that monitors uterine activity. These devices are attached by wires to a tabletop monitor.

Internal foetal monitoring is done when the baby's heart rate is difficult to find or if the baby repeatedly moves away from the external monitor. A scalp electrode is fastened to the baby's head with a small hook or suction pad and connected to the external monitor. The contractions can still be monitored externally. The EFM provides a visual digital display of the foetal heart rate, and a sound bleep which can be switched up so that the heart rate can be heard. Some women and their partners find this reassuring.

The mother is advised to adopt an upright position in a chair or on the bed as she needs to be fairly still while this monitoring is done. If the mother or baby moves during this time, the monitor may need to be readjusted. Some hospitals have radiotelemetric monitoring equipment, which allows a woman to move around and change position while being monitored.

Many hospitals routinely monitor the foetal heart rate for 20 minutes when the woman is admitted to the labour ward. This provides the staff with a good baseline from which to assess the foetal heart rate and uterine activity as the labour progresses. The woman is then monitored at intervals

Below An electronic foetal heart monitor may reassure a labouring mother that all is well with her unborn baby.

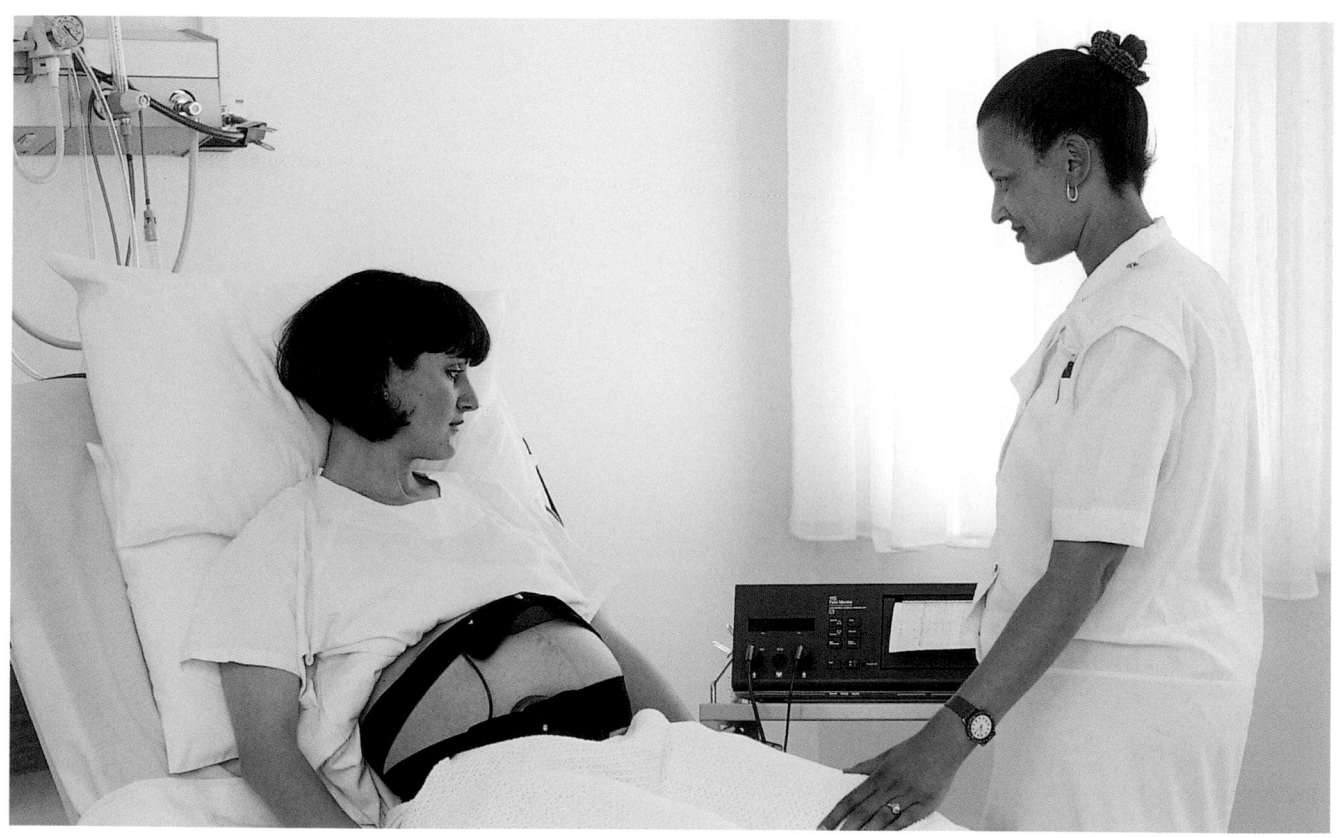

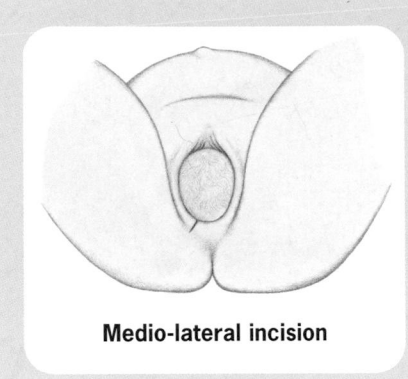
Medio-lateral incision

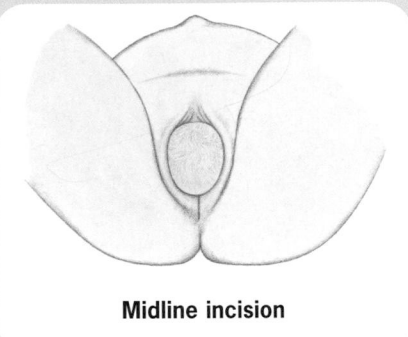
Midline incision

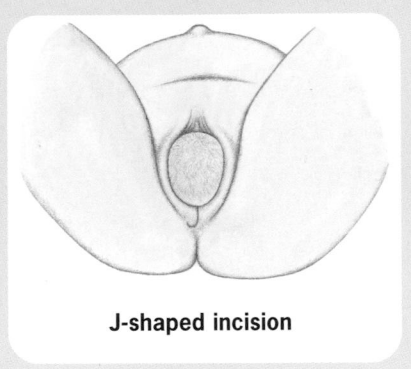
J-shaped incision

Above An episiotomy is performed at the height of a contraction in second-stage labour, when the perineum is stretched thin.

during the labour, either by electronic foetal monitoring or with the foetal stethoscope.

Continuous electronic foetal monitoring is usually done if a woman has opted for a full epidural or if Syntocinon is used to induce or augment the labour. Other reasons include a baby that is considered to be at risk or if the mother has a medical problem, such as high blood pressure. Current research shows that the continual use of electronic foetal monitoring in labour does not guarantee a better outcome. Research has also shown that there is a greater likelihood of further intervention for a labouring woman receiving continuous electronic monitoring.

Episiotomy

An episiotomy is a surgical cut made into the perineum (the skin and tissues between the vagina and anus) to enlarge the opening of the vagina to help ease the birth of the baby. Research over the past decade has proved that routine episiotomy is not

required for most births. There is also controversy over whether an episiotomy is preferable to a natural tear.

A debatable reason for doing an episiotomy is when the doctor or midwife feels that the perineum is likely to tear as the baby's head is born. There is the belief that a surgical cut is easier to repair, causes less pain and heals faster than a naturally occurring one. But studies have shown that when a tear occurs, it may be less painful and heal faster than an episiotomy, and not the other way around. Women with tears have also been found to resume sex sooner and with less pain than women who have had an episiotomy.

In the past, it was also believed that episiotomies prevented some degree of damage to the pelvic floor. However, recent studies on the effects of episiotomy on the pelvic floor show that the presence or absence of an episiotomy does not affect a woman's perineal function. In fact, one British study strongly suggested that exercise is the most common

factor in restoring a woman's normal pelvic floor strength after childbirth.

Steps to avoid an episiotomy

1. If a mother is encouraged to ease the baby's head out slowly during pushing, using a position aided by gravity and where the perineum is supported, it is possible to minimize tearing or the need for episiotomy.
2. Avoid giving birth flat on your back. An

An episiotomy may be performed if the baby:

- is in the breech position (bottom first, not head) and is born vaginally. (Most breech babies are born by Caesarean section)
- is premature and cannot tolerate prolonged pushing against the mother's perineum
- is in distress and needs to be born immediately
- is very large, as assessed by scan (this is very controversial)
- needs easing out by forceps.

upright position (for example, being raised on pillows into a semi-reclining position) is much better than lying almost flat and will let gravity help to stretch the vagina evenly and slowly.

3. Try to avoid sustained breath-holding during pushing; use gentle expulsive, spontaneous pushing without excessive straining to ease the baby down. By preventing excessive straining during pushing, you can reduce the over-stretching of the pelvic floor.

4. Massaging the perineum with natural oil for six weeks before your due date can improve the pliability of the skin and underlying tissues. This massage also helps women become familiar with their anatomy and accustomed to stretching sensations felt during the birth.

5. Epidurals often increase the need for episiotomy. With a fully effective epidural, the pelvic floor may be very relaxed and the baby's head may not completely turn into the best birthing position. Sometimes the mother is unable to push effectively. When this happens, the doctor may need to use forceps to help the baby out. An episiotomy is done to make enough room to put the forceps in position. The likelihood of this happening is reduced in women who have a partial epidural during labour. Many episiotomies could be avoided if caregivers were more patient and gave the mother time to push in her own way.

What to ask in general

- Why is this procedure being done?
- What is involved?
- How will this affect me, my baby and my labour?
- What are the risks and benefits?
- What are the alternatives?
- What will happen if I wait?

Intravenous therapy (IVT)

Many hospitals prefer to limit the amount of food or drink you ingest while you are in labour. Their justification for this is to make sure your stomach is empty should you need to have emergency surgery. The concern is that, should aspiration (vomiting and inhaling the vomitus into the lungs) occur, it could have dire consequences for the mother. This may be given as a reason for routine IVT. Research, however, seems to suggest that this age-old practice often does more harm than good, and

Perineal Massage

Perineal massage is the gentle stretching and massaging of the skin and tissues around the vagina and perineum. It is good to massage your perineum during pregnancy since this is where you will feel pressure and stretching as your baby is born. Massage will keep your perineum soft and elastic and may well reduce your risk of a tear or episiotomy. Perineal massage is not routine in the UK.

1. If you have had a previous baby and experienced a tear of the perineum or an episiotomy, the scar tissue is not as elastic as the rest of the perineum, so concentrate on that area.

2. Do not massage the perineum if you have an active herpes lesion or vaginal infection, as this may spread the infection. Do not massage around the urethra because you are more susceptible to infection during pregnancy.

3. Try a daily treatment from around 36 weeks. A nice warm bath before you begin will help you relax and it will also ensure that your perineum is soft and pliable. You may need a mirror, or you may need to ask your partner to participate.

4. Sweet almond or vegetable oil or your own body secretions are a good lubricant. Dip your thumbs into the oil before inserting 3–4cm (1.5–2in) inside your vagina, and then press your perineum

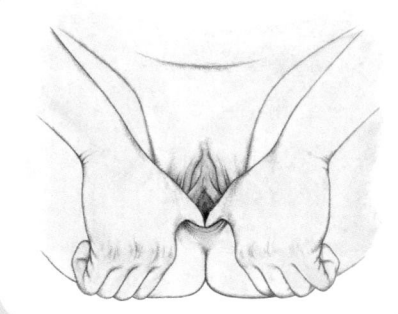

toward your rectum and to the sides. Gently stretch the opening until you feel a slight burning or tingling. Maintain the pressure for about two minutes until the area becomes a bit numb. Easy does it; keep massaging and maintaining the stretch and pressure for three to four minutes.

withholding food and liquids from a labouring woman is not necessary.

Other reasons include inducing or augmenting labour. The most effective way of doing this is to administer synthetic oxytocin to the mother via a drip.

Should you request an epidural, having a drip is mandatory. The same applies if you are having surgery. Whatever the emergency, the drip allows immediate access to a vein if medication is necessary.

A glucose drip can be given to increase the mother's blood sugar levels as well as keep her hydrated. However, drinking clear fluids in the form of water or clear fruit juice can easily do this, too. Being on a drip may restrict your movement and can often heighten your sense of being a patient and your perception of pain. Always ask if it is really necessary to have a drip in place if your labour is progressing smoothly, and tell your caregiver if you prefer to take your fluids orally.

Complications

Foetal Distress

If your baby starts to show signs that he is not tolerating labour, and foetal distress is a concern, your caregiver may decide to deliver your baby immediately by Caesarean. Early signs include a faster, irregular heartbeat or a heartbeat that does not recover well between contractions. One of the clear signs that your baby may be struggling is the passing of the first stool, known as meconium. This will be seen in the amniotic fluid and is one of the reasons for breaking the 'bag of waters'.

Placenta praevia

This is a condition where the placenta has implanted over, or slightly over, the cervix. A sign would be painless vaginal bleeding with no apparent cause, and may occur during rest or sleep as well as during activity after the seventh month of pregnancy.

The location of the placenta can be seen on an ultrasound scan and most caregivers will show the mother exactly where the placental site is.

Depending on the severity of this condition, treatment may involve bed rest or very little activity. Your caregiver is most likely going to opt for a Caesarean section to deliver your baby.

Placental abruption

A torn placenta occurs about once in 200 pregnancies. It is more likely to occur in the third trimester of pregnancy or during labour. This condition is more common in women who have had more than one pregnancy, or those who have a poor nutritional status. Signs and symptoms include abdominal pain and tenderness, vaginal bleeding, and a rigid, hard uterus. This is a serious condition and if these symptoms are present after you have had a fall or a blow to the abdomen, you must contact your caregiver immediately, and go straight to the hospital. This is a life-threatening situation for the foetus, as extensive separation of

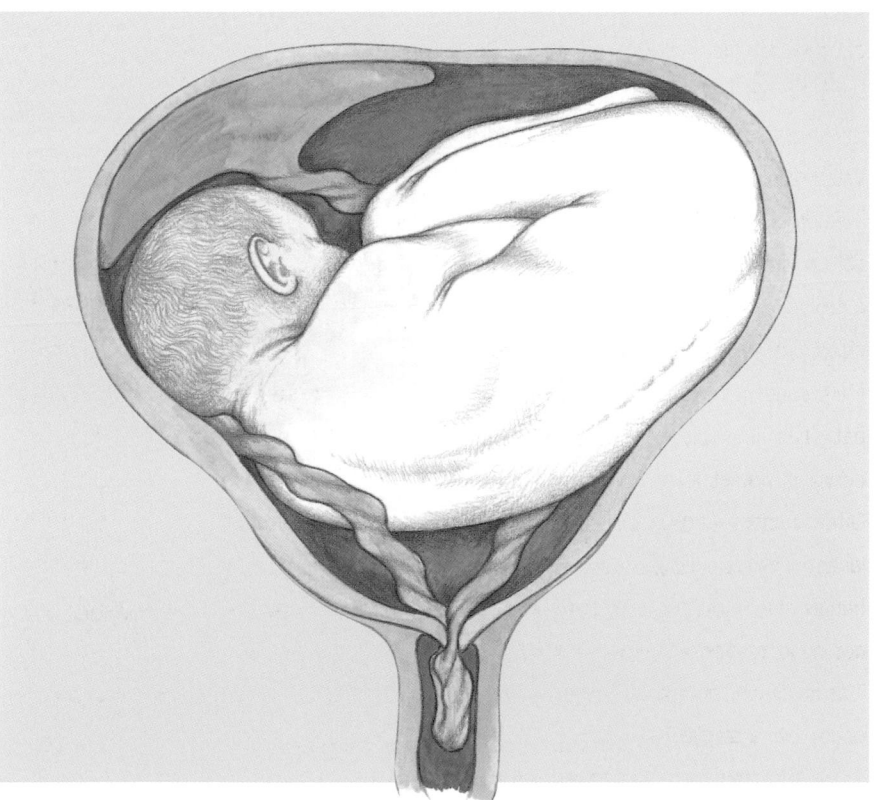

Above *A baby lying with its shoulder presenting, cannot be delivered vaginally and would need to be delivered by Caesarean section. The risk of prolapse cord is higher should the waters break.*

the placenta will deprive the baby of oxygen and cause foetal distress. Treatment depends on the severity of foetal distress, and how far the labour has progressed. An emergency Caesarean section is the most likely way the mother will deliver.

Cord prolapse

This occurs when the baby's umbilical cord is washed out in front of the baby's head and is one of the greatest obstetrical emergencies, requiring immediate intervention.

When the umbilical cord prolapses, there is a high risk of the baby's oxygen supply being cut off or impaired, as the cord becomes pinched between the head of the baby and the mother's cervix. When this occurs, a Caesarean will be performed immediately. If an epidural is not in place, the operation will be done within minutes under general anaesthesia.

Rupturing membranes when the head is still high in the pelvis is the main cause for a prolapsed cord and one which all obstetricians and midwives should guard against. Membranes should not be ruptured if the baby has not engaged and if the mother's cervix is not at least 2cm (0.8in) dilated. Other factors that predispose to a prolapsed cord are twin pregnancies, as the babies may be lying in various positions and not head or bottom down into the pelvis. This is termed an unstable lie and can also occur with a single pregnancy.

An exceptionally long umbilical cord is also more likely to prolapse.

This is a very serious and frightening event for any mother. It is a rare complication and

in 99.8 per cent of cases it does not occur. If detected early the baby can be safely delivered with no further complications.

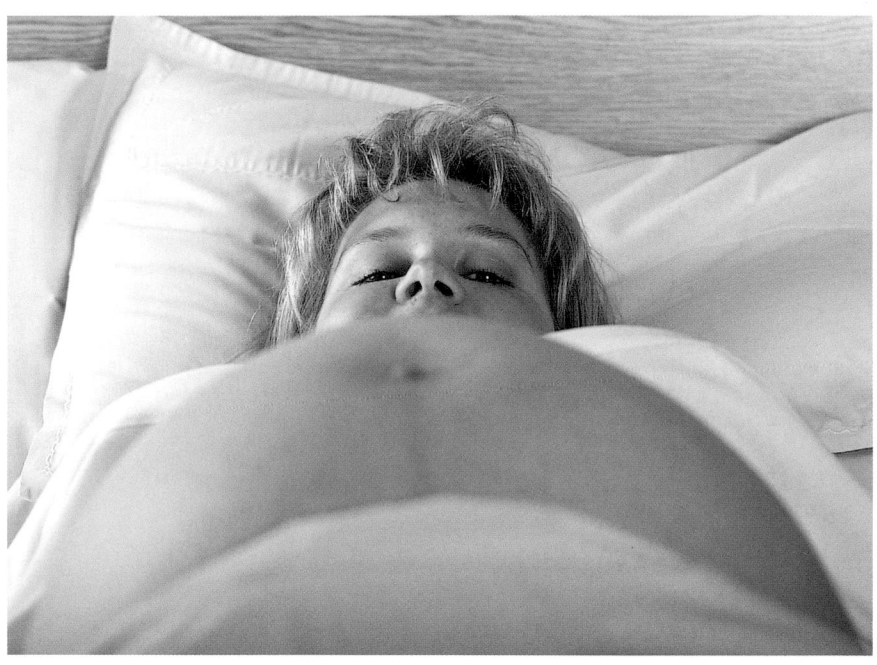

Overdue

Working out a due date is not an exact science because we usually do not know the precise date of conception and, even though you may have regular periods and cycles, the date you actually ovulate is only an approximate one.

For every extra day a baby stays in the womb, the chances of a harder, more difficult labour increase. The placenta, which feeds and nourishes your baby, only has a certain life span and it may not be able to continue supporting the baby over an extended period. The placenta should be capable of supplying your baby with sufficient nutrients up to 42 weeks. It is impossible to know which babies are at risk.

If a pregnancy goes much beyond its due date, postmaturity and possible placental insufficiency pose some risks to the unborn child. The baby may lose fat stores and, as a result, her skin will become red and wrinkly and look 'oversized' for her body and it may begin to peel. Other risks include a longer labour, due to the size of the baby and the inability of the skull bones to mould as they would normally in a term baby. This may mean a more traumatic labour and birth for both mother and baby. The risk of still birth doubles by the 43rd week and you will be induced if you had not started labour by this point. Babies whose due date comes and goes are monitored very closely. It is imperative that you agree to have medical intervention if there is any sign of foetal distress.

Caesarean birth – the safety net of birth

Obstetrics today is a lot safer due to better knowledge, safer practices and the advent of antibiotics and basic hygiene. Technology has brought with it many benefits but also potential risks. Caesarean section was formerly only performed on mothers who had died during birth, but improved surgical practices and safer anaesthetics make it a safer procedure. Still, it carries with it a four times higher risk of maternal death, and a 10 times higher risk of infection than vaginal birth. In both cases, the risks are small but women need to know that a Caesarean involves major abdominal surgery. Birth by Caesarean means a baby is delivered from the mother's uterus through an incision of about 15cm (6in) into the abdomen. It may be done electively for personal or medical reasons or as an emergency when the safety of the mother or baby is in question before or during labour. In some countries, elective Caesarean sections for non-medical reasons are not allowed. It may be performed under general, epidural or spinal anaesthetic.

The birth of your baby is an event that you will always remember and, even if you are not planning a Caesarean, it is worth learning everything you can about it.

Elective Caesarean

This is a planned Caesarean. You will know in advance the day and time your baby will be born. You may opt for an elective Caesarean for personal, non-medical or medical reasons.

Below Ask to see your baby soon after her birth, if possible. You may offer her the breast, if discussed with your doctor beforehand.

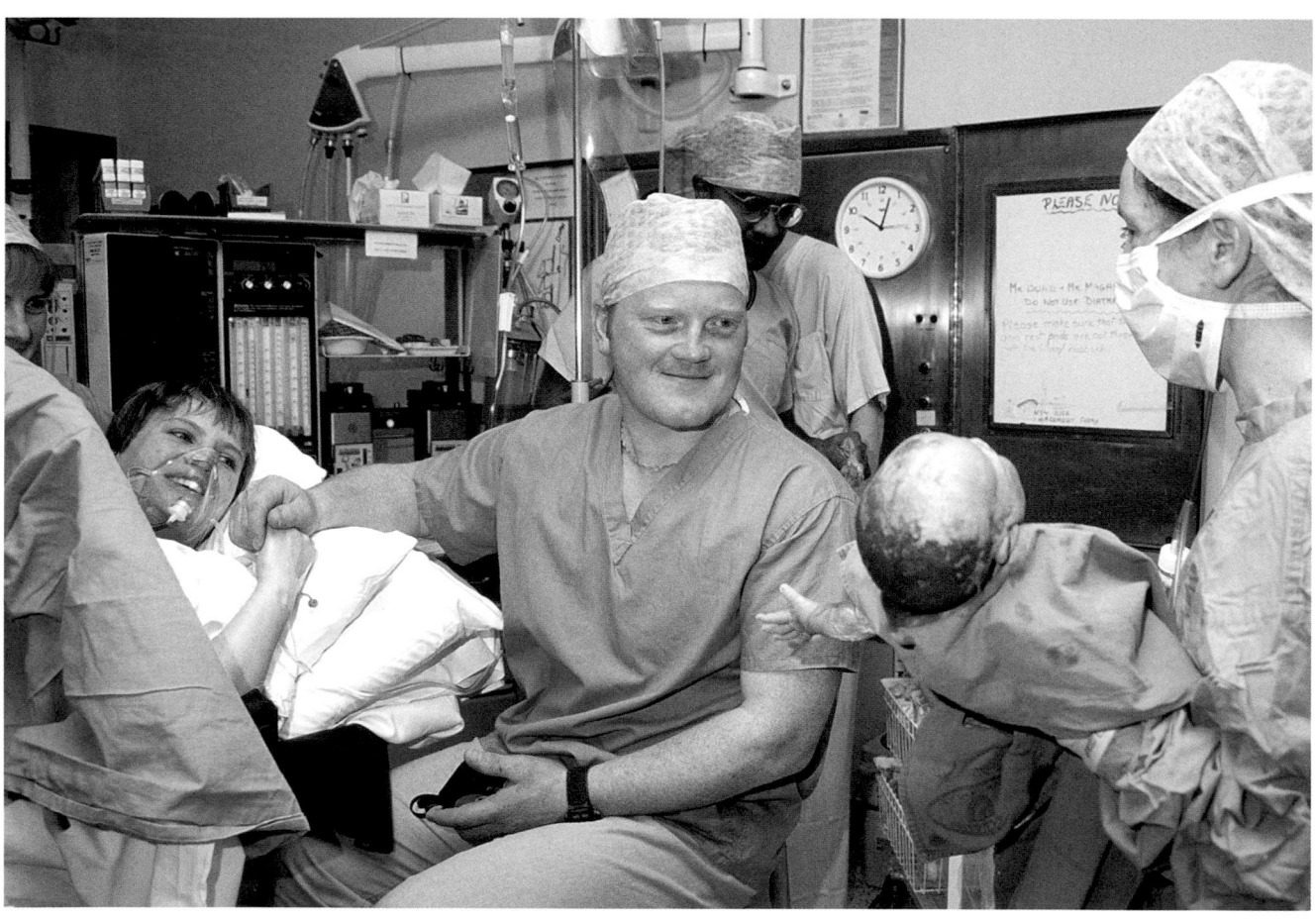

You may have an elective Caesarean if you have any one of the following conditions:

- pre-eclampsia or diabetes
- you have had previous birth complications
- your placenta may be lying low or even blocking the cervix
- you are expecting more than one baby
- your baby is in a breech position
- your baby is in an abnormal position (such as transverse)
- cephalopelvic disproportion – sometimes a baby is too big for the mother's pelvis and just will not fit through. Many feel that it is impossible to judge this until a woman goes into labour with her first baby.

Emergency Caesarean

This may happen if a complication occurs during labour or even before labour starts. It is considered an emergency if:

- your baby's cord prolapses (comes out before the baby)
- your baby starts showing signs of distress – low heartbeat, meconium in the amniotic fluid
- your labour is not progressing (this may not be a true emergency)
- any life-threatening situation such as pre-eclampsia, diabetes, previous scar rupturing, placental abruptio.
- maternal distress.

What to expect in an emergency Caesarean

An unplanned, emergency Caesarean delivery can be very stressful for the mother. The experience may be perceived as intrusive. Unfamiliar and unexpected procedures occurring in rapid succession can be very

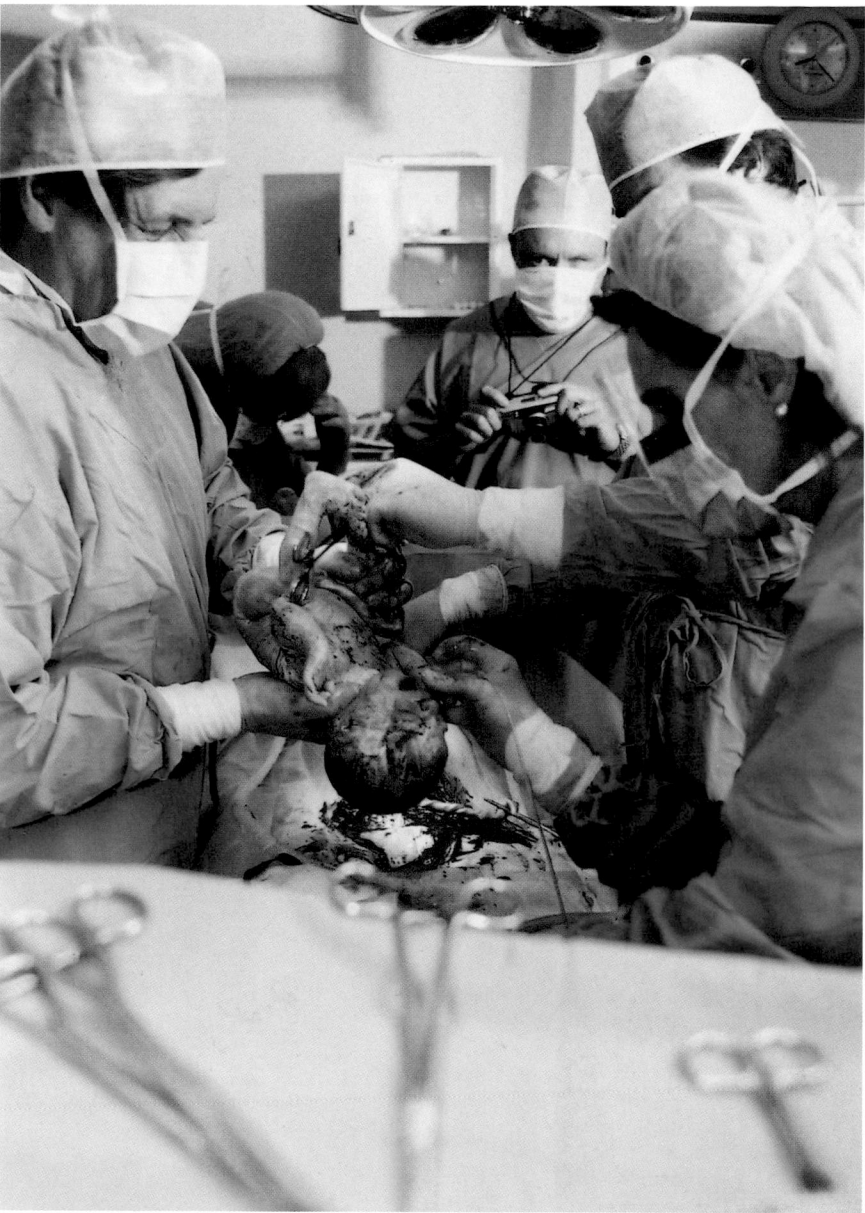

frightening. It is important for all pregnant women to familiarize themselves with the reasons for Caesarean delivery, as well as the procedures that will be done.

Discussion with caregivers is vital. Even if the mother feels that she is not in control, gaining knowledge will decrease her stress. When inquiring about childbirth education classes, be sure to check if Caesarean birth is discussed.

Above *Hearing yout baby's first cry will be like music to your ears.*

What you need to know about Caesarean birth

Even if you are planning a vaginal birth, you should always make some kind of plan in case you end up in theatre. Talk to your caregiver as to what kind of anaesthetic you would prefer, who will be allowed in theatre with you and if you can play your own choice of music. Ask how soon you can hold and breast-feed your baby.

If you have had a spinal block or epidural you will not feel anything from the nipple line down, except for a feeling of 'someone rummaging in a drawer'. You are likely to feel tugging and some pressure as the baby is eased out. As your sensation returns, you will start to feel pins-and-needles and warmth in your legs. You will be given pain relief, and this is administered via the drip.

If all is well, you can request to see your baby immediately. It is usual, however, for her to be given straight to the paediatrician for the usual checks and the Apgar test (see p138). Once she has been given the all-clear, she will be brought to you. She will be warmly wrapped as it can be very cold in theatre. You may want to request in your birth plan that you wish to have support from staff when holding your baby. There is no reason to doubt your ability to breast-feed your baby. Some moms even breast-feed their babies in theatre. This must be negotiated before the day!

After surgery

You will not be able to leap up and out of bed quickly to tend to your baby. Remember you will have had major abdominal surgery and you will need help in lifting and carrying everything. You will be encouraged to get out of bed very soon after your operation. Take it easy and remember hospital staff are there to help you.

Below Holding your baby after a Caesarean is beneficial and the start of bonding.

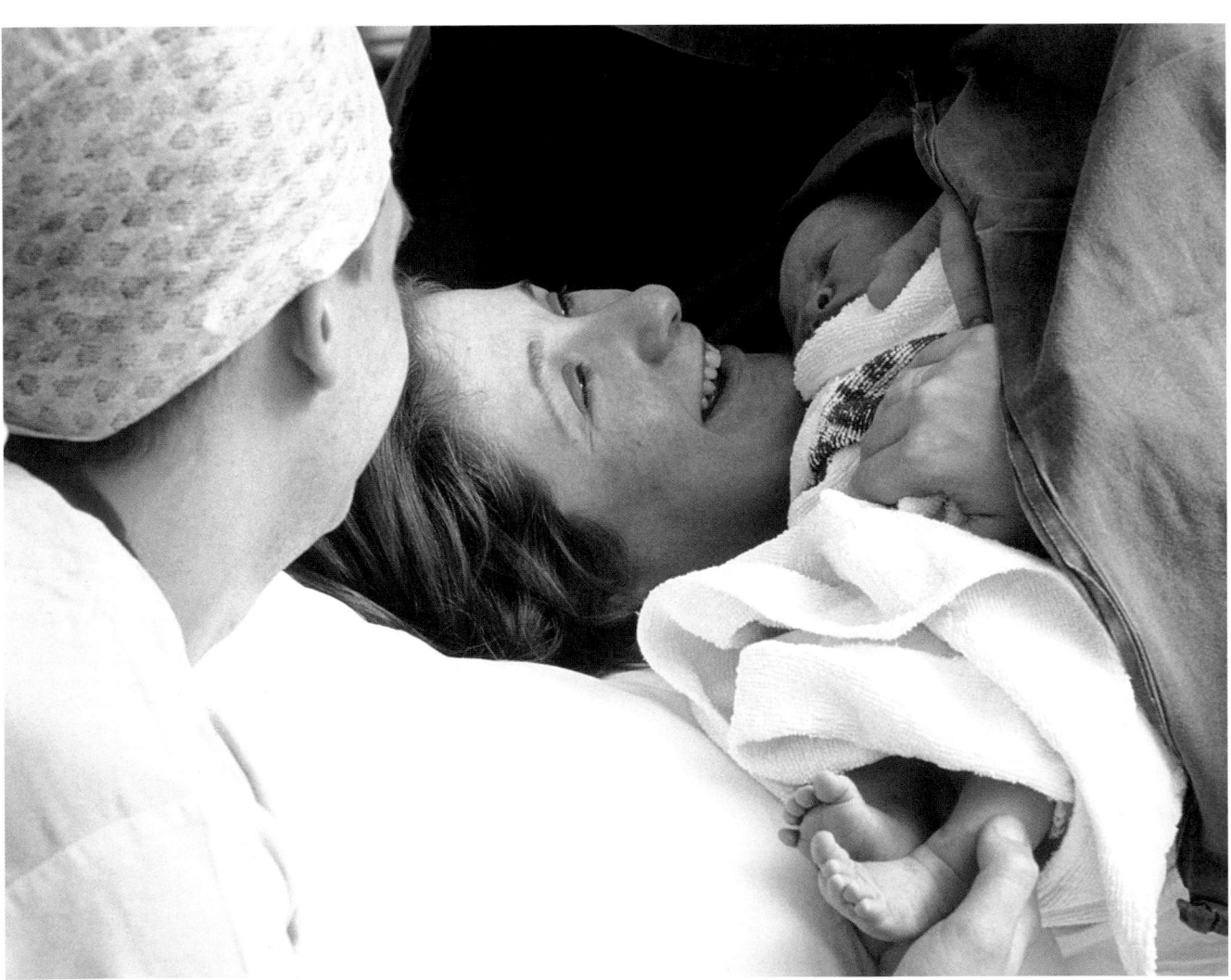

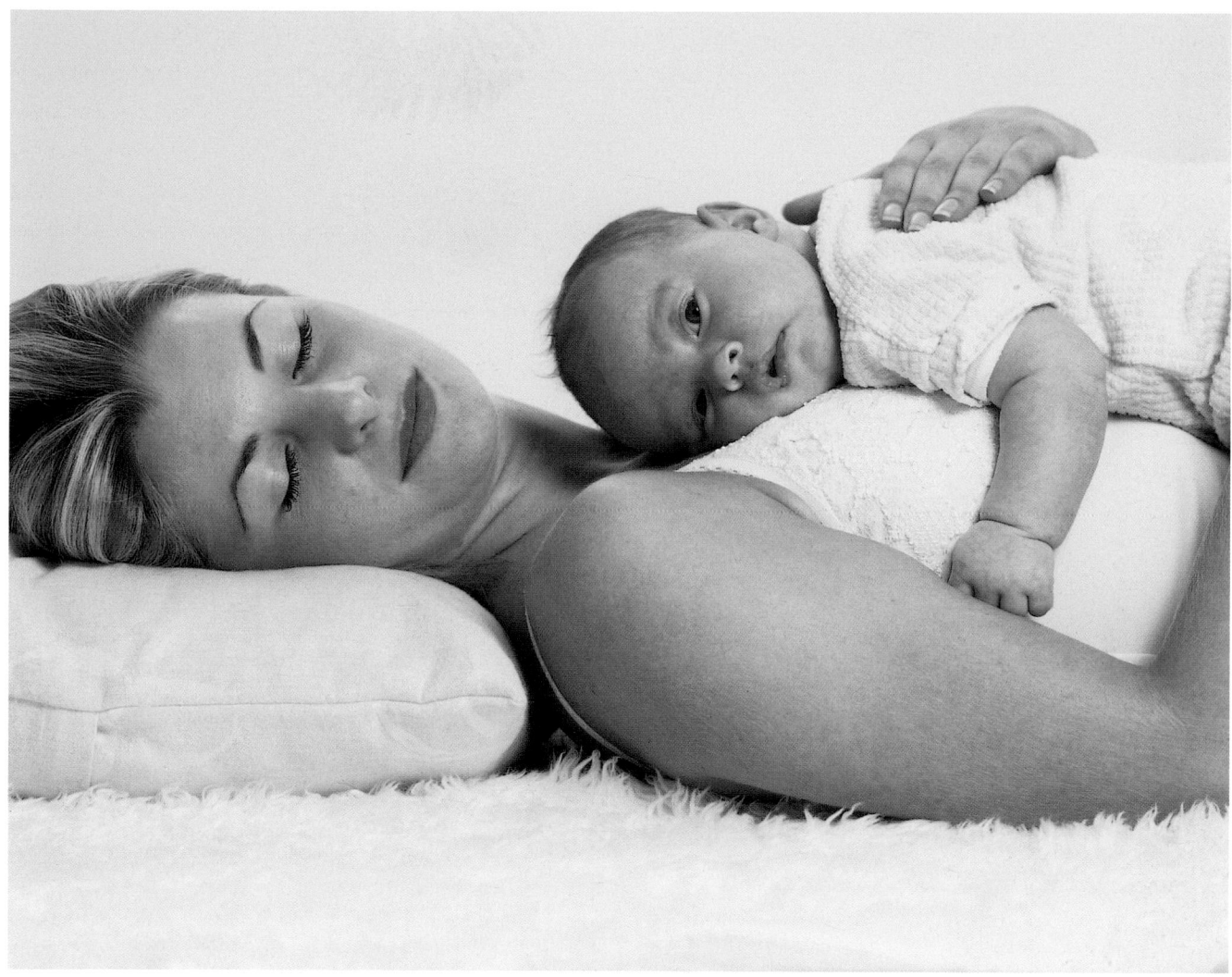

Above Babies are very sensitive to smell, so do not wear strong perfumes in the early days as your baby adjusts to the smells of his mother, father and the new environment.

Your movements will not be restricted for very long. Try to do some simple leg movements as well as deep-breathing exercises. When you get up for the first time, hospital staff will help you if you feel you cannot manage on your own. Be sure to stand as upright as you can and do not slouch. Use a pillow to support your tummy when you cough, laugh or sneeze. Move slowly and you will be walking as normal in a few days.

If all is well, you may be allowed to go home within a few days. This may be longer if there are any complications or if you feel that you are not coping. Check with your health insurance provider as to how much time they will cover.

Depending on the reason for your Caesarean, you may be able to try for a vaginal birth with your next pregnancy. This must be in consultation with your doctor. Most doctors believe that if you have had two Caesareans, further deliveries should be by Caesarean. This should be discussed once you are pregnant again, as new circumstances may arise.

You may have felt disappointed if plans changed during labour and you had to deal with something you were unprepared for. That is why being informed, open-minded and above all flexible about your options is so important. It is the safe passage of you and your baby through birth that is the most vital issue. You can still have a most fulfilling birth experience as long as you are aware what is happening and involved in decision-making on the day. Remember this is not only an operation, but also the birth of your baby.

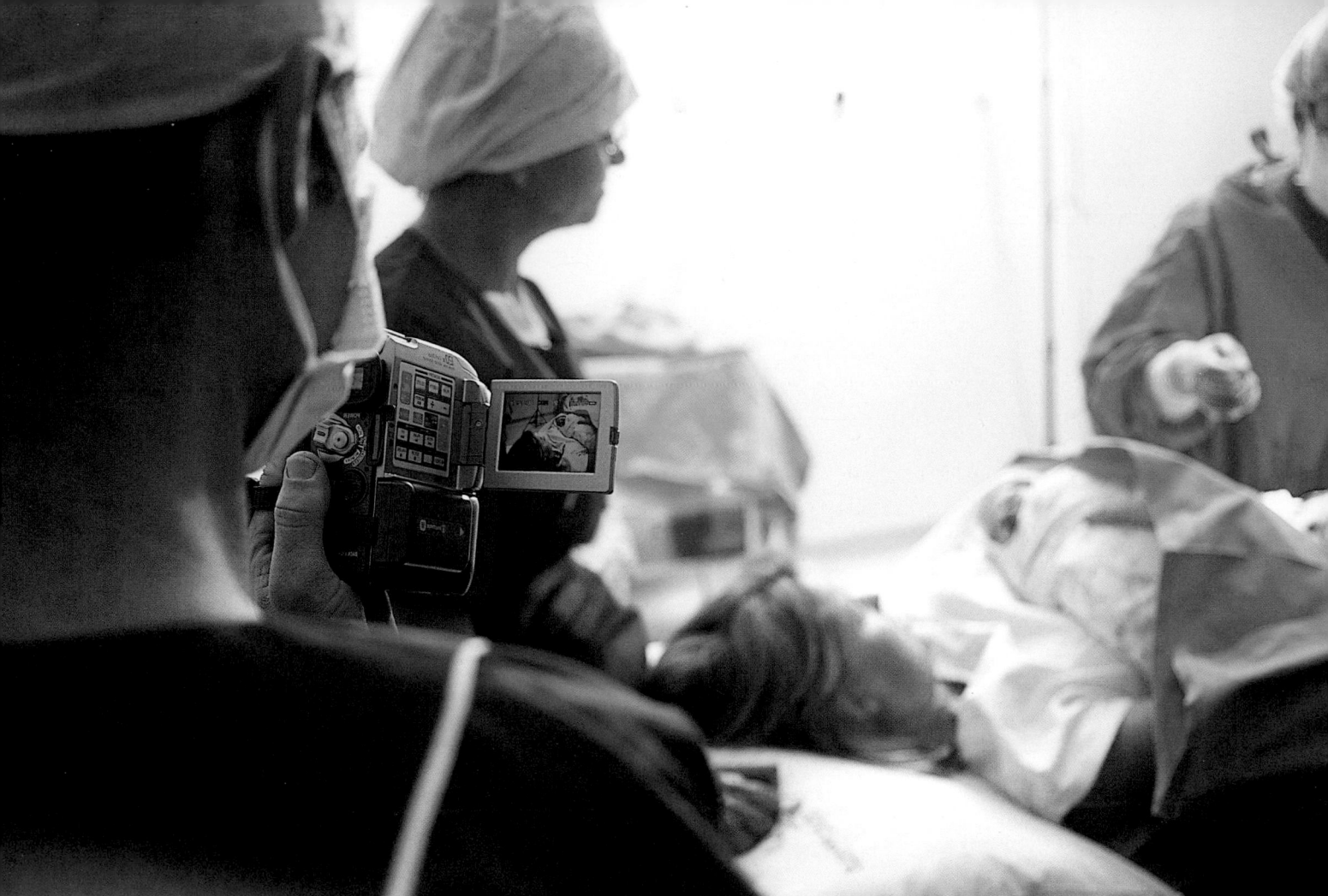

The first 24 hours

The moment of birth is spectacular and, in most cases, an overwhelming experience for a woman as well as for her partner. It is very exciting and emotional, and the moment is etched into the minds of most women. Birth heralds the start of a bond with your child. Not every new mother feels undying love for her newborn; love takes time to grow. Research shows that the first few moments of bonding between mother and child, as well as the first few hours after birth, are vital in establishing a foundation for love to grow as well as the success of an everlasting relationship between them.

THE FIRST FEW MOMENTS OF BONDING ARE VITAL IN ESTABLISHING A FOUNDATION FOR LOVE

Once your baby is delivered, you may be given an injection of synthetic oxytocin in your upper thigh, which you may or may not be aware of. This injection will cause the uterus to contract, which assists in the speedy delivery of the placenta and membranes shortly after the baby. It will also reduce the risk of excessive blood loss.

Once given this injection, the placenta is usually delivered within 15 minutes of the birth; however, it will take longer if you did not receive the injection. As slight traction is applied to the part of the cord that is still attached to you, you will feel a little discomfort as your uterus is 'massaged and rubbed', causing it to contract even more.

Your vaginal area will be sponged down with an antiseptic solution or warm water, and checked for any tears internally and externally. It is normal for you to feel tender and a little swollen. Your doctor or midwife will use a finger and a piece of gauze to feel inside the vagina. If necessary, this is when you will be stitched up. If you have an epidural in place, you will not need local anaesthetic. Should you gain feeling in your lower body, your doctor will inject local anaesthetic into the tissues of the perineum and vagina before you are stitched. If you feel anything at all, ask your doctor to wait a little longer until you are completely numb.

Initial bonding

Research has shown that a mother's core temperature will increase once her baby is placed on her abdomen, and the baby will not get cold if he lies skin-to-skin against his mother with a light towel covering both of them. A small cotton cap is usually placed on your baby's head. Experience has also shown that a period of extended, uninterrupted skin-to-skin contact between mother and baby, with him given an opportunity to suckle at the breast, creates a sensitive time for parents to explore their baby. They can channel their excitement and curiosity into new stirrings of love and attachment that started in the pregnancy. If the baby is healthy, all attempts should be made to allow the new parents private time with their newborn before the baby is whisked away for routine medical procedures.

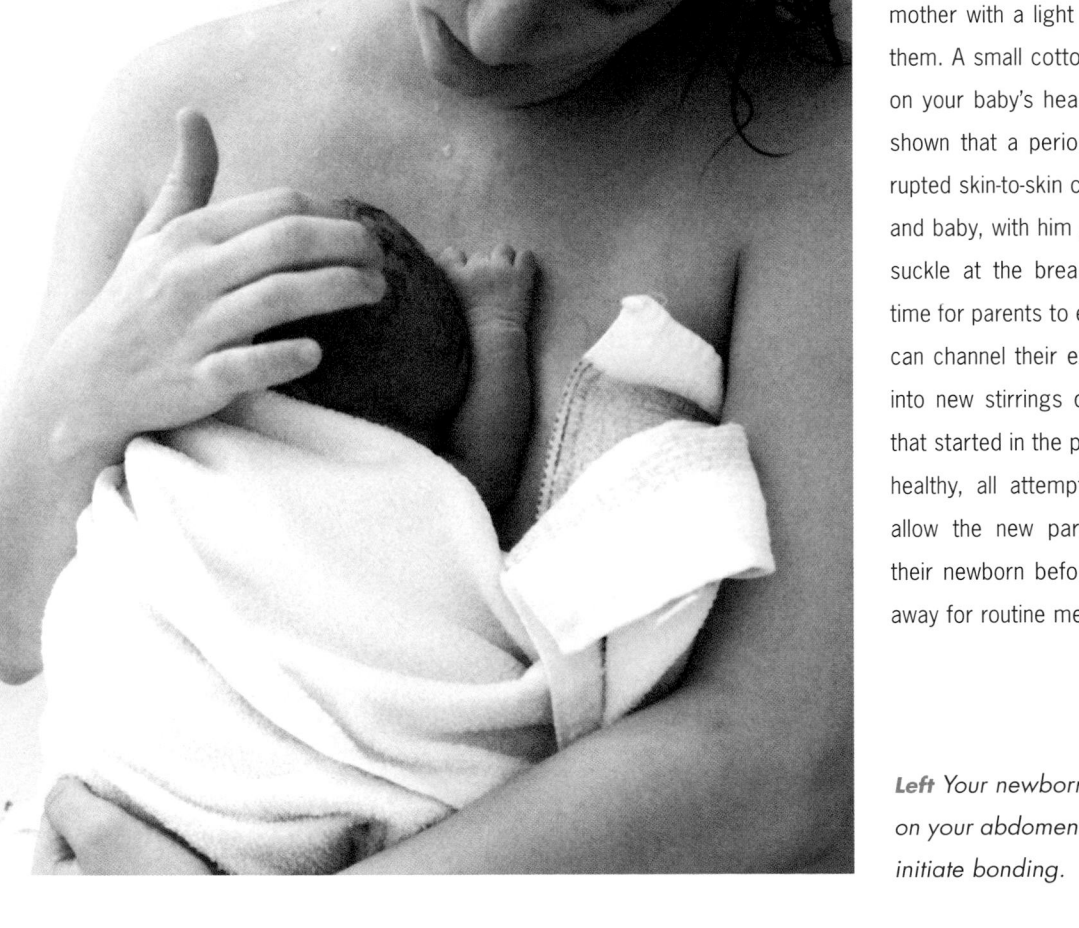

Left Your newborn baby will be placed on your abdomen soon after the birth to initiate bonding.

Your baby's first checkup

Your baby's breathing passages may be cleared of excess mucus with a thin plastic tube known as a 'suction catheter'. An Apgar score (*see* below) is given as a quick assessment of the baby's condition. This is done at one minute after birth and then again at five minutes.

Depending on what you requested, your baby may be removed from you and taken to a special area within the room that has a warm panel above the working area. Here your infant's length and head circumference will be measured, and his weight recorded. At this stage, it is usual for your baby to be given a vitamin K injection into the thigh muscle, which is necessary for normal clotting of the blood. This is a routine precaution and there is no need for alarm. If your baby needed a little boost of oxygen, it would be given at this point as well. If all is well, your child will be returned to your arms fairly quickly.

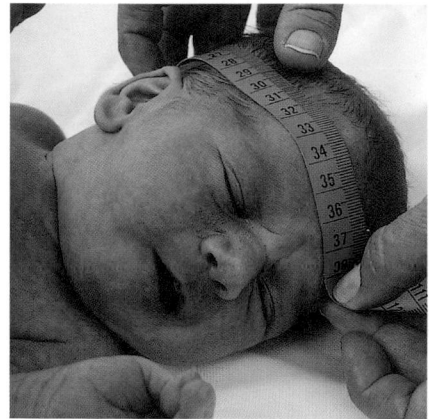
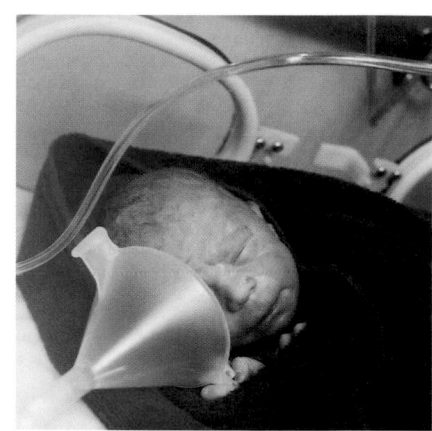
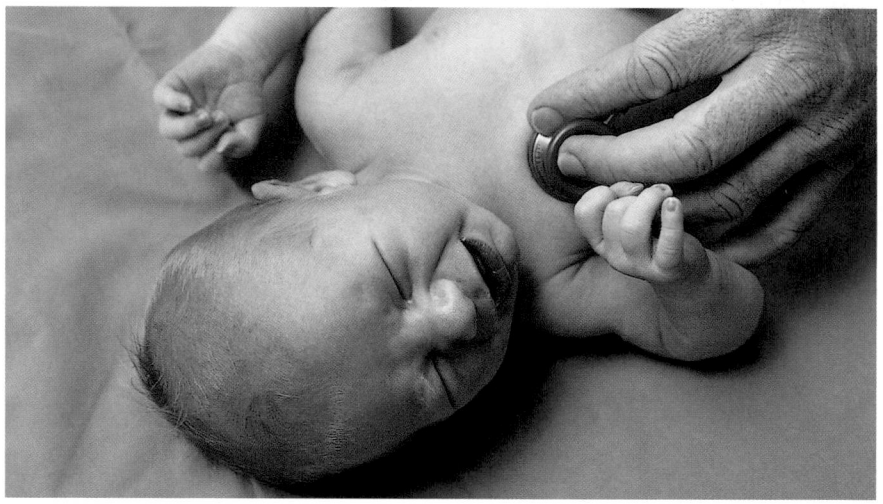

Above Your baby's heart rate will be checked for a strong, regular beat.
Top left The circumference of the baby's head will be measured.
Top right Sometimes a baby needs a boost of oxygen.

The Apgar score is a clinical assessment of a newborn baby immediately after birth. The checks are based on five vital signs:

A = **Appearance** or colour. A pink skin colour is an indication of healthy lung functioning and that your baby is getting enough oxygen.

P = **Pulse** or heart rate. This shows if her heartbeat is regular and strong.

G = **Grimace** or response to stimulation. Facial expressions and responses show how alert she is to stimuli.

A = **Activity** or muscle tone. Moving her limbs around shows the tone and health of her muscles.

R = **Respiratory** effort or breathing. Normal breathing shows the health of her lungs.

Each vital sign is given a score of 0, 1 or 2. A score of 2 is normal, a score of 1 is mildly abnormal and a score of 0 is severely abnormal. The individual scores are then added together to give a score out of 10.

Dedicated to dads

Do not leave your partner alone to telephone family and friends. Enjoy this special time with your new family. This time can never be recaptured once it has passed.

- Be sure to tell her how proud you are of her, especially if she is feeling a little disappointed in the way she gave birth.
- She may want you to be with the baby should it be necessary for your infant to be placed in an incubator. She needs the reassurance that you are representing your family when she cannot.
- Check that the identification bands have been put on your baby before she leaves the labour ward.

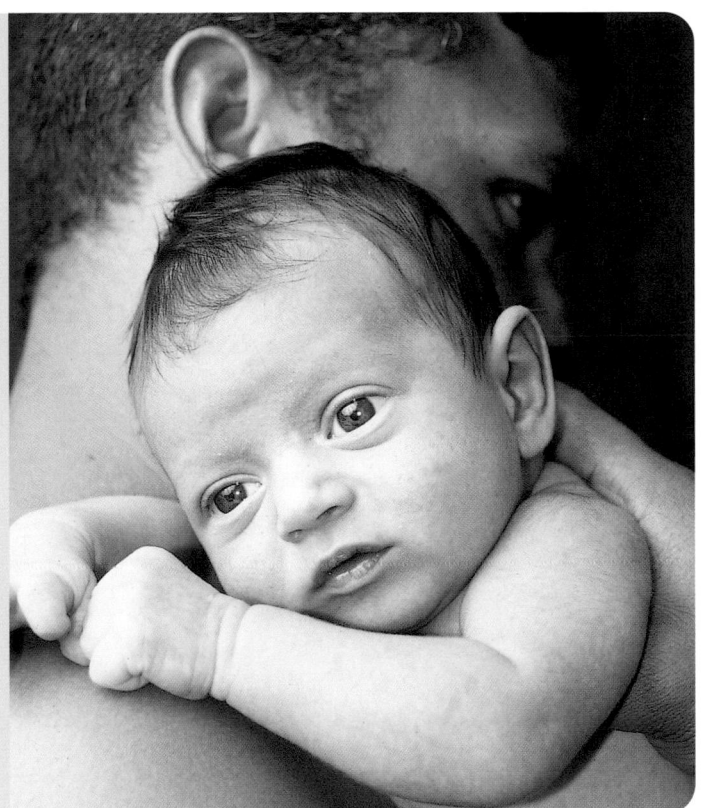

While the midwife takes care of your baby, your doctor will focus on you. In the case of a Caesarean birth, these procedures will be carried out in theatre by the paediatrician.

Ideally you should recover in the same room in which you gave birth. (If the ward is busy, you will be moved to another room.) The soiled linen will be removed from your bed and you will be made comfortable. Before you go to the recovery ward, you will be washed if you are unable to walk, or allowed to take a shower if you can get up. Your vital signs – blood pressure, pulse and temperature – will be checked and you will be asked if you have passed urine. If you have an epidural catheter in place, it will be removed. Your intravenous drip and urinary catheter, if you have either in place, will be left in place for six to 12 hours.

You and your partner will be offered something to drink and perhaps something light to eat. If you and your baby are well, it is very likely that you will be left alone with your partner and your baby for about an hour, sometimes a little longer. Different hospitals have different rules. (Part of your birth plan should include details of what you would like to see happen if all is well after the birth.) Your midwife may dim the lights and close the door. She will leave you with a bell just in case you need assistance. You and your partner can now enjoy some quiet time with your new family member.

The first two hours after birth are optimal for parent-infant bonding. Your baby is usually alert and may want to suckle at the breast or may be more interested in just looking at you and everything around her. It

is very likely that you will be captured by your newborn and very curious about her body. Should you be one of those mothers who do not fall in love at first sight, don't despair. Love takes time to grow and you will fall in love with your baby, even if it takes a little time. Handling and touching your baby will enhance this process. Do not worry if you feel confused by the aftermath of birth. It can take a little time to settle into the reality of becoming a mother.

For nine months you and your baby have been inseparable. After your baby is born, you are separated for the first time. Some women do not want to let their babies out of their sight. Others are happy to have their babies in the nursery while they rest and recover. It all depends on your baby's needs and your choice.

Rooming in

'Rooming in' means that after your baby is born, she will stay with you at your bedside in the hospital. This is beneficial for the following reasons:

- your baby can get to know her parents
- she has constant access to feeding
- it gives you the chance to practise your mothering skills while still under the wing of the nursing staff
- you will learn to identify your baby's needs and cries
- you can 'tune in' to your baby much faster
- a newborn baby feels more at ease as she hears her mother's voice, identifies her by smell, feeds frequently from her breast, hears the beating of her heart and has her needs met immediately

- When you handle and touch your baby, it promotes the release of the 'mothering hormone' prolactin, which helps get breast-feeding off to a good start.

If you have had a long and difficult labour or perhaps a Caesarean, you may not feel physically capable of caring for your baby in the beginning. You may even need to rest for a day or so before taking on the full-time care of a baby. The full magnitude of becoming a parent might only impact on you now, and you might want to step back and rely on the professional help around you. If you already have children, you may want to

Below Once you are moved to the post-natal ward, your baby will be left with you; this is known as 'rooming in'.

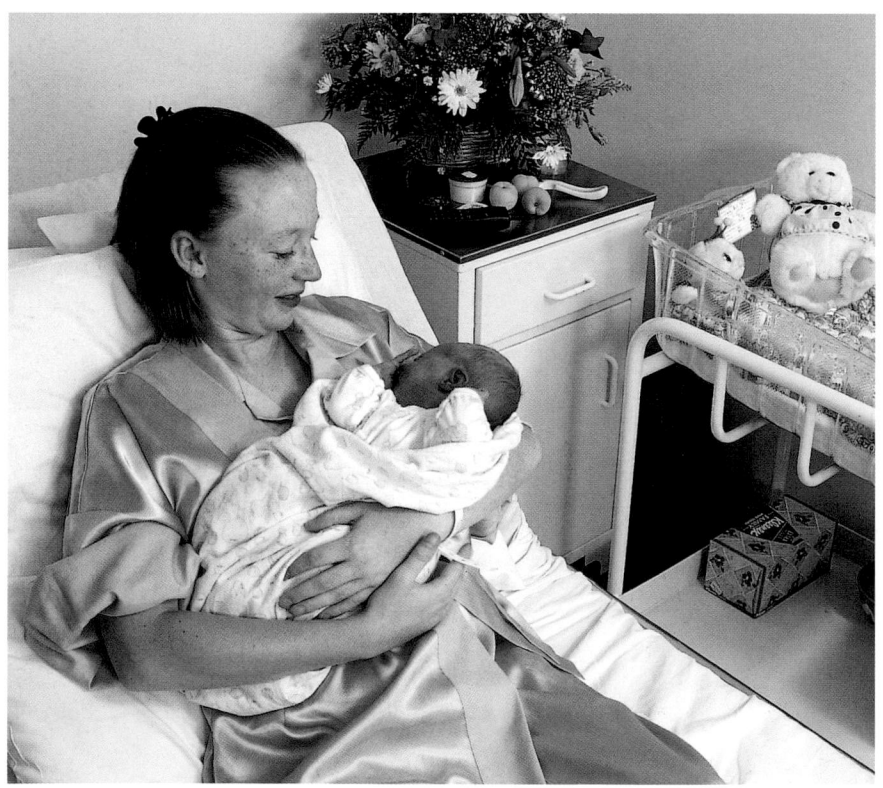

be nurtured before going home to take care of your children.

There are different ways of rooming in, and a rooming-in policy should be flexible, according to the family's needs. You should be allowed to choose the way you wish to do this. You may want your baby with you only some of the time. Most mothers would probably make use of both systems of care initially, taking more responsibility as their confidence grows. Explore your options by taking a tour of the maternity ward before the big day.

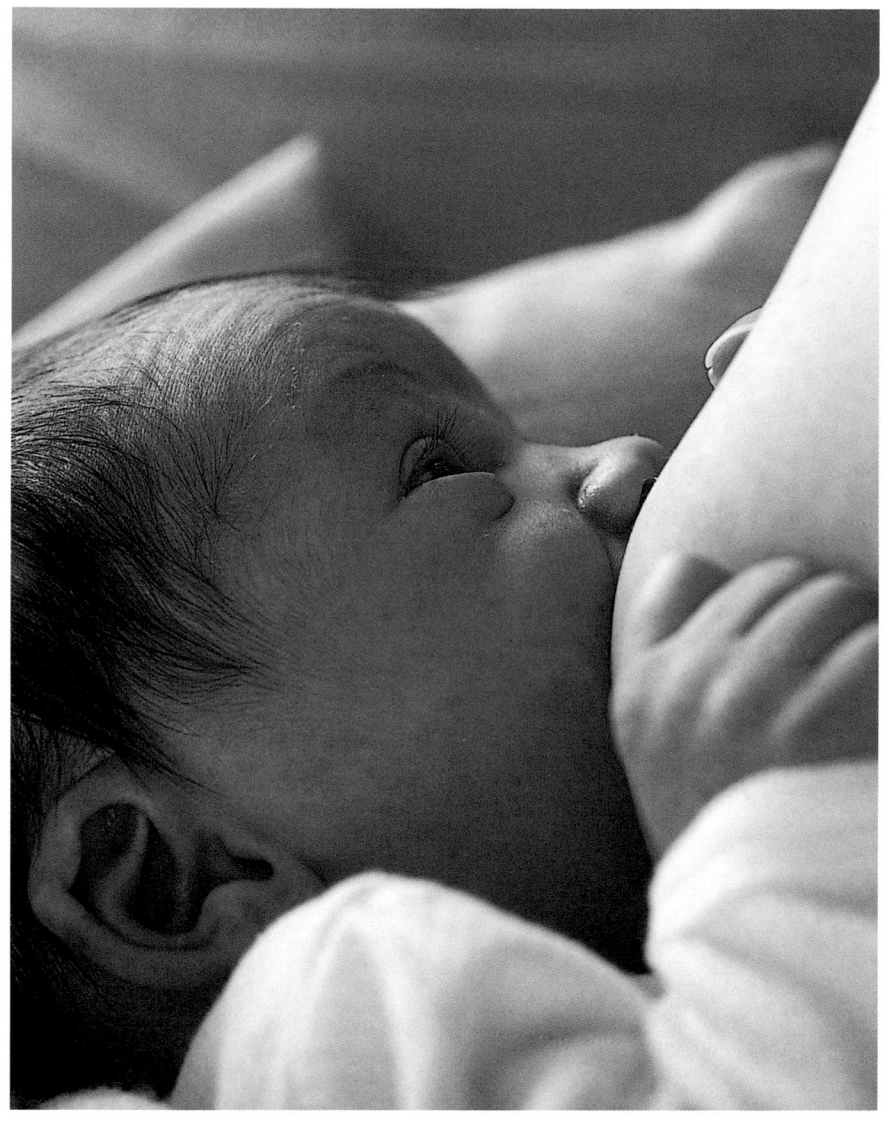

Left *Make sure your baby's body is facing your body when feeding. This makes it easier for your baby to swallow and to latch correctly.*

or short during pregnancy, the nipples will become erect and ready when the baby is about to feed. The nipples have very delicate nerve endings which make them sensitive to touch. This is a common complaint of women during pregnancy. There is no need to 'toughen' them by scrubbing or cleaning them vigorously. This is NOT recommended! No creams or lotions and no prodding or pulling is necessary – just wear a comfortable, well-fitting bra. The best way you can prepare for breast-feeding is to attend a breast-feeding education class before your baby is born.

There are very few reasons why breast-feeding may not work for a woman, unless:

- it does not appeal to her or she finds it distasteful
- she feels that breast-feeding is inconvenient and that bottle-feeding will better suit her lifestyle needs
- she plans on going back to work before six weeks
- she has had breast surgery and has damaged milk ducts.

Breast-feeding

Many women worry that breast-feeding will not work for them or that there is a particular regime that has to be followed in order to prepare for breast-feeding. It is important that you carefully consider the feeding method you choose for your baby. Knowledge and information, skills and good support all contribute to building your confidence. The size and shape of your breasts have nothing to do with whether or not you will be able to breast-feed. Contrary to what you will be told, there is nothing special you have to do in order to prepare your breasts for feeding. They prepare themselves. The raised area on the nipple, called 'Montgomery's tubercles', secretes a fluid that lubricates and protects the nipples from drying out. The breasts become more vascular and the nipples become larger and usually lengthen as the pregnancy progresses. This occurs so that the baby can suckle with ease. Although your nipples may look flat

Newborn appearance

Your baby's appearance may surprise you at first glance. She may not even resemble anyone you know, never mind being your offspring! In the days and weeks of early postpartum (following childbirth), she is going to change so much. When you have your baby to yourself, open up the blankets and examine her from head to toe.

Weight

The average weight of a full-term baby falls in the range of 3–3.4kg (7–7.5 lb). He or she measures approximately 48–53cm (19–21in) in length.

Eyes

Your baby's face may be a bit puffy and swollen from the pressure of the birth canal. Swollen eyelids protect the eyes from harsh light. Babies' eyes are usually a deep blue colour and the pupils are very large at birth. They can focus at a distance of about 20cm (50.8in). She may have a squinting appearance in the first few days. This is due to the small eye muscles being immature. It may appear worse due to the folds of skin in the corners of the eyes.

Top Your baby will be weighed immediately after birth.
Right It is normal for a baby to develop a 'sucking blister' from feeding.
Far right Your baby's eyelids are swollen to protect the eyes from harsh light.

Ears

These look a bit like crumpled cauliflowers and will straighten out within a few days. Any hair that is on them will rub off very quickly. Remember that your baby can hear you and recognizes your voice from the start.

Head

If forceps or the ventouse was used during delivery, there may be some bruising on your baby's face or on top of her head. These marks will disappear within a few days. Swelling may take a little longer to go down. If your baby was delivered vaginally, she may have an egg-shaped head. Her skull bones are not fused at the time of birth and, in fact, will overlap or ride over each other when the pressure of the vaginal walls presses on her head. If you run your fingers over her head gently, you will feel slight

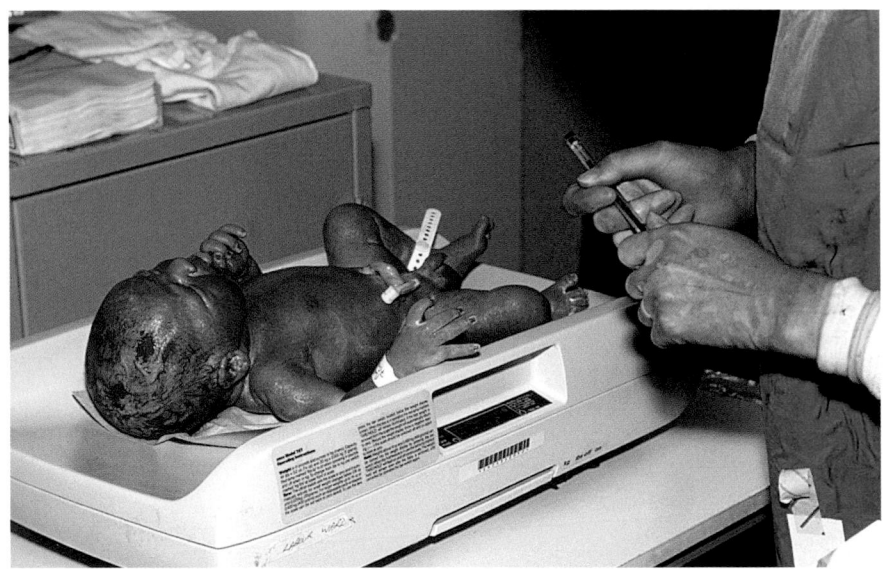

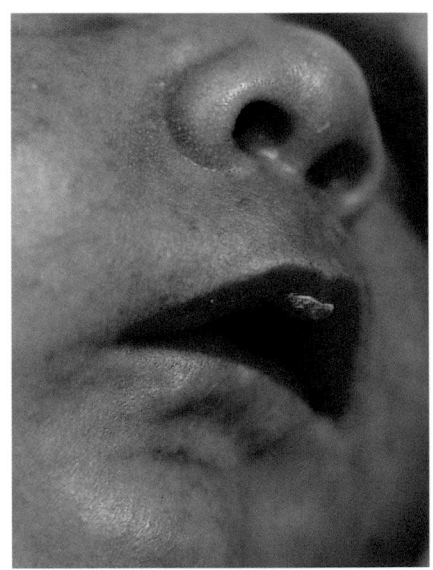

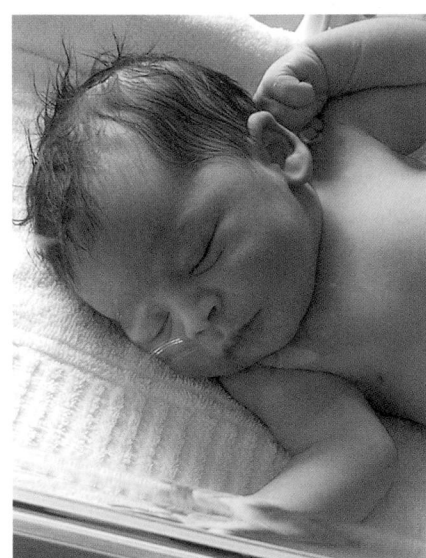

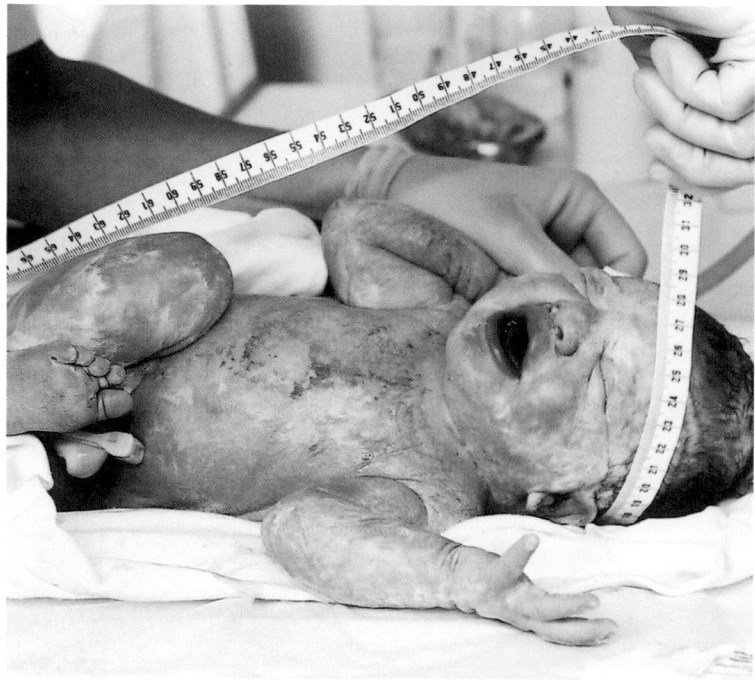
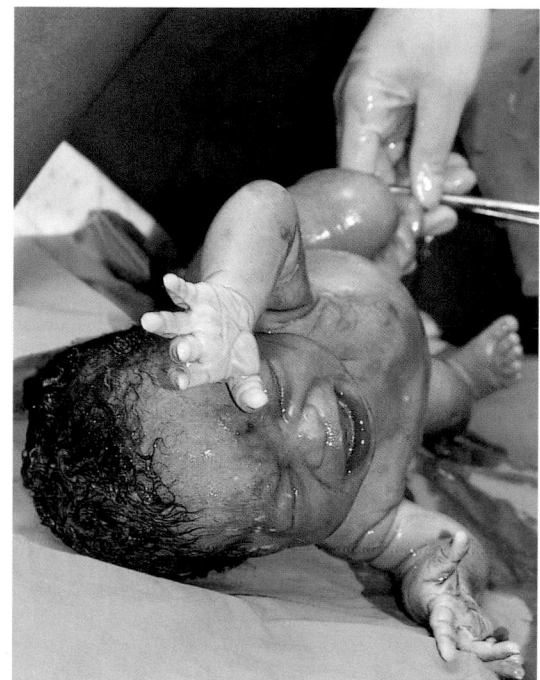

Above left Your baby will be covered in a cheese-like substance called vernix. *Above right* The umbilical cord contains three blood vessels but no nerves, so your baby does not feel pain when it is cut.

ridges where this has happened. This is called 'moulding' and is normal.

There are two soft spots on a baby's head called fontanelles. These are areas where the skull has not yet fused together. These will fuse within six weeks to 18 months. 'Stork bites' are light pink patches on her forehead, especially her eyelids. These are flat, dilated capillaries that will fade as your baby grows. They are also found in the nape of the neck. Your baby may have a lot of hair on her head or none at all.

Body

Lanugo is the name given to the fine, fuzzy, downy hair that you will see on your baby's body. This kept your baby warm *in utero* and will rub off before you take your baby home. It is very prevalent in early or premature babies and not as evident in full-term babies.

Vernix

The white cheese-like substance found on your baby's body and in the creases is known as vernix. Vernix protects your baby from her watery environment and helps lubricate the vaginal passage at the time of birth. Her skin may be a little wrinkled, especially if she was a little over her due date, but she will soon shed this and her new beautiful skin will appear.

Genitals

The genitals of newborns are often swollen and the skin is darker in colour. Swollen breast tissue is also normal, which is due to the mother's hormones that have passed to the baby during pregnancy. The testes in a boy may or may not have descended, but they should be in place within six weeks. This will be checked at the six-week checkup.

Umbilical cord

The length of the cord is about 50cm (20in). The cord holds three blood vessels but no nerves. Before the cord is cut, it will be clamped in two places. This is not painful for the baby. This cord is long enough for the baby to stay attached to the mother and still find his way up her abdomen to the nipple.

Recent research has shown that a baby will instinctively start to look for his food source within 20 minutes after delivery and will 'leopard crawl' up the mother's abdomen to the nipple.

This process can be interfered with if the mother has had certain pain-relieving drugs during labour. The bit of cord that is left at the baby's naval will shrink and dry up soon after birth, and will fall off within seven to 14 days.

Newborn reflexes

Long before birth, your unborn baby has been getting ready for life outside the womb. During her development, she was unable to survive outside the womb, but once she has left her shelter she can never go back. This tiny being comes programmed with a set of reflexes that will ensure her survival and 'hook' her parents in so that they cannot help but feel protective of her.

Moro or startle reflex The baby throws out her arms, stretches out her hands and fingers, and crys out as if startled. She then draws her limbs closer to her body as if trying to cling to something to stop herself falling. This reflex occurs as the baby detects the change in equilibrium (feels itself falling).

Rooting reflex The baby opens her mouth and turns her head toward a stimulus touching the cheek, usually her mother's breast, in search of food. This is diminished by five to six months and disappears by one year of age.

Grasp reflex A newborn will grasp an object placed in her palm, cling briefly and then let go. It is present in both hands and feet in babies of normal gestation and disappears by four months.

Stepping reflex When a baby is held well supported, with one foot touching a surface, she will step with one foot and then the other in a walking motion. This disappears by two months and the baby will not make attempts to step until she is ready to walk.

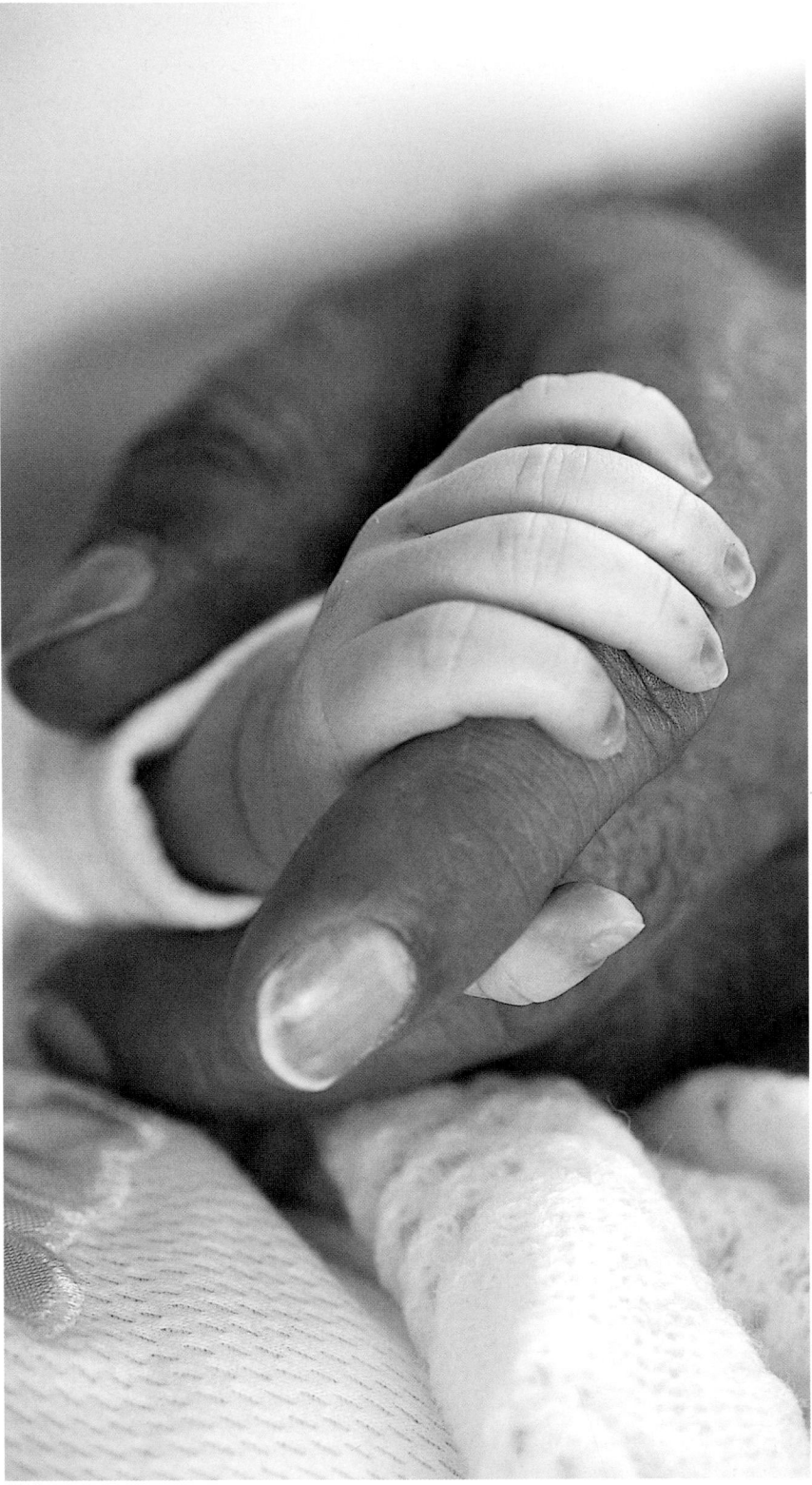

Above *Your baby will briefly cling to anything that is placed in his hand, which shows that his grasping reflex is fine.*

Tonic neck reflex A baby turns his head sharply and assumes a fencing position. He arches his back and stretches out all the muscles on the front side of the body while flexing the muscles on the other side. During labour, when the baby does this, it helps him 'swim' down the cervical canal. Later in his infancy, this reflex will enable him to use one arm to reach for a toy while supressing the other arm.

Spinal cord reflex If the baby is stroked along his spinal cord, his entire body will straighten up in the direction of the stroke. His trunk will move back and forth in 'squirmy' movements if there is enough touch stimulation along the spinal cord. In this way, the baby helps himself wiggle down the birth canal as the pressure of the walls of the vagina stroke his back.

Yawning Under natural delivery circumstances, the baby gives a few massive yawns shortly after birth. This reflex action ensures a deep intake of oxygen to the lungs. The breathing and yawning process begins naturally, long before the cord stops pulsating. Sometimes this slow yawning does not occur and the midwife will try to get the baby to breathe as quickly as possible. This is indicated by crying.

Diving The diving reflex really stands the baby in good stead. Up until the age of about six months, the baby is able to stay under water without inhaling water into the lungs. A small flap of skin closes off the top of the trachea and any water taken in will be swallowed and pass into the stomach.

Smiling Smiling is unique to our species and researchers are convinced that there is a reflex smile. It appears as early as three days after birth. It is fleeting and may not even be recognized as a smile. It can be initiated by the sound of a high-pitched voice – usually the mother's – tickling of the baby and the passing of wind. It seems to appear as a form of startle response – a surprise reaction.

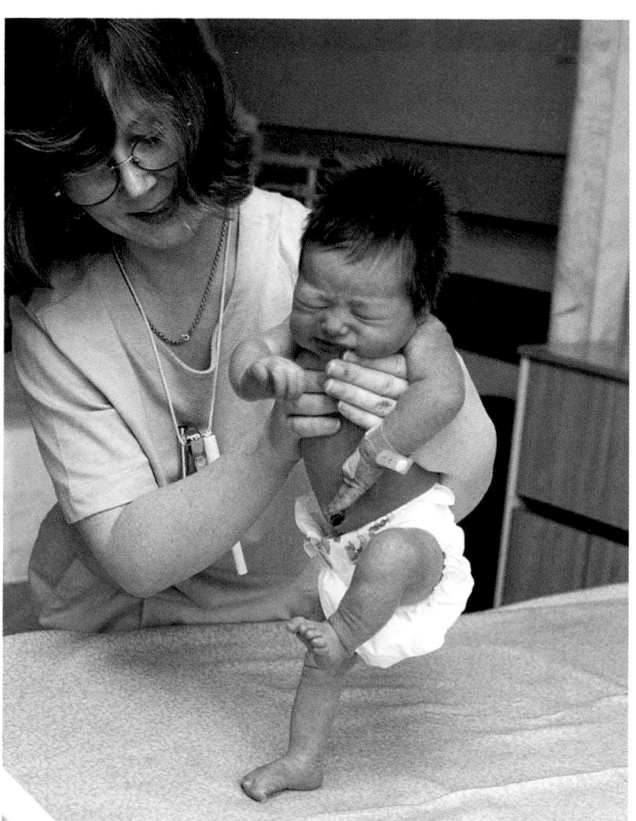

Above right The midwife will hold your baby upright and check her stepping reflex.
Right Your baby will yawn shortly after birth to take oxygen into the lungs.

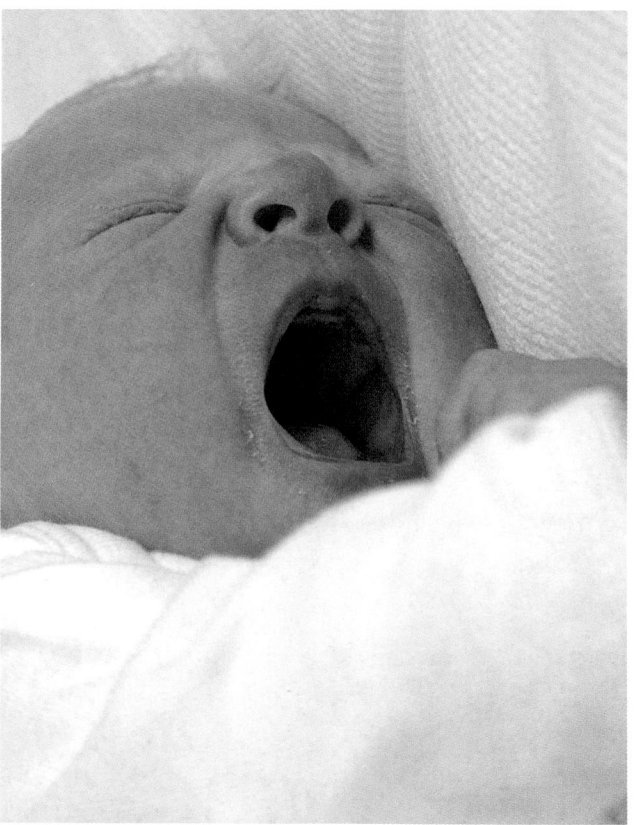

Postpartum

Many women think that the discomforts of pregnancy come to an end once the baby is born, but there is a period of recovery before you 'bounce back'.

Vaginal birth

Even if you did not tear or have an episiotomy, the vagina stretched a great deal to accommodate your baby's head and it is normal to feel tender. It should take about six weeks for the tissues to return to normal. If some perineal tissue tore during the birth or if you have had an episiotomy, it will take about a week for the stitches to dissolve and for the area to start healing fully. Sitting may be uncomfortable and passing a bowel movement may be particularly painful.

Recovery from vaginal birth

Once the birth of your baby is over, you may be surprised to experience a bit more discomfort. Your body has to adapt and adjust to the fact that it is no longer pregnant and the effects are not all immediate.

Bleeding after birth

Irrespective of whether you had a vaginal birth or a Caesarean, you will bleed heavily for the first few days after your baby is born. This discharge (lochia) is the blood from the 'wound' where the placenta was attached to the wall of the uterus. The discharge will initially be heavy with blood clots and will gradually change colour and consistency, and become less profuse as you recover from the birth.

After birth pains

Your uterus stretched extensively over the nine months of pregnancy in order to accommodate your growing baby, and it will take about two weeks for it to return to its original size and place. Every time you breast-feed you will feel contractions as the uterus sweeps itself clean and gets rid of any 'leftovers' from the birth.

Perineal health

- An ice pack placed on the perineum in the first 24 hours after birth significantly reduces the swelling and bruising.
- After that, warmth either from a hot lamp placed near the perineum or from sitting in warm water is very soothing.
- It is very important to keep this area clean and as dry as possible during its healing phase.
- If you notice any bleeding or pus (sign of infection) oozing from the site of the episiotomy or tear, or if the swelling worsens significantly, you must call your doctor or midwife.
- Whether you have had an episiotomy or a tear, or you have given birth without any perineal trauma, Kegel exercises (see p85) will help you regain the support and tone of the pelvic floor.
- Drink plenty of water to dilute your urine and prevent any stinging; it will also prevent constipation which could cause extra discomfort in the perineal area.
- If you find that sitting down is painful, cover an inflated swimming ring with a clean pillow case and sit on that. It will take some of the pressure off a very delicate spot.

- If you still feel pain with sex some months after the birth or if you experience urinary incontinence, you should see your doctor or midwife.

It could take anything from three to five months for your body to recover from pregnancy. One of the first things you will notice is the decrease in the 'bloated' feeling you have become so accustomed to. Your sudden weight loss can be put down to the extra water you were carrying during your pregnancy. Pain in the joints may still bother you for a while and you will continue to perspire more than usual, especially when breast-feeding. Your bladder will also take a while to return to normal, so those regular visits to the toilet are not yet a thing of the past. Remember, you may still look about five months pregnant immediately after birth, but do not panic – this is normal.

Recovering from a Caesarean section

The stitches from the Caesarean section will dissolve slowly over a period of days. When body gases move around under the wound it can feel uncomfortable, as can passing urine and having a bowel movement. It is also normal to feel pain under the ribs. This is due to trapped air in the thoracic area, post surgery. When you cough, sneeze or laugh, keep a pillow handy to place across your abdomen. This provides support to the wound site.

You will be instructed on how to care for your wound before you leave the hospital. Bath and shower as normal, and try to use nonperfumed products that will not irritate your skin. Your wound may weep for a while, but if any gaping, or pain and redness, and a bad smell occur, contact your doctor immediately. Your lochia will be the same as if you had given vaginal birth; it is bright red to start with, becoming muddy brown to clear over three to six weeks.

Give your body time to heal and take things slowly. You should not drive for at least 10 days to three weeks. Do not start normal exercise before six weeks, although walking is recommended. Take time to ease into your role as a new mother and know that there will be good and bad days.

Rest is vital, especially after a Caesarean. Your abdomen may not look exactly like it did before you fell pregnant and there may be a slight bulge of skin over the top of the scar, but do not despair. Make sure your diet is adequate and get back to exercise as soon as your doctor gives you the green light. Your scar will be below your panty line and covered by pubic hair, and it will shrink and fade over time.

Below *A nurse will tend to your wound from the Caesarean section.*

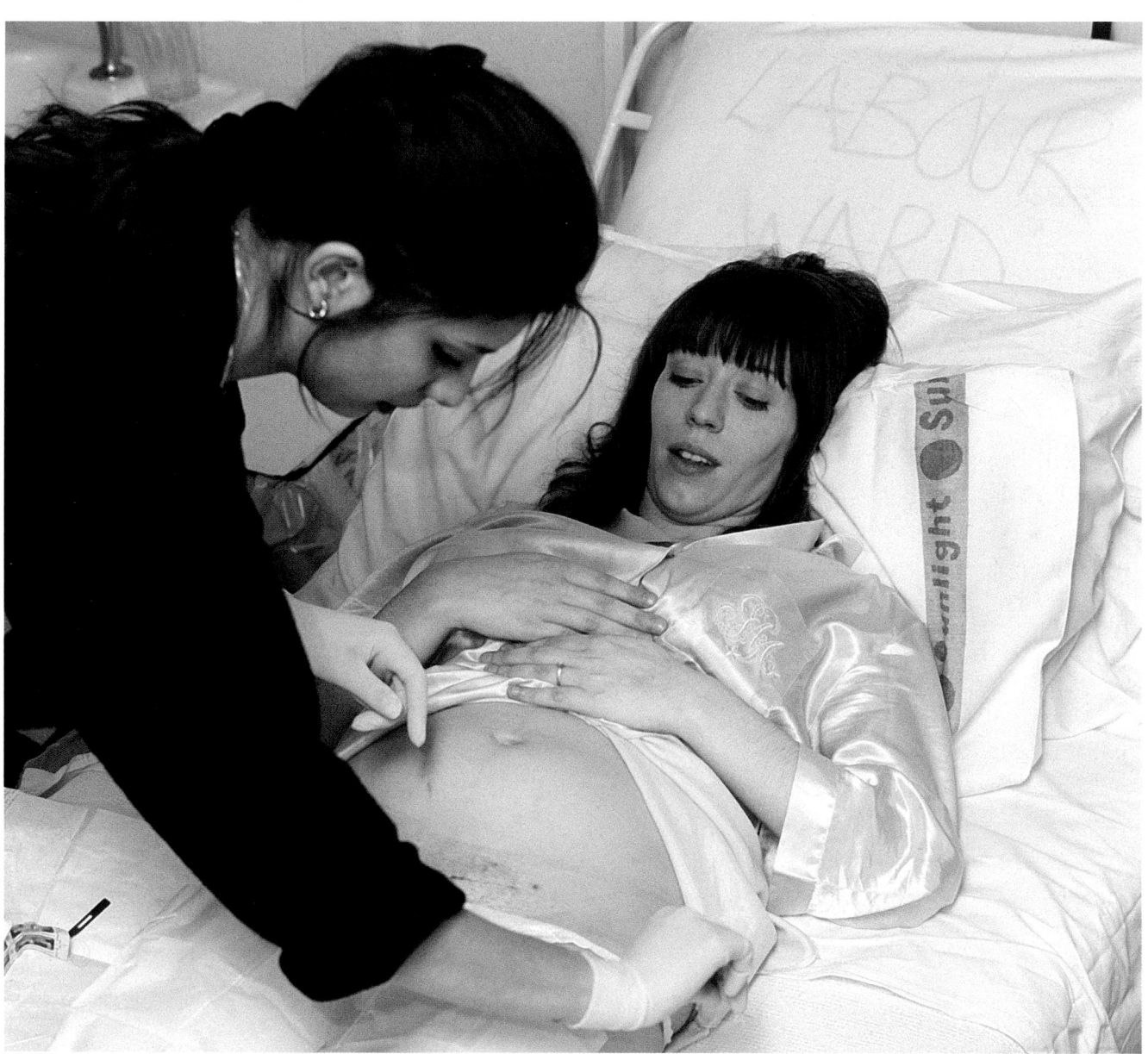

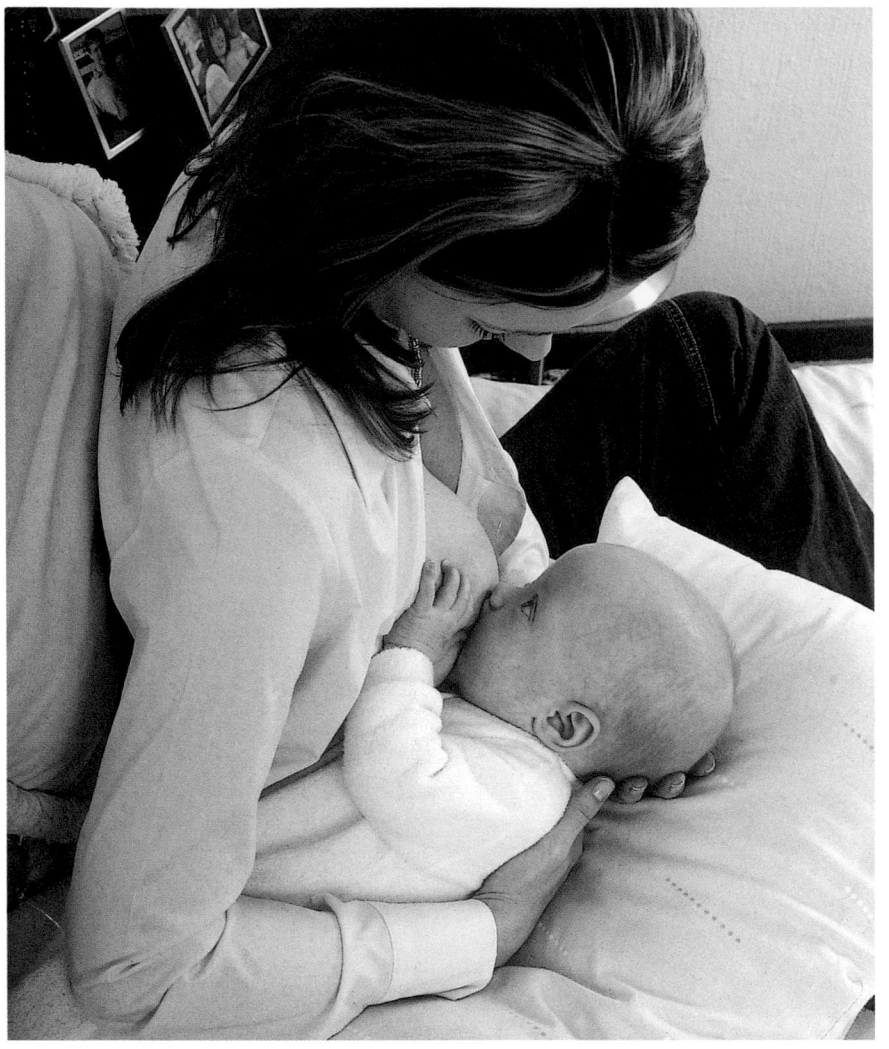

Emotional pain

It can be a shock when the responsibility of caring for a new human being dawns on you. The realization can cause you to feel a bit down for a few days, although not all women experience this. If you still feel sad and depressed after three months, seek counselling as you may be suffering from postnatal depression. Seek help sooner rather than later, as this condition can be very successfully treated.

Tips to feeling good

- Eat regular, nutritious meals.
- Sleep as often as you can – always try to sleep when the baby sleeps.
- Learn to prioritize.
- Be intimate with your partner – making love will probably be the furthest thing from your mind but when you are ready, go slowly and use extra lubrication.
- Relax and put your feet up as often as you can.
- Use your slow, deep-breathing techniques, especially if things are getting too much and you need to keep calm.
- Ask for help from your family when you are feeling overwhelmed.
- Look after yourself and make sure that you take time out for yourself – every day.
- Give yourself time to adjust to this new 24-hour, seven-days-a-week job.

Breast discomfort

For about three days after your baby is born your breasts will produce colostrum – a rich, creamy 'milk' full of nutrients and antibodies. As your milk comes in, your breasts may prickle and the skin on the breast may feel taut. Breast-feeding should not be painful – and if it is, it could be that your baby is positioned incorrectly when placed at the breast. It is vital that this be corrected immediately or it could lead to cracked and bleeding nipples, and engorged breasts. If your breasts become engorged, try to

Above If you do feel breast discomfort, you may need to support your baby on pillows, and turn his body to face you.

express milk. Use ice packs or warm compresses to ease sore breasts. Make sure that you are well supported when you are feeding and bring the baby up close to the breast rather than leaning forward into your baby. Support your baby on pillows and turn your baby's body to face you. This will also prevent any back strain.

Bonding

When your baby is born, nature has a few tricks up her sleeve to help you love and adore this little offspring, if not immediately, then certainly over time. At the time of birth, the new baby will have a very high level of adrenaline and will be very alert and receptive to her mother's voice and contact.

These high levels of adrenaline are necessary for the survival of the baby had it been born 'in the wild'. The baby's pupils will be very large and she will look very appealing as you make eye contact for the first time. This is how your baby makes you fall in love with her. Most of the time the mother is not even aware of how her baby's pupil changes are affecting her, but as they dilate and take in their surroundings, the mother responds by pulling the baby closer and nearer to her as she cuddles and coos. The oxytocin and endorphins surging through your body create a state of arousal that can make you more receptive to forming an attachment. Your behaviour is strongly affected by your baby. Your pupils are also wide, your sense of smell is sharp and clear, and your ears pick up every sound. When the placenta is delivered, the hormone cortisol ensures that your nurturing and protective instinct takes over.

Your first opportunity to get close is immediately after birth. Newborns are often awake and alert for a few hours after birth, so keep this precious time just for the three of you and once you go home, ask people to give you a few days before they start visiting. You never know how you are going to feel when you see your baby for the first time. You may fall in love instantly or you may feel quite numb and only learn to love this little being over time as you get to know her. The secret is to spend as much time as you can together.

Cuddling, kissing and prolonged gazing helps to form a bond between parent and baby. The sense of touch is the most powerful in human bonding. Studies have shown that babies who are touched, cuddled and stroked do not just grow, they thrive. Touching promotes feelings of wellbeing for mother and baby and will allow your baby to venture out into the world with self-confidence later. Touching and holding her

Left Eye contact is a very important aspect of bonding with your little one.

not only develops trust, but also enhances your baby's developing self-esteem. All mothers instinctively touch their babies. Baby massage can alleviate many of the discomforts that adapting to the outside world brings. Find out about baby massage classes.

Your baby's response

Many mothers report that they feel really close to their infants when the baby looks at them and holds their gaze. Eye contact is one of the most powerful ways of communicating. One of the first things your newborn baby will do is look for your face. He will take in every curve and your face will be imprinted on his mind. He will recognize you much sooner than you think.

A newborn baby recognizes his mother's and father's voice from when he was in the womb, and he will turn toward you when he hears your voice. Your baby gets to know you from your voice, so talk to him a lot. Turn off the television or radio when talking to him so that he does not have difficulty distinguishing your voice from background noise. A young baby listens intently to his mother's voice and will respond to it willingly. When you talk to your baby you may find yourself making exaggerated facial expressions. There is a good reason for this. Even at a young age he will start to mimic those expressions. Give him a few seconds – it takes a while for him to react.

Your baby gets to know you from your smell, so allow lots of skin contact and

Below *Breast milk is the best nutrition for your baby, and you should make every effort to breast-feed.*

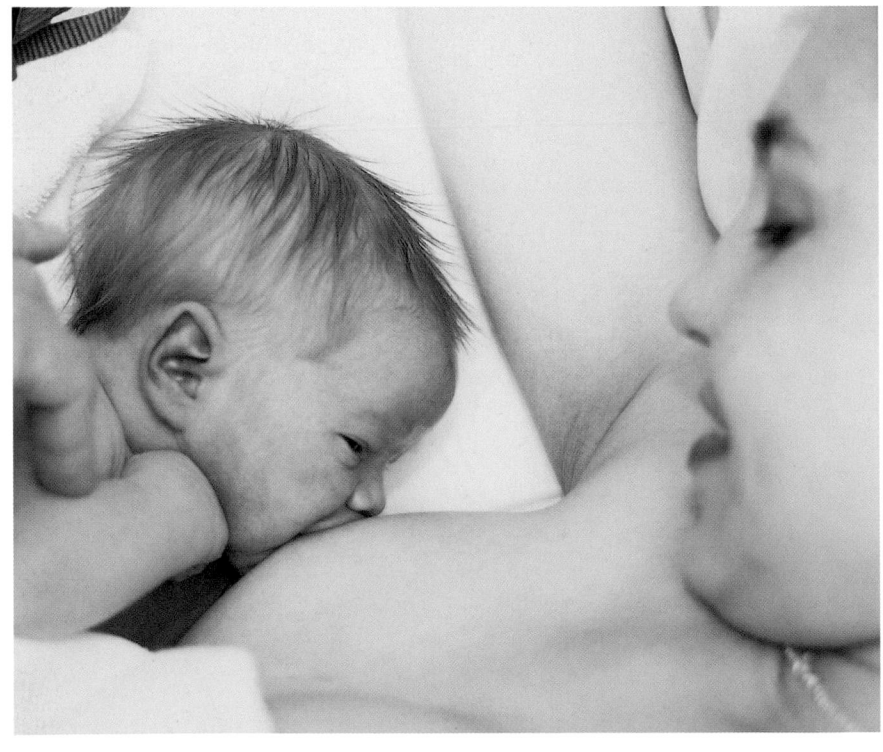

nuzzling at the breast. Your baby can identify the smell of your breast and breast milk over another woman's. In the early days, try not to overpower your body smell by wearing strong perfumes or deodorant. Let your baby get to know your smell by letting him lie directly on your skin. This is great for new fathers to do as well.

Your baby will learn to identify each one of you separately. Mothers also have some extraordinary abilities. According to research, mothers can identify their babies purely by smell within six hours after birth. Babies take about 45 hours to imprint their mother's smell, which is more likely to occur if your baby is with you for an extended period immediately after birth.

Nutrition

Breast milk contains every single nutrient and is the perfect food in every way for your baby. There is no better 'brain food' and every attempt should be made to breast-feed.

There are many other advantages to breast-feeding besides nutrition. Babies feel comfort and love at the breast, and a special closeness develops when a mother feels good about her body providing everything her baby needs. Breast-feeding and skin-to-skin contact releases hormones in the mother, helping the uterus to contract, stimulating the milk supply and helping the mother to relax and tune in to her baby's cues.

Even in the absence of breast-feeding, touching and skin contact with your baby initiate the mothering instinct.

Whether you breast- or bottle-feed, use this time to talk to your baby, stroke her and hold her close.

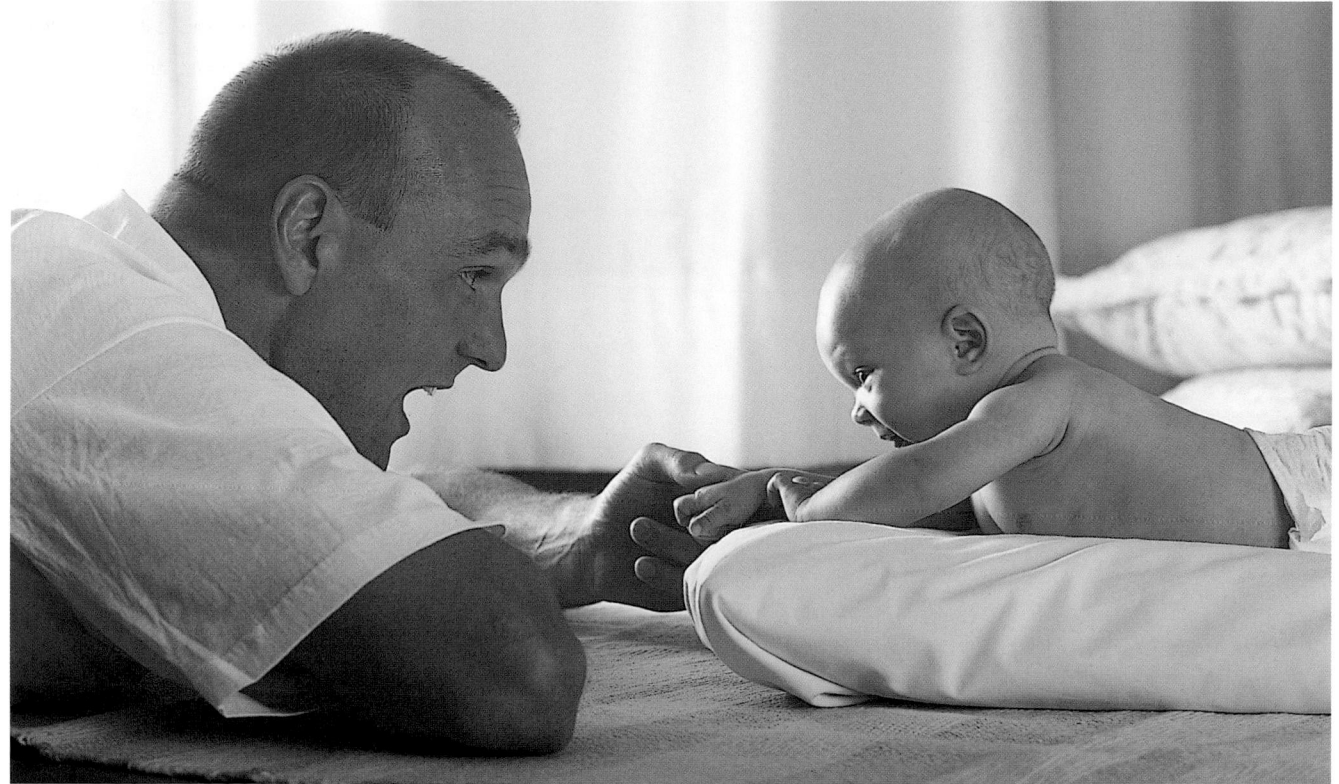

Dedicated to dads

Coming home from the clinic after the birth of a baby should be a happy experience. It is particularly significant for a first-time mother to be able to return to the surroundings of her home feeling safe and secure, among her familiar things and all the comforts that make her home special. Remember that she left home as a 'single entity', and now returns home as a mother with a baby. This and other issues make her somewhat apprehensive about coming home, even though it is something she has been looking forward to. A little consideration and planning will show her that you care and that you too have mixed feelings about bringing your baby home.

Tips for homecoming

You will probably be given a list of things to bring to the clinic. Try to make sure you bring what she has asked for.

- Taking a baby car seat is imperative – your baby should always be safely strapped into a car seat from the very first trip. Under no circumstances should a baby be held by anyone in the front passenger seat!
- Do not just grab the carry cot and proudly head for the exit. Remember, she cannot walk as fast as you and may interpret this as insensitivity to her condition. Say your goodbyes to the nursing staff and leave as a family.
- Get her and the baby settled and offer to make her a cup of tea, coffee or some other refreshment. Frozen dinners are a godsend at a time like this.
- Ask family to bring dinner when they come to visit the baby. Do not invite your friends over right away. In fact, limit visitors on the first few days.
- Encourage visitors to make their own tea AND to clean the cups and saucers. Sometimes men forget that it is the small, practical things you do for your partner that score substantial points and make her feel loved.

Glossary

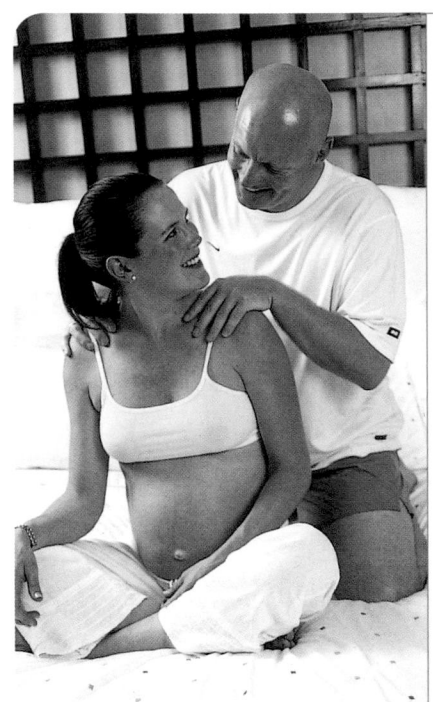

Alpha-fetoprotein (AFP) is a protein that circulates in the baby's blood before birth, and escapes into the mother's blood; it may be used to test for neural-tube defects and Down's syndrome.

Amniocentesis An invasive diagnostic test carried out in early pregnancy to detect the presence of genetic abnormalities in the foetus, more specifically Down's syndrome.

Amniotic fluid The liquid in which the foetus floats. It protects the baby throughout pregnancy and is contained in the amniotic sac.

Anaemia A deficiency in red blood cells or haemoglobin in the blood, resulting in breathlessness, tiredness and pale skin.

Braxton-Hicks contractions These painless, 'practice' contractions prepare the uterus for labour.

Breech position Position of a baby who is presenting bottom or feet first instead of head first.

Caesarean birth The delivery of a baby through an incision in the mother's abdominal wall and uterus.

Cephalic The name given for the position of a baby who is head down in the uterus.

Cervix Circular muscles at the 'neck' of the uterus, which act like a drawstring. The cervix is tightly closed throughout pregnancy and opens up or dilates during labour.

Colostrum The first milk produced by the breasts at the time of birth and for a few days after the birth. It is concentrated and contains many antibodies to protect the new baby.

Contraction The tightening of the uterine muscle fibres during labour. As the muscle fibres tighten, they become shorter, causing the uterus to open.

Coombes Test A test used to confirm the diagnosis of antibody induced anaemia, which suggests rhesus incompatibility.

Down's syndrome A genetic disorder causing mental and physical handicaps.

Dilation (stretching to enlarge) as in the uterus stretching to open.

Dura mater The toughest and outermost

of the three membranes covering the brain and spinal cord.

Embryo The name given to a developing baby in the first eight weeks of gestation.

Engagement The descent of the baby's head into the pelvis. Usually occurs in the last four weeks of pregnancy.

Fertilization The union of male and female germ cells whereby reproduction takes place.

Foetus The name given to a developing baby from eight weeks of gestation to birth.

Folic acid A naturally occurring B vitamin that is vital to the proper growth of cells. A deficiency of folic acid when cells around the spine of the baby are dividing and growing can result in a neural-tube defect.

Fontanelles The two soft spots on a baby's head where the skull has not yet fused together. These will fuse within six weeks to 18 months.

Fundus The name given to the top of the uterus. It is measured to date a pregnancy.

Gestation The period of time, in weeks, from the last menstrual period to the birth of a baby.

Haemoglobin The colouring pigment of red blood corpuscles and the agent whereby oxygen is taken up in the lungs and carried through to the tissues.

Human chorionic gonadotrophin (HCG) A hormone that is only produced during pregnancy and that forms the basis of all pregnancy tests.

Hypertension The medical term for high blood pressure.

Induction A procedure by which labour is started artificially.

Ketones Chemicals in the blood that indicate the body is low in blood sugar.

Lanugo The soft downy hair that is present on a newborn baby's skin.

Leucocytes The white blood cells.

Ligaments Tough, fibrous tissue connecting one bone to another.

Lightening This is when your baby starts to move snuggly into the pelvis in the ninth month of pregnancy.

Linea nigra The dark line running from the navel to the pubic hairline. It is visible from about the fifth month of pregnancy.

Lochia The discharge consisting of blood from the 'wound' where the placenta was attached to the wall of the uterus.

Meconium The first stool produced by a newborn baby. It is made up of secretions of the bowel and swallowed substances while the foetus is *in utero*.

Neural tube The structure that develops into the brain and spinal cord. Incomplete development results in a neural-tube defect.

Occiput Crown of the baby's head.

Oedema Excessive swelling due to fluid retention in the tissues.

Oxytocic drugs These drugs are the synthetic form of the hormone oxytocin, and is given to a mother to accelerate labour or to speed up the delivery of the placenta.

Pelvic floor muscles The sling of muscles that surround and support the bladder, vagina and rectum.

Perineum The tissue and skin between the vagina and anus.

Premature baby A baby that is born before 37 weeks of gestation.

Postpartum The period following childbirth. It is usually a challenging and exhausting time for new mothers.

Rubella German measles.

Show A plug of mucus in the cervical opening during pregnancy which will come away during labour, often as the first indication that labour may soon begin.

Small for dates babies If a foetus appears unusually small or large, an ultrasound will be conducted which will determine whether the baby is due on the date originally calculated. If your due date is accurate, the baby is said to be small (or large) for dates.

Spina bifida A gap in the baby's vertebrae, leaving the spinal cord partially exposed.

Symphysis pubis joint It holds the pelvis steady when using the legs. If the ligaments have stretched or softened too much, it will not do its job properly, causing strain on other pelvic joints, and resulting in pain.

Teratogenic Substances that can prove harmful to a developing foetus.

Trimester (i.e. a third) The months of pregnancy is divided into three sections of roughly equal length: the first, second and third trimesters.

Triple test This test is done at 16–18 weeks, and measures three hormones from the baby and placenta: alpha-fetoprotein, chorionic gonadotrophin and estriol. Changes in these hormones may indicate an increased risk of spina bifida or Down's syndrome.

Ureters The tube that transports urine from the kidneys to the bladder or cloaca.

Vernix The white cheese-like substance that protects the baby's skin before birth, and provides extra lubrication during birth.

Index

pushing and birth **119**

pyelonephritis 64

R

rash 62

recti muscles 54, **86**

reflexes (newborn) 144–145

relaxation 92

rhesus (Rh) factor 27

rhesus incompatibility 27

rooming in **140**

rooting reflex 144

S

saddle block 103

salmonella 74

screening ultrasound scans 19

sexual intercourse 66

sexually transmitted diseases (STDs) 29

show (labour) 113, 154

skin changes 62

smiling reflex 145

smoking 77

sodium 72

spina bifida 19, 154

spinal cord reflex 145

squatting position **99**

stepping reflex 144, **145**

strength training 82

stretch marks 62

stretching 82

stripping the membranes 124

substances in moderation 75

sugar 75

surgery, after 135

swelling 63

swimming 82

symphysis pubis joint 53, 154

Syntocinon drip 124

syphilis 29

T

teeth and gums 15, 61

tension and labour 93

teratogens 31, 74, 154

tests and scans 19–22

   screening tests 19

   diagnostic tests 20

tonic neck reflex 145

tool kit, self-help 106–107

toxoplasmosis 74

Trans Cutaneous Electrical Stimulation

   (TENS) **97**

transition **118**

treadmill **81**

trimesters of pregnancy 34–51

triple test 19, 154

true labour 113

U

ultrasound scans **18, 20**

   diagnostic 20

   screening 19

umbilical cord 132, **143**

upright position **98**, 99

ureters 55, 154

urine tests 11, 16, 17, 34

V

vacuum extraction **126** see also

   ventouse

vaginal birth 146

vaginal birth after Caesarean (VBAC) 111

vaginal birth, recovery 146

vaginal bleeding 64

vaginal discharge 63, 117

vaginal fluid loss 64

varicose veins 61

ventouse **126** see also vacuum

   extraction

vernix caseosa 42, 50, **143**, 154

visualization 93

vitamin A 72, 75

vitamin B 72

vitamin C 25, 71, 72

vitamin D 72

vitamin K 72,

vitamin K injection 138

vomiting 27, 60

W

walking 81

warning signs and symptoms 64–65

   bladder infection 64

   contractions 64

   decreased foetal movement 65

   excessive swelling 64, 153

   severe abdominal pain 65

   vaginal bleeding 64

   vaginal fluid loss 64

water birth 110, **111**

weight 15

weight gain **69**, 70

weight loss 112

Y

yawning reflex **145**

yoga **81**

Z

zinc 72

Further reading

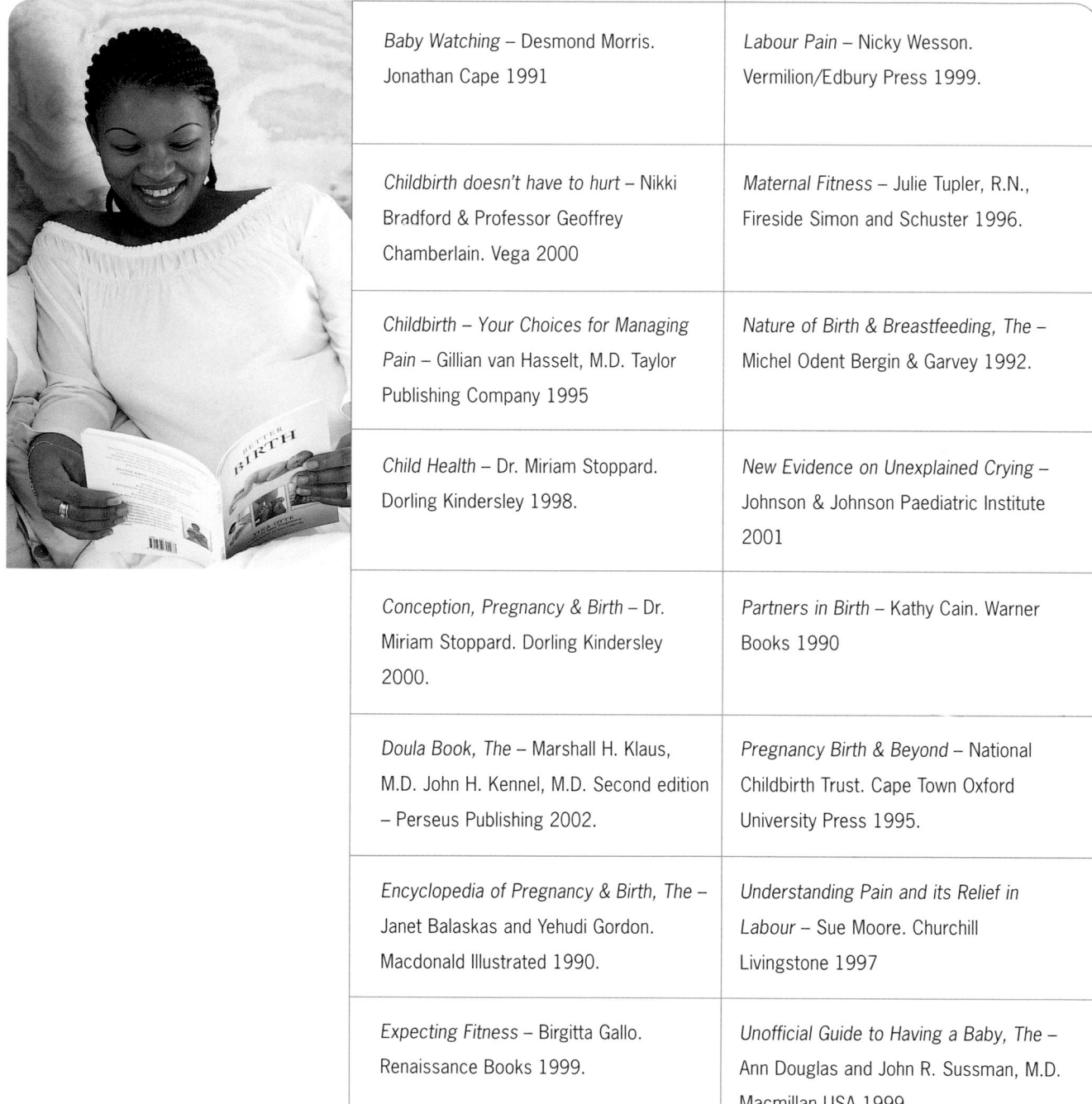

Baby Watching – Desmond Morris. Jonathan Cape 1991	*Labour Pain* – Nicky Wesson. Vermilion/Edbury Press 1999.
Childbirth doesn't have to hurt – Nikki Bradford & Professor Geoffrey Chamberlain. Vega 2000	*Maternal Fitness* – Julie Tupler, R.N., Fireside Simon and Schuster 1996.
Childbirth – Your Choices for Managing Pain – Gillian van Hasselt, M.D. Taylor Publishing Company 1995	*Nature of Birth & Breastfeeding, The* – Michel Odent Bergin & Garvey 1992.
Child Health – Dr. Miriam Stoppard. Dorling Kindersley 1998.	*New Evidence on Unexplained Crying* – Johnson & Johnson Paediatric Institute 2001
Conception, Pregnancy & Birth – Dr. Miriam Stoppard. Dorling Kindersley 2000.	*Partners in Birth* – Kathy Cain. Warner Books 1990
Doula Book, The – Marshall H. Klaus, M.D. John H. Kennel, M.D. Second edition – Perseus Publishing 2002.	*Pregnancy Birth & Beyond* – National Childbirth Trust. Cape Town Oxford University Press 1995.
Encyclopedia of Pregnancy & Birth, The – Janet Balaskas and Yehudi Gordon. Macdonald Illustrated 1990.	*Understanding Pain and its Relief in Labour* – Sue Moore. Churchill Livingstone 1997
Expecting Fitness – Birgitta Gallo. Renaissance Books 1999.	*Unofficial Guide to Having a Baby, The* – Ann Douglas and John R. Sussman, M.D. Macmillan USA 1999.

Author's acknowledgments

I have been dealing with childbearing couples and child-rearing families for over 20 years, and it is in these amazing people that I have found the inspiration to write about pregnancy and birth. Thank you all for sharing this most significant event with me.

Although I have had many mentors who have shaped and guided me through my years of writing and teaching, for this book, I would like to make special mention of Dr Marinda Taha and Sr Jo Murphy. Thank you for taking the time to ensure that the content of this book is accurate and up-to-date.

Also to my editor, Leizel Brown, who has made sense out of my 'too many words' and still managed to let me say what needed to be said – only better!

A loving thank you to my husband Ralph whose unwavering belief in me makes me strive to new heights. Lastly to my two beautiful daughters Natasha and Nicole who have, through their births, ignited in me a flame of love so intense that I cannot let go of the desire to tell mothers-to-be about the unbelievable journey they are about to embark on, whether it is their first child or their fifth.

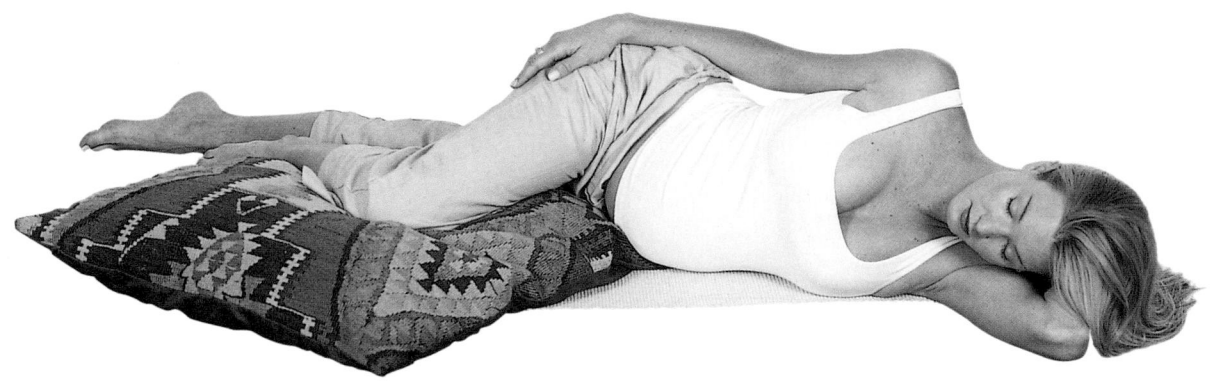

Photographic credits

All photographs © **Alchemy Publishing/Media24 South Africa** with the exception of the photographers and/or their agencies listed below:

Cover	galloimages/gettyimages.com	81 (left)	www.imagesofafrica.co.za	112	Mother & Baby/Eddie Lawrence
4	PhotoAccess	81 (right)	PhotoAccess	114	Digital Source
8	Mother & Baby/Ian Hooten	82	Mother & Baby/Ian Hooten	121 (bottom)	Mother & Baby/Ruth Jenkinson
10	Philips Medical Systems	87	PhotoAccess	123	Mother & Baby/Ian Hooten
11	Mother & Baby/Caroline Molloy	90	Mother & Baby/Ruth Jenkinson	124	Mother & Baby/Ruth Jenkinson
14	Mother & Baby/Caroline Molloy	92	www.imagesofafrica.co.za	127	www.imagesofafrica.co.za
17	Mother & Baby/Ian Hooten	94	Mother & Baby/Ruth Jenkinson	132	Mother & Baby/Frances Tout
18	Welma Viljoen	95	www.imagesofafrica.co.za	134	Mother & Baby/Ruth Jenkinson
22	Mother & Baby/Eddie Lawrence	97 (left)	www.imagesofafrica.co.za	137	Mother & Baby/Lucy Tizard
25 (top)	www.imagesofafrica.co.za	102	www.imagesofafrica.co.za	138 (top left)	www.imagesofafrica.co.za
27	PhotoAccess	104	www.imagesofafrica.co.za	142 (top)	Science Photo/Antonia Reeve
30	Science Photo/Ian Hooten	105	Mother & Baby/Ruth Jenkinson	142 (bottom right) Kurt van Vrede	
61	www.imagesofafrica.co.za	106	www.imagesofafrica.co.za	145 (top)	Mother & Baby/Eddie Lawrence
72	www.imagesofafrica.co.za	107	www.imagesofafrica.co.za	147	Mother & Baby/Toni Revan
73	Science Photo/David Munns	109	Mother & Baby/Ruth Jenkinson	149	Mother & Baby/Paul Mitchell

On The Trail Of
The
CELTS
In Britain

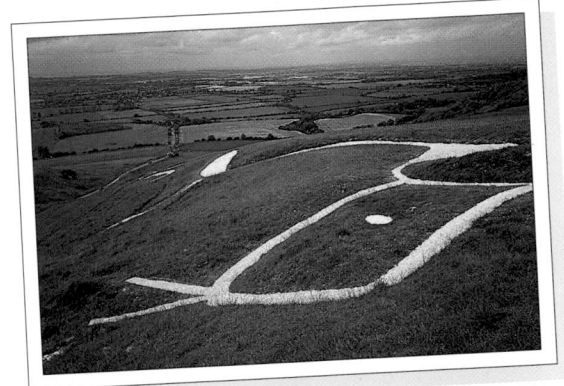

Peter Chrisp

W
Franklin Watts
NEW YORK • LONDON • SYDNEY

© 1999 Franklin Watts
First published in Great Britain by
Franklin Watts
96 Leonard Street
London EC2A 4XD

Franklin Watts Australia
14 Mars Road
Lane Cove
NSW 2006
Australia

ISBN 07496 3227 5

Dewey Decimal Classification 941.01
A CIP record for this book is
available from the British Library

Printed at Oriental Press, Dubai, U.A.E.

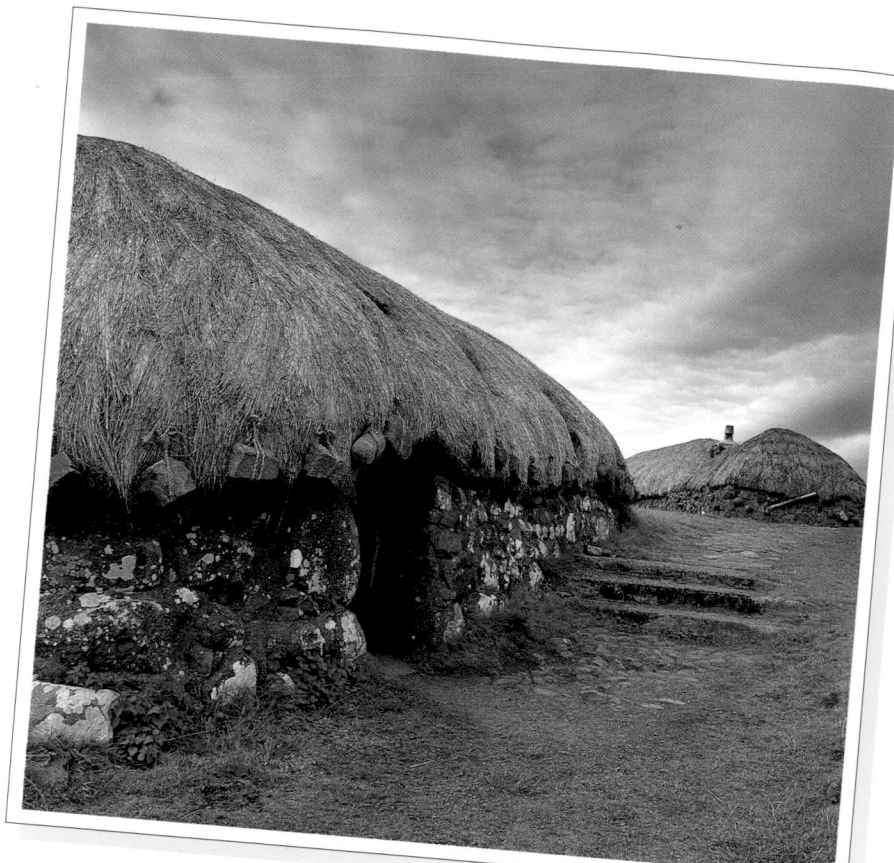

Planning and production by Discovery Books Ltd
Editor: Helena Attlee
Design: Simon Borrough
Consultant: Tim Copeland
Artwork: Stuart Carter, Mike Lacey,
Stefan Chabluk

Photographs: All pictures are by Alex Ramsay
except: Lesley & Roy Adkins Picture Library:
pages 11 (bottom), 19 (bottom); The British
Museum: pages 5 (both), 14 (left), 17 (bottom), 23,
26 (top); Colchester Archaeological Trust: 24-25
(all); Colchester Museums: page 21 (bottom);
Crown Copyright: reproduced by permission of
Historic Scotland: 12-13, 13, 17 (top); The Scottish
Crannog Centre/Barry Andrian: 14-15 (main
picture), 15; The Stock Market: page 27.

CONTENTS

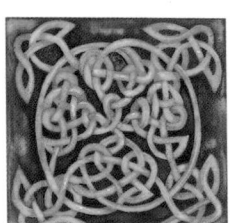

WHO WERE THE CELTS?

Two thousand years ago, Britain was home to a people called the Celts. There were Celts in many parts of Europe.

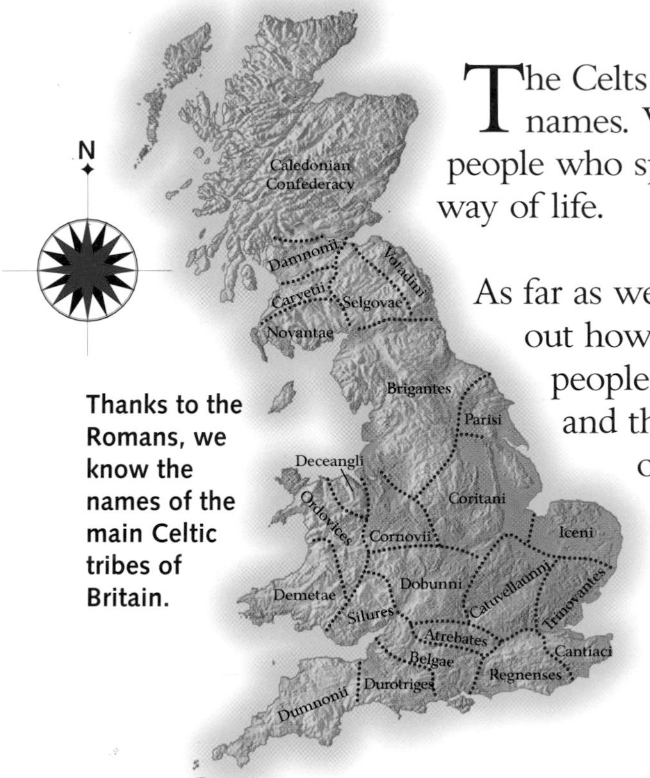

The Celts belonged to many different tribes with different names. We use the name 'Celt' as a label to describe people who spoke similar languages and followed the same way of life.

As far as we know, the Celts did not write books. To find out how they lived, we rely on the writings of other people, especially the Romans. The Romans visited and then invaded Britain, and they wrote descriptions of what they saw. The problem with Roman writers is that they looked down on the Celts as backward savages, so their accounts were not always accurate. Luckily, we have another way of finding out about Celtic life in Britain, through archaeology.

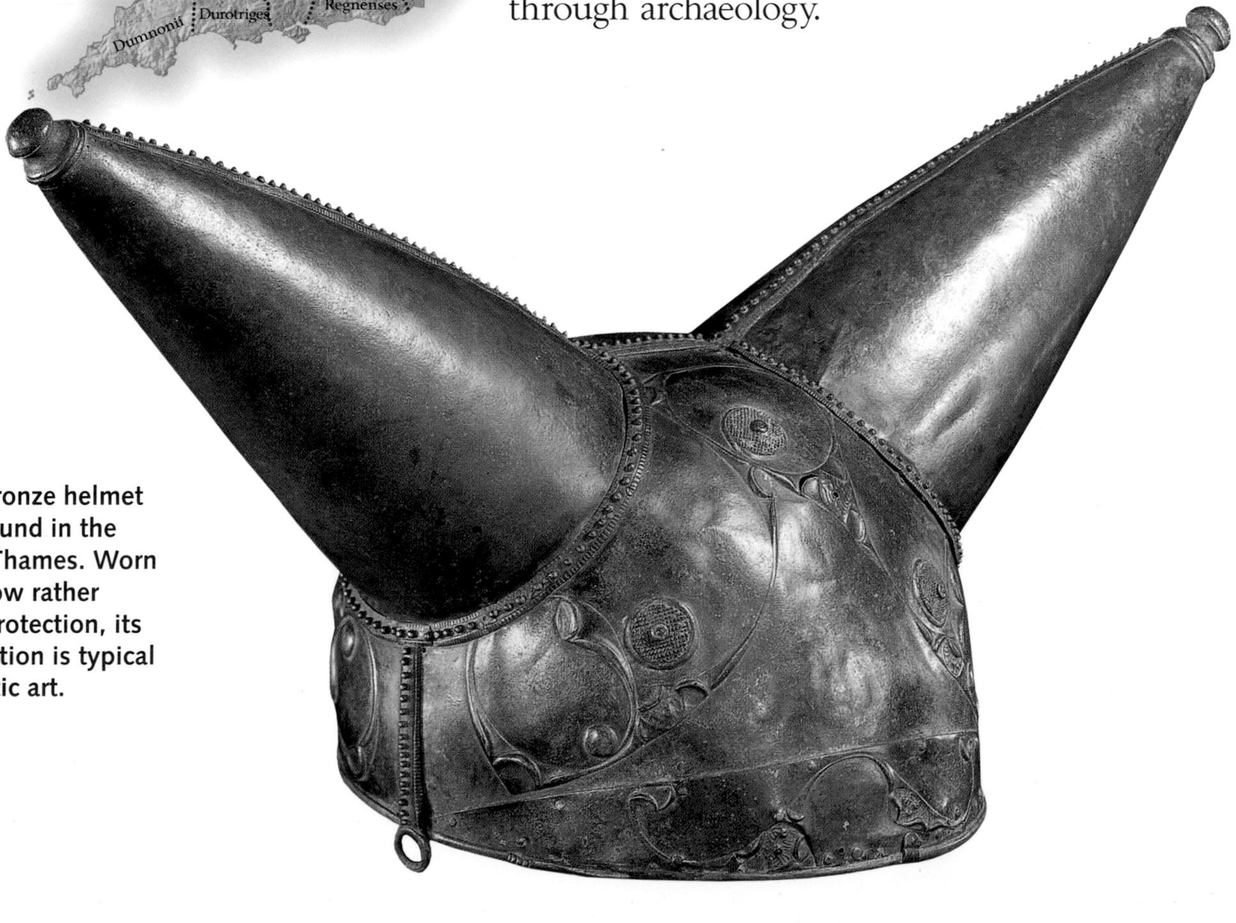

Thanks to the Romans, we know the names of the main Celtic tribes of Britain.

This bronze helmet was found in the River Thames. Worn for show rather than protection, its decoration is typical of Celtic art.

4

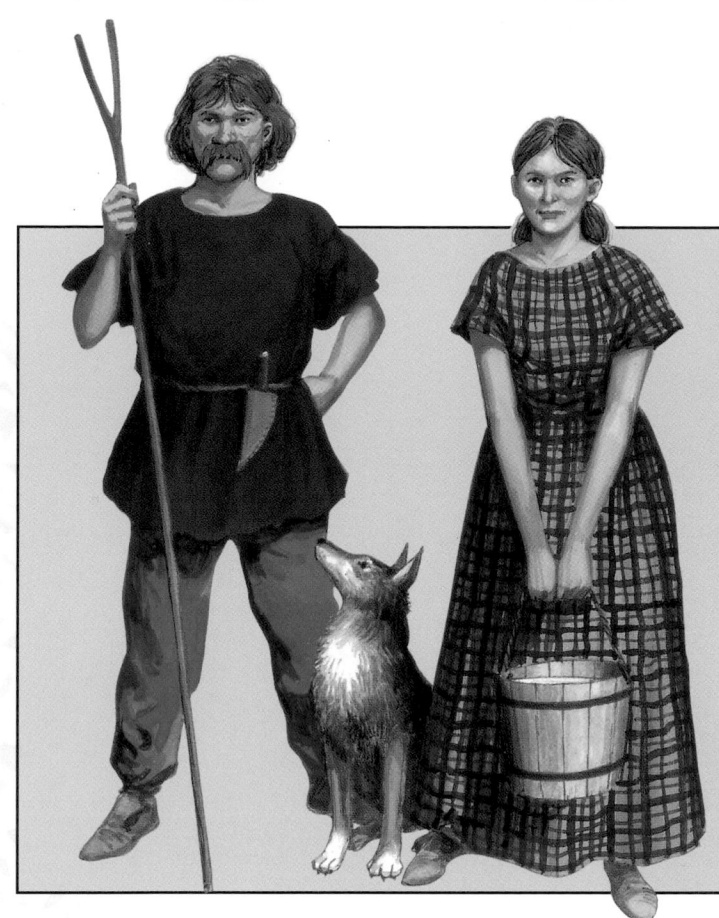

CELTIC CLOTHES

The Celts wore striking clothing, with shirts and trousers dyed in various colours. They used brooches or belts to secure their clothes. Diodorus of Sicily was a Greek who lived in the Roman Empire. He described the Celts in these words: 'Some of the men shave the beard, but let the moustache grow until it covers the mouth. When they are eating, they often get their food tangled in their moustaches!'

Archaeology is the study of things left behind by people who lived in the past. The Celts of Britain have left all sorts of evidence for archaeologists to study.

There are Celtic hill-forts, chalk pictures on hillsides and the remains of buildings. There are also many chance finds of beautiful Celtic metalwork, from rivers and fields.

GAMES

Rich Celts relaxed by playing board games. These glass gaming pieces were found in a chieftain's grave at Welwyn. They were probably used in games like draughts.

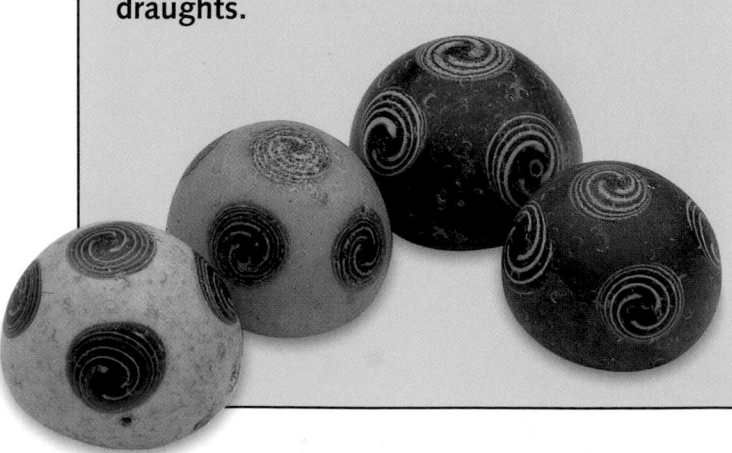

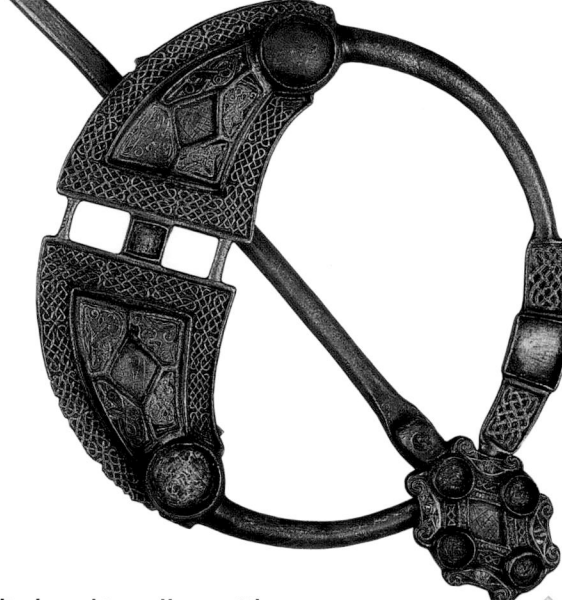

The Celts loved jewellery with inlaid patterns. This brooch was used to fasten a cloak.

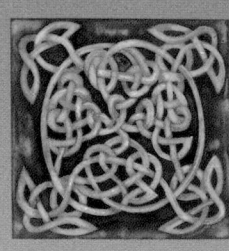

CELTIC DEFENCES

The most spectacular remains of the Celts are the hundreds of hill-forts that they built in many parts of Britain.

Although they are called 'forts', they were more like defended villages, or small towns. Inside, there were often dozens of round-houses (see page 9).

Maiden Castle in Dorset is one of the biggest hill-forts in Britain. It has massive defences made up of a series of tall earth banks and deep ditches. Archaeologists have discovered that the banks originally measured 25m from top to bottom. The ditches were even deeper than they are today.

The fact that people needed to build such strong defences shows us that warfare between the tribes was common. We are also told

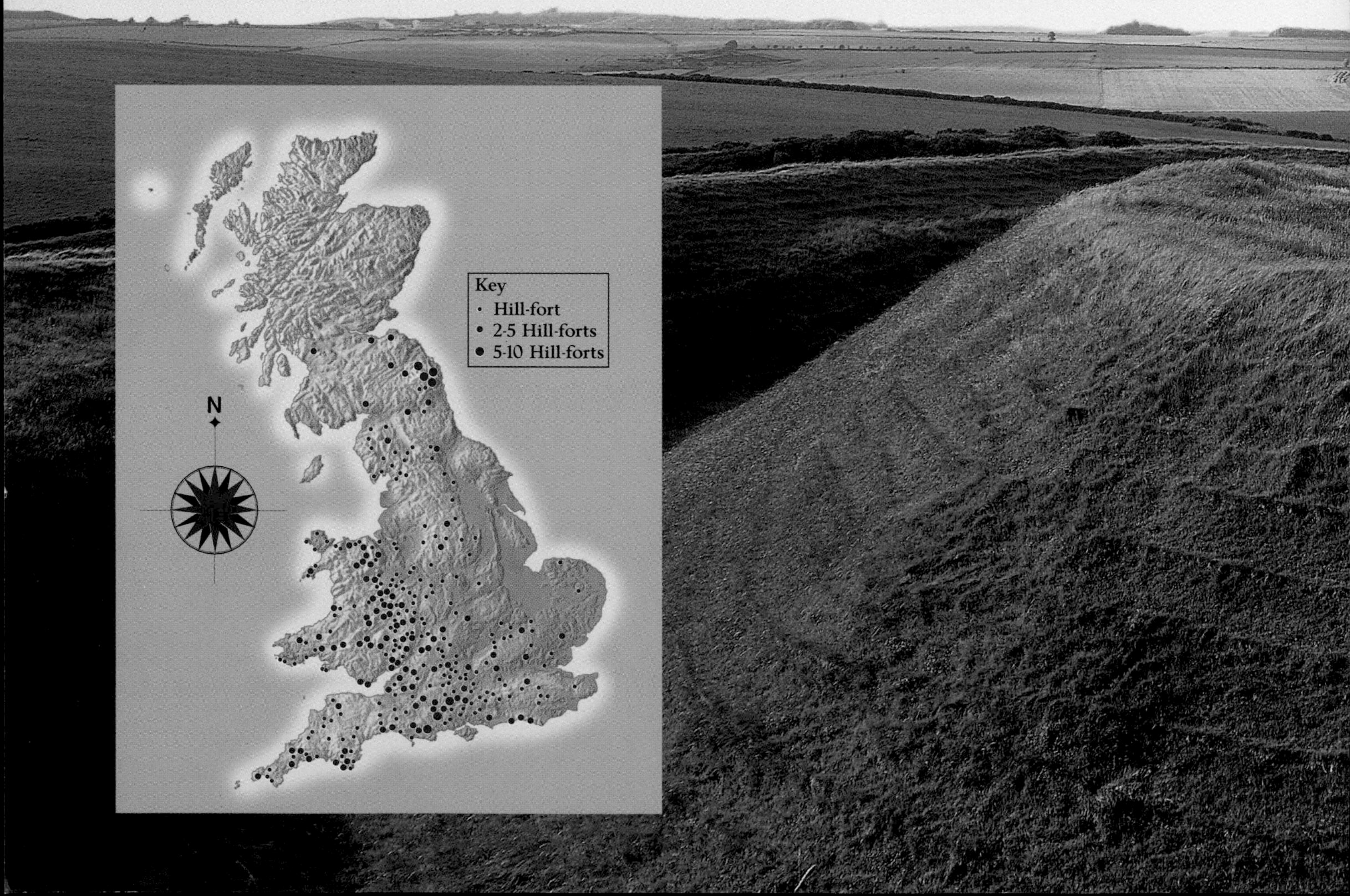

Imagine trying to run up the banks at Maiden Castle with a hail of pebbles pouring down on you. This fort must have been very difficult for enemies to storm.

Key
· Hill-fort
• 2-5 Hill-forts
● 5-10 Hill-forts

N

this by Strabo, a Roman writer who said of the Celts, 'the whole race is war-mad, high-spirited and quick for battle.'

Archaeologists also discovered a pit holding more than 20 thousand pebbles at Maiden Castle. All the pebbles had been brought up to the castle from the seashore and so they must have had a special use. They were probably used as ammunition to fire out of a leather sling at attackers.

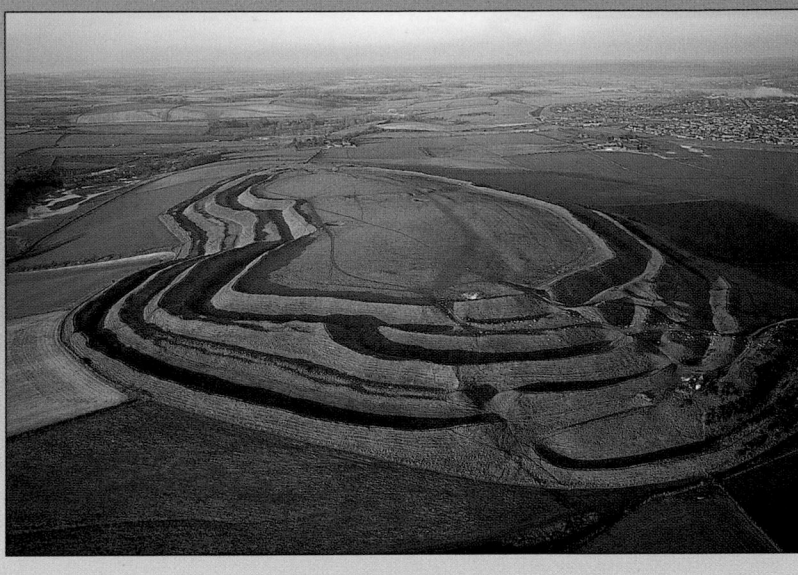

This picture shows what the whole of Maiden Castle looks like.

At the hill-forts of Bredon Hill in Worcestershire and Stanwick in Yorkshire, archaeologists have found collections of human skulls. They may have been collected as trophies by the winners of a battle.

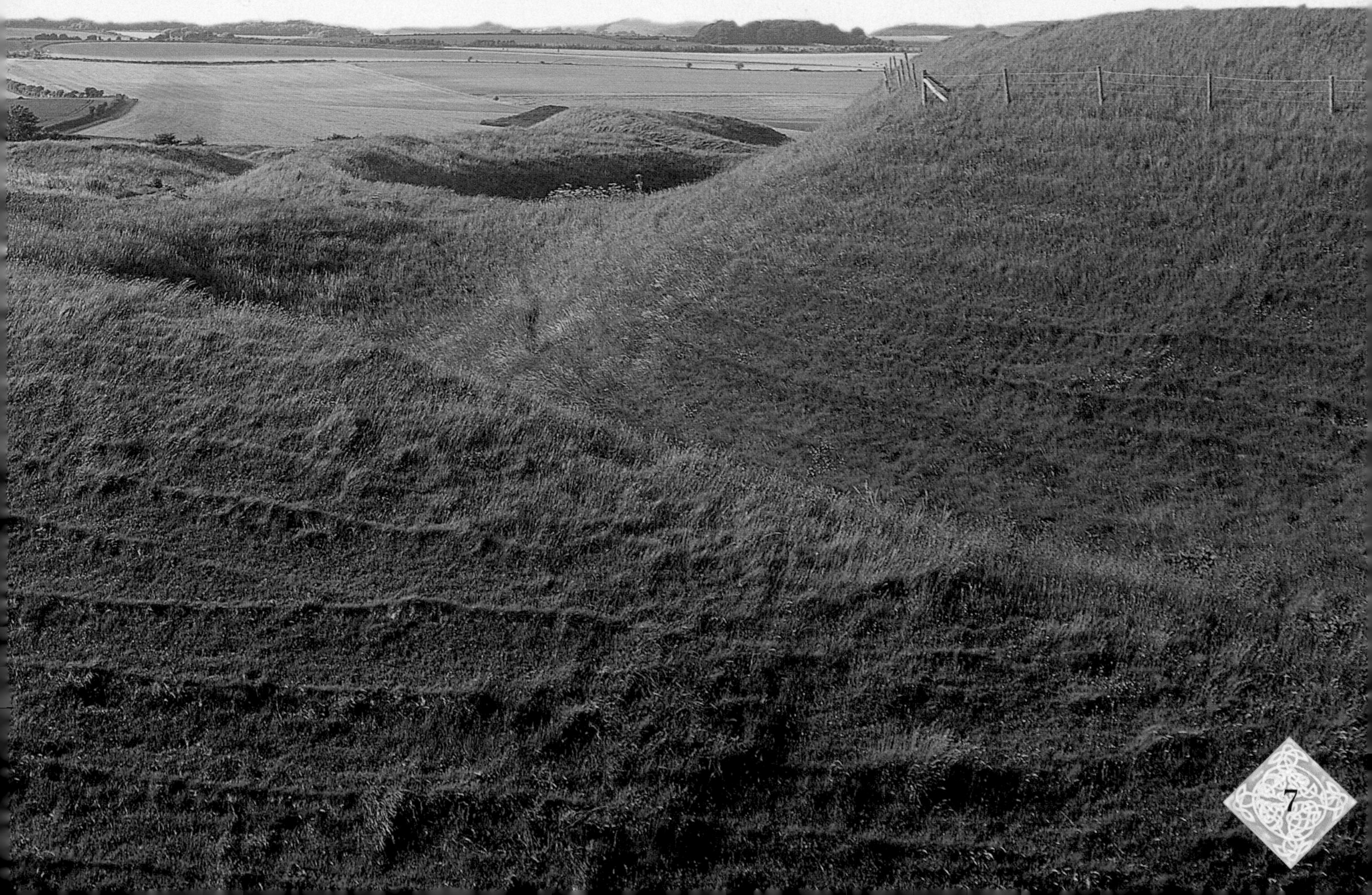

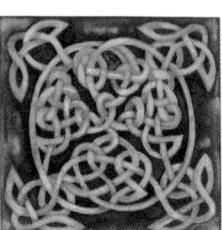

WOODEN DWELLINGS

In Celtic times, the south and east of Britain was thickly wooded. The Celts of the lowlands used wood to build their homes.

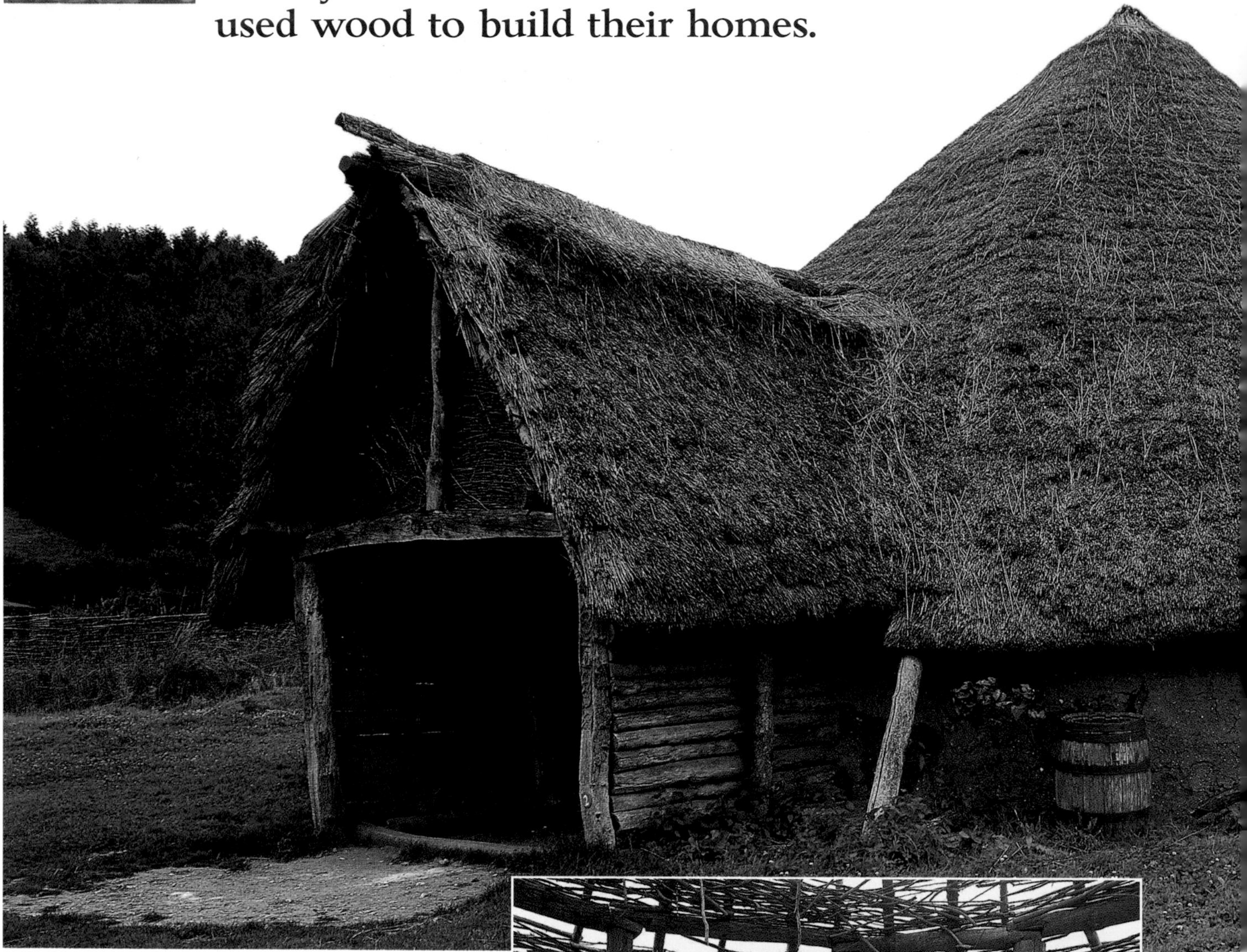

Wooden buildings rot. Usually the only traces of Celtic houses are the holes left by the wooden posts that held them up. By studying the size and position of the post-holes, archaeologists can imagine what the building once looked like.

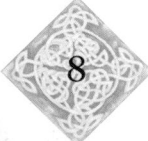

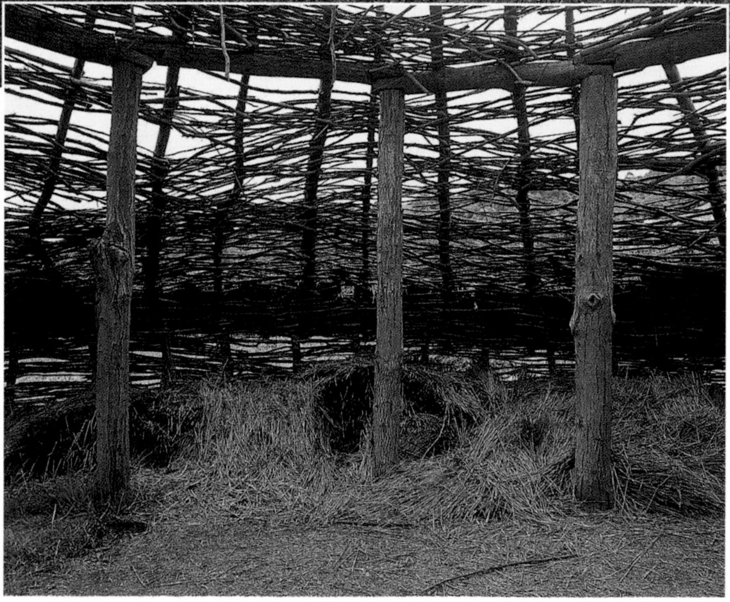

8

Here you can see the posts that held up the enormous sloping roof.

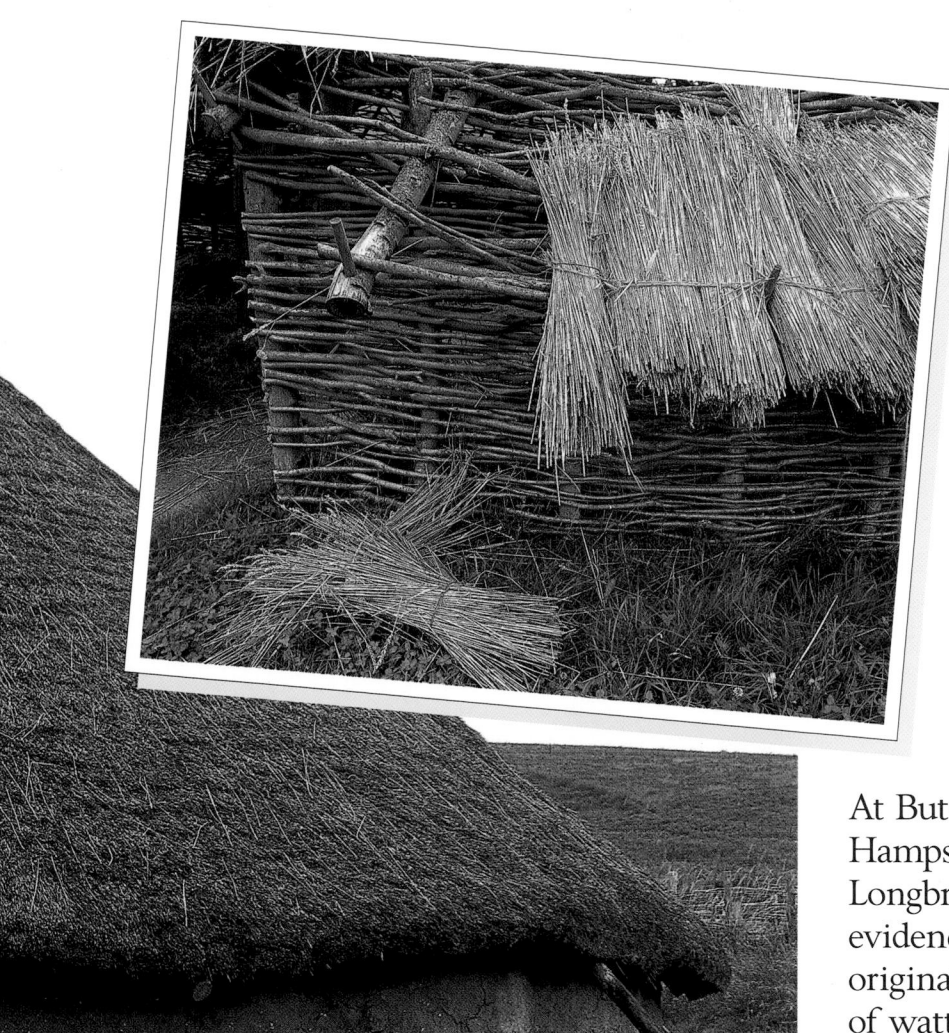

The roof was thatched with straw, from wheat grown on the farm.

In 1960, a Celtic house was discovered in Wiltshire, at Longbridge Deverill Cow Down. The house had burned down, leaving the blackened bases of the posts visible in the ground. The circular building was 15m in diameter, which makes it the biggest Celtic house ever found in Britain. Its size suggests that it must have been the home of someone rich and powerful.

At Butser Ancient Farm, in Hampshire, they have rebuilt the Longbridge round-house, using the evidence that they found on the original site. The outer wall is made of wattle which is plastered with mud, to keep the wind out. The tall sloping roof has been thatched. It took 15 tonnes of straw to cover it.

◀ This is a modern reconstruction of a Celtic round-house, at Butser Ancient Farm in Hampshire.

COOKING

The Celts cooked their meals on an open fire in the centre of their homes. Archaeologists have found a lot of evidence of Celtic cooking, including hearths, animal bones, burnt grains, and bronze and iron cooking pots still coated with soot from the fire.

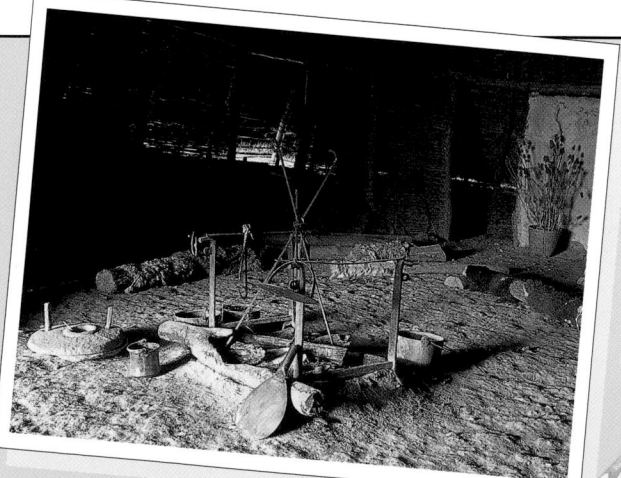

The hearth at Butser.

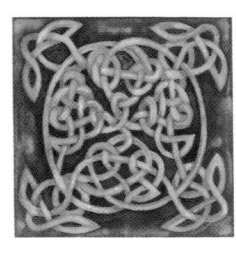

STONE SETTLEMENTS

On high ground or moorland there are few trees. Celts living in these places built their homes from stone rather than wood.

Here you can see one of the rooms in a house at Chysauster, with the courtyard behind.

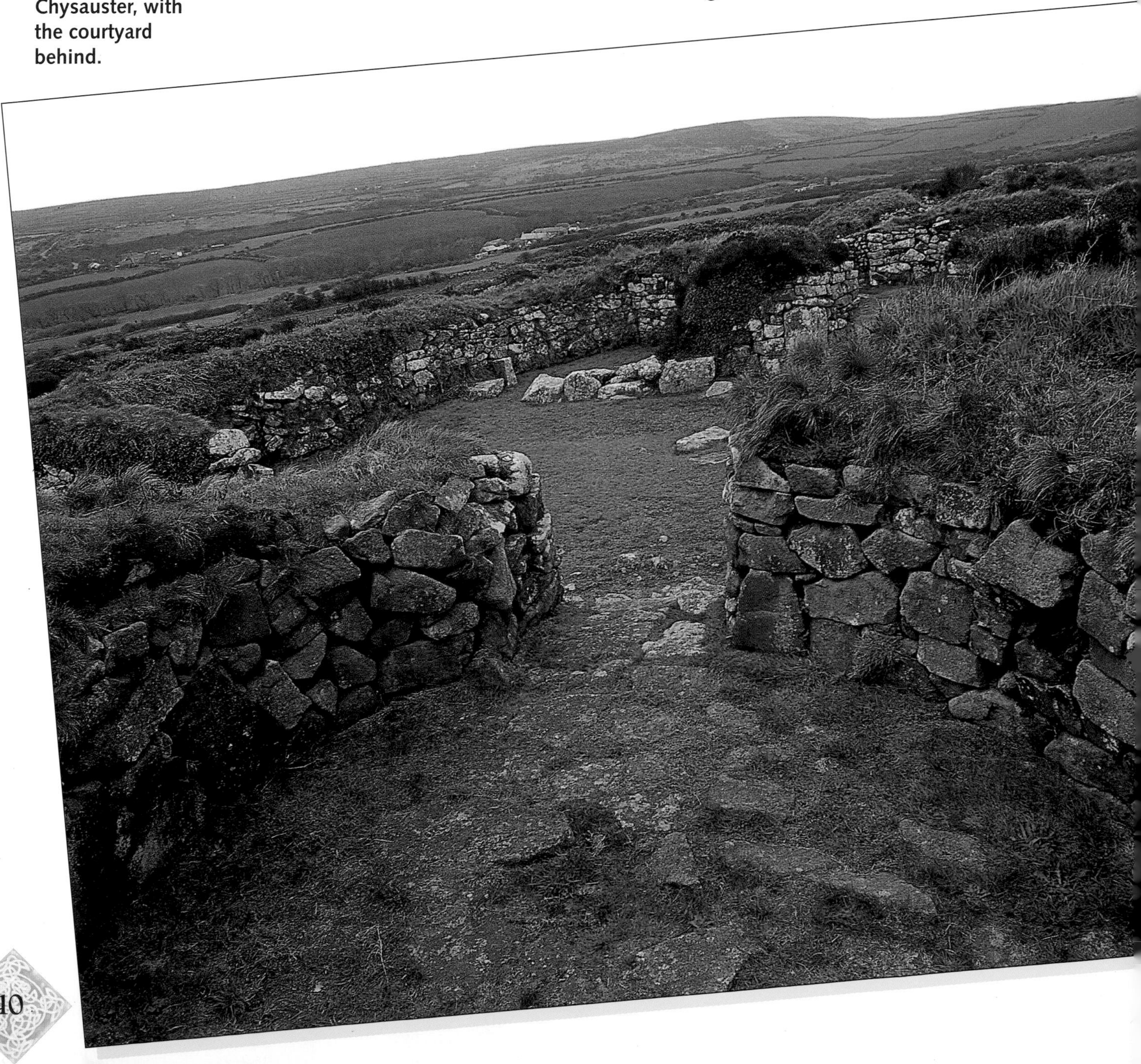

At Chysauster, on the windswept moors of Cornwall, you can visit a Celtic village with nine stone houses. Although the roofs of the houses have disappeared, the walls are still between two and three metres high.

Each house has a central courtyard, with rooms off it, surrounded by a massive wall. The thick wall provided shelter and protection for the people and their animals. A long entrance passage faces east or north-east, away from the usual direction of the wind.

In the middle of some rooms, there is a stone with a hole in it. This was a socket for the pole which held up the roof. Each room was like a separate hut with its own tall roof, thatched with straw or covered with grassy turves. The family probably lived in one room, while other rooms were used for the farm animals and for storing food.

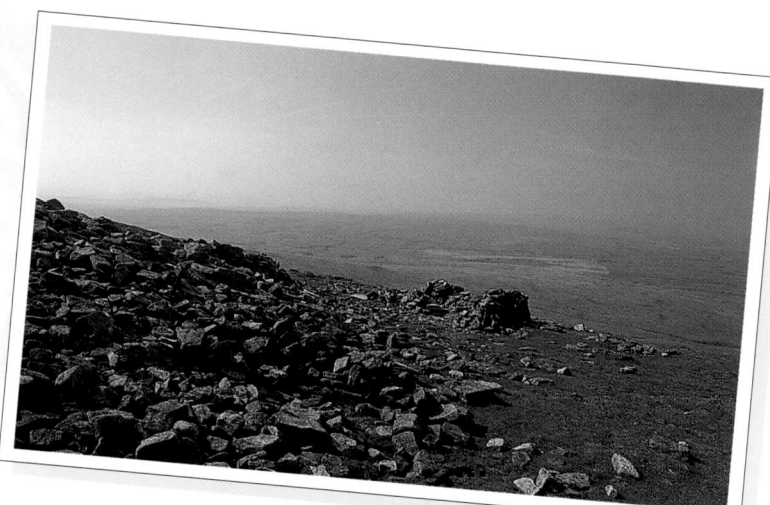

Ingleborough was the site of several stone houses. Unlike wood, stones do not rot away. They provide vital clues for archaeologists.

Ingleborough in Yorkshire is the highest hill-fort in the country. There are no trees in this area, but there was plenty of stone that the Celts could use to make houses. The remains of twenty round-houses have been found. The wood for making roofs had to be carried all the way up from the valley below.

SPINNING WOOL

Celtic clothes were usually made from wool. In Celtic houses, archaeologists often find small round weights, made of bone, clay or stone, with a hole through the middle. These are 'spindle whorls' and they were used for spinning wool. Each whorl was fastened to the end of a stick, called a spindle. Wool was tied to the spindle, which was then spun in the air, twisting it into thread.

This woman is on a reconstructed Celtic site. She is dressed as a Celt, and has learned to spin wool using a weighted spindle.

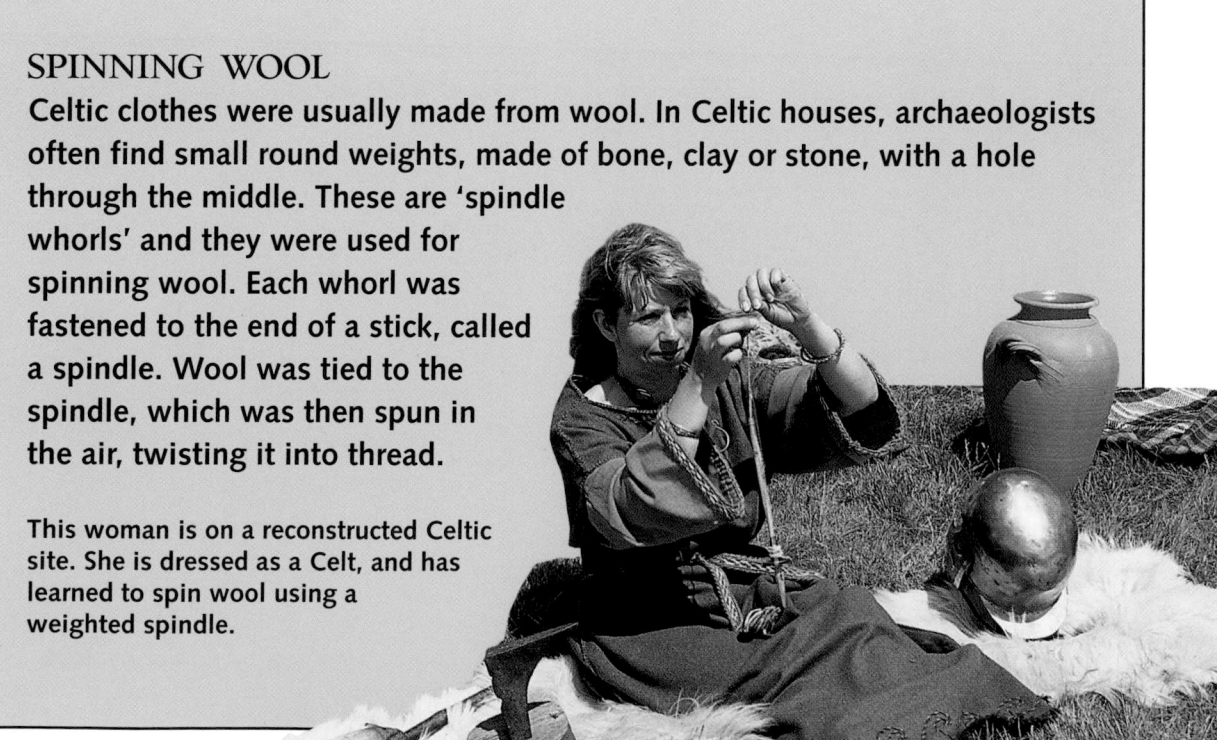

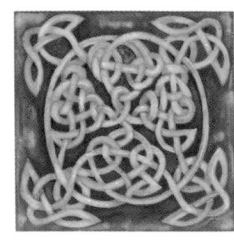

CELTIC TOWERS

In the north of Scotland and on the Scottish islands, people built stone tower-houses for themselves called brochs.

This broch is at Dun Carloway on the island of Lewis. You can see that it has an inner and an outer wall, with a space in between. There are stairs inside the space, leading to upper levels. Inside the broch, a ledge sticks out of the wall about 2m above the ground. This may have supported an upper floor or a walkway.

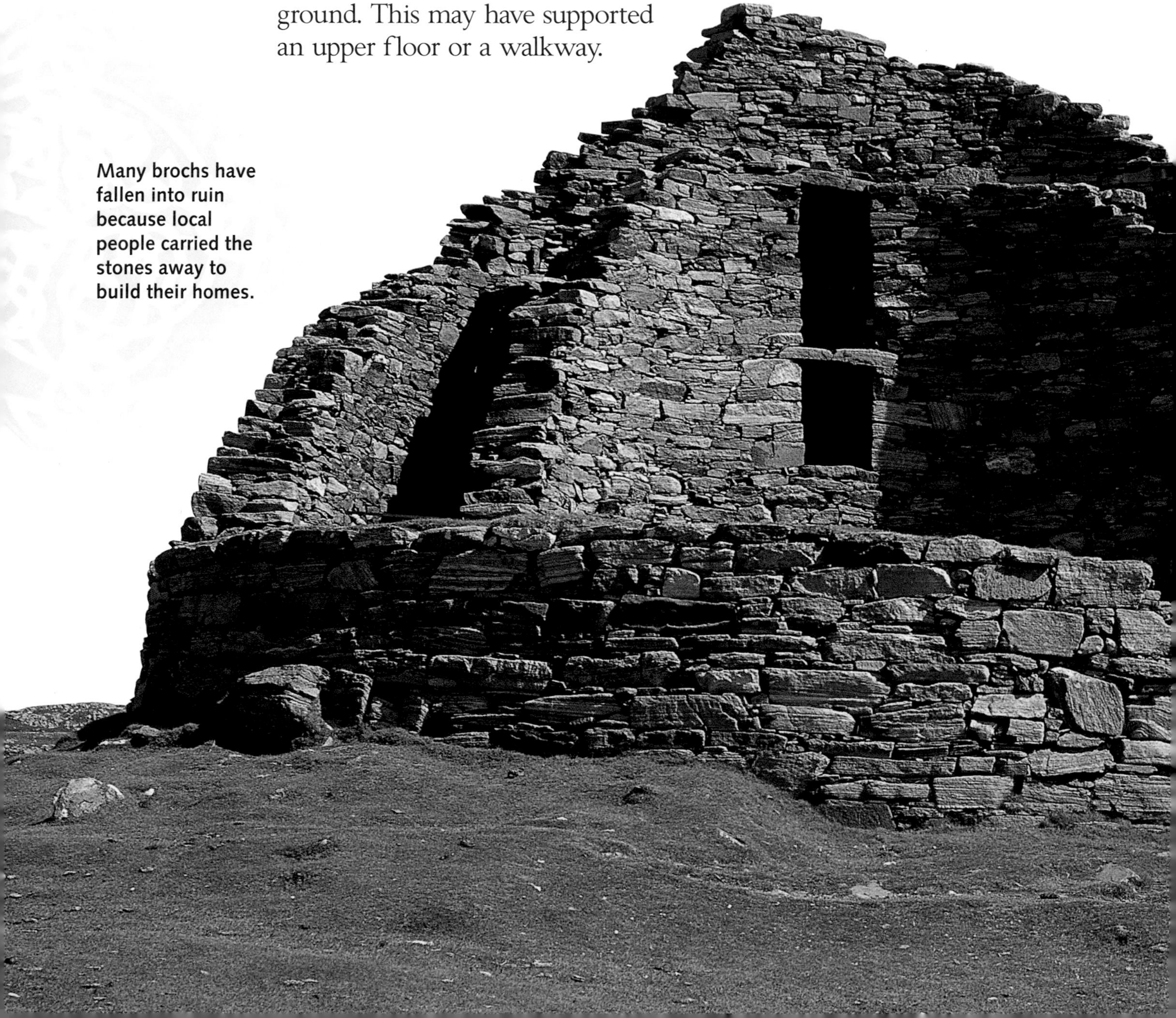

Many brochs have fallen into ruin because local people carried the stones away to build their homes.

The best preserved broch is on Mousa, a tiny island off Shetland. It is 13m high with curving sides - a sturdy shape. With only one little door as an outside opening, the people who lived here were well-protected against attack. The houses must have been very dark inside.

Archaeologists can only guess at how the brochs were used. Some believe that the ground floor was used for storage and for sheltering animals in winter. They think that people lived on the upper floor. No one can be sure of the truth and there is still a lot of disagreement among archaeologists about the way that the Scottish Celts lived in their brochs.

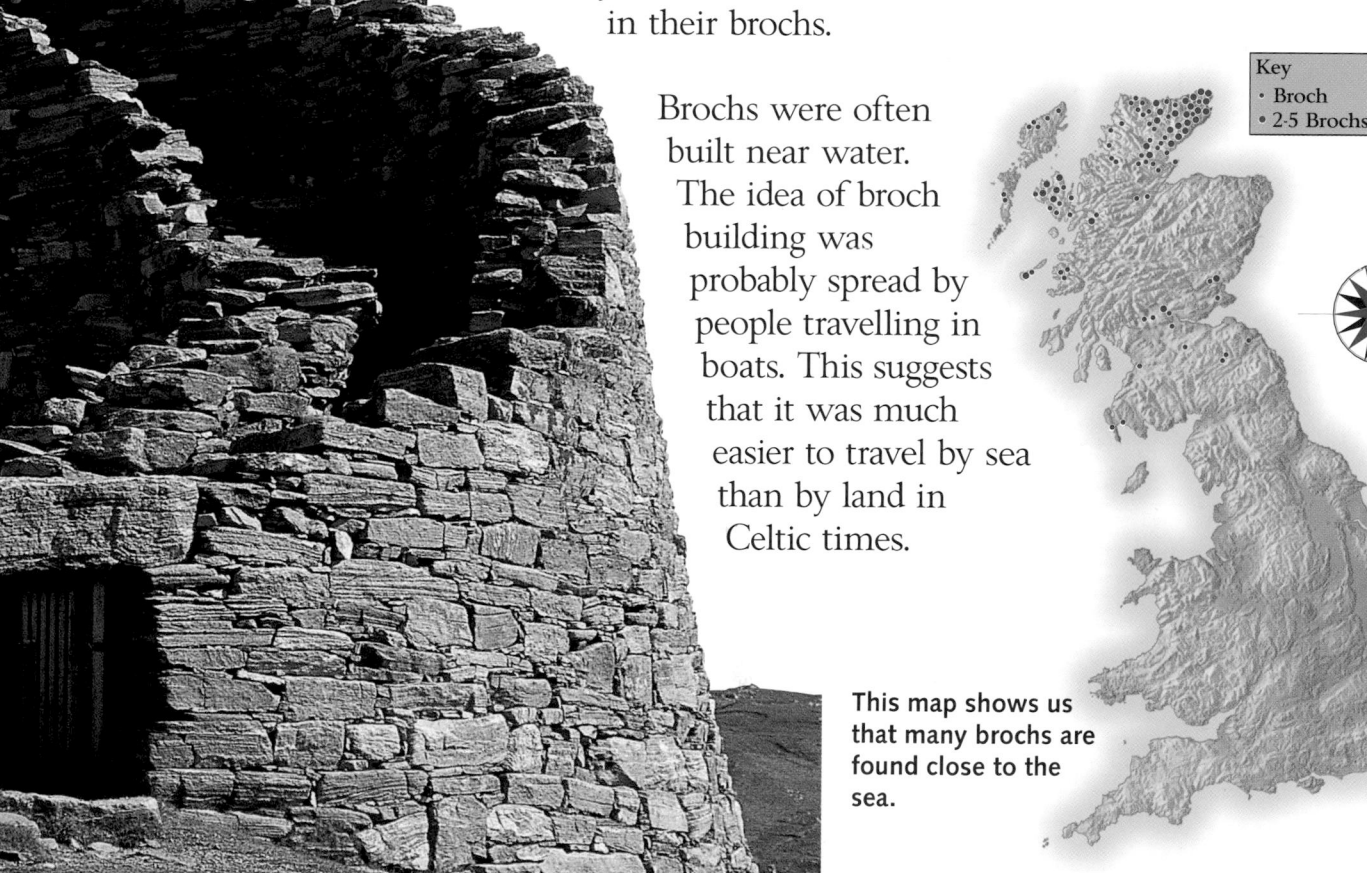

The Mousa broch is one of the best preserved ancient buildings in Britain.

Brochs were often built near water. The idea of broch building was probably spread by people travelling in boats. This suggests that it was much easier to travel by sea than by land in Celtic times.

Key
· Broch
● 2-5 Brochs

N

This map shows us that many brochs are found close to the sea.

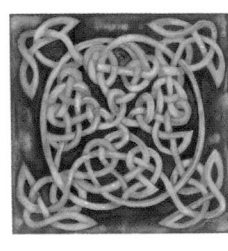

LIVING ON WATER

Brochs were not the only strange structures lived in by the Celts. In the Scottish Highlands, some people lived on artificial islands called crannogs.

There were once 18 crannogs on Loch Tay. Now they have all sunk below the water or become overgrown with plants. Archaeologists have spent many years finding the crannogs and studying them. They often had to work under the water, which was very difficult and uncomfortable.

By studying the evidence, archaeologists have learned that the crannogs were made by driving wooden posts into the bottom of the loch. Rocks, branches and turf were dropped between the posts. These formed a solid base for the crannog.

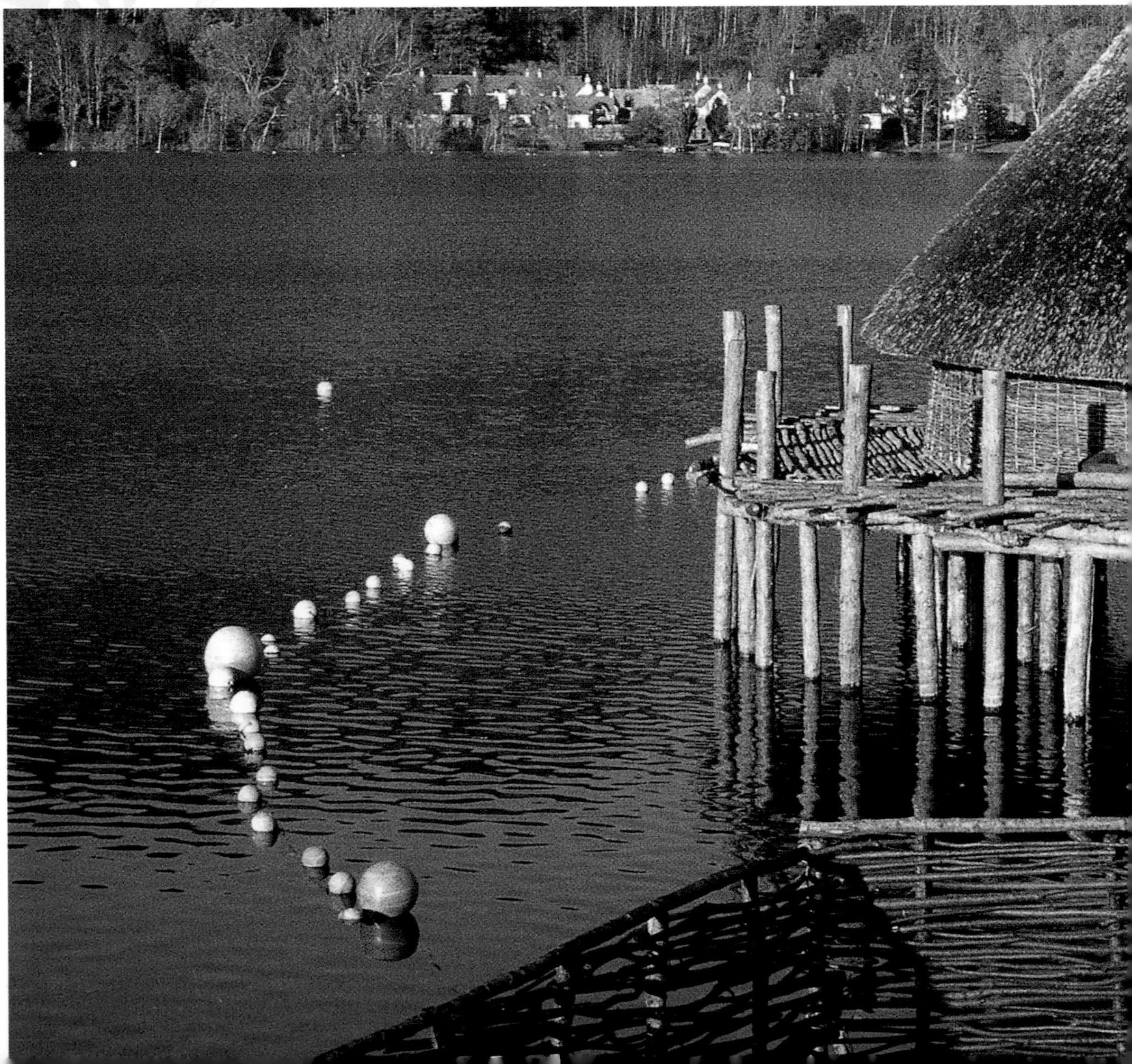

This is a modern reconstruction of a crannog on Loch Tay.

Between 1995 and 1996, a team of archaeologists built their own crannog on the loch. They spent a year building the base. Then they built a big round-house on top.

Archaeologists wanted to find out why the Celts went to so much trouble to live on water. One possible reason was for protection from attack, either by other people or by wild animals. Wolves and bears still roamed Britain in those days. Also, the crannog house stands out against the water. The people who lived in such a place may have wanted to show their neighbours that they were rich and important.

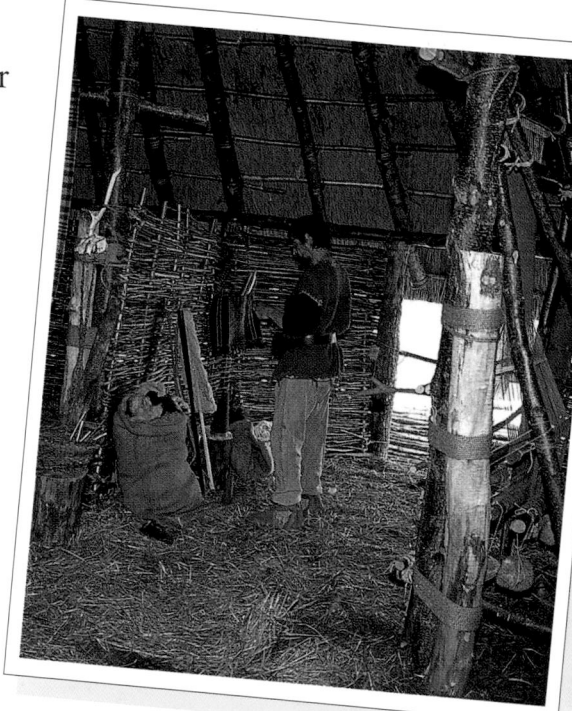

▲ The archaeologists have filled the crannog with reconstructions of household items, including a loom for spinning wool, on the right.

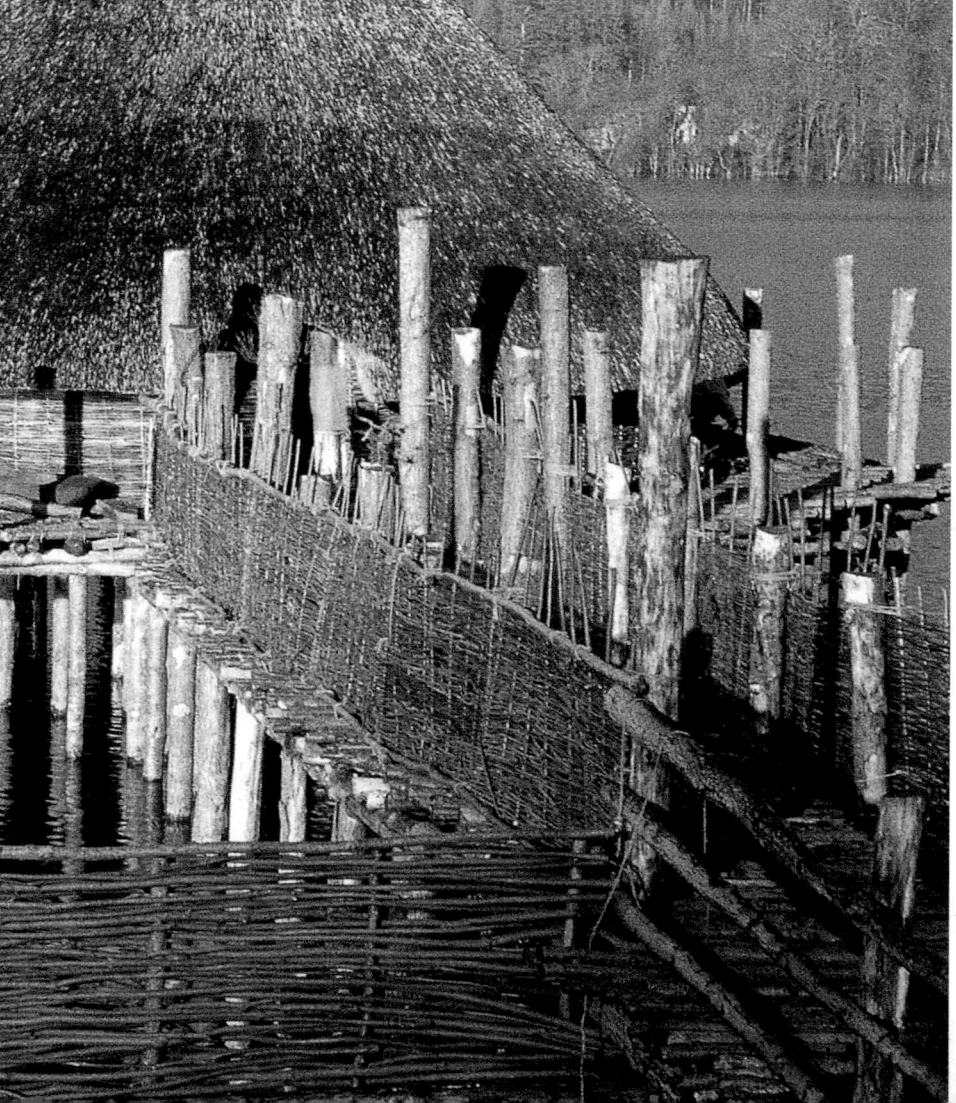

Wood can last for thousands of years under water. Many wooden objects were found in Loch Tay. The biggest was a boat which had been hollowed out of an oak tree. Grains, seeds, nuts and animal droppings were also found. Archaeologists have been able to use this evidence to find out about the food the Celts ate and the kinds of animals they kept. They even found a broken butter dish with the greasy remains of butter in it.

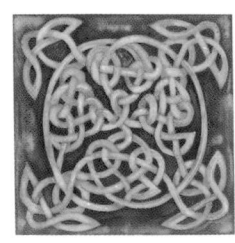

MYSTERIOUS TUNNELS

In Cornwall, stone-lined tunnels called 'fogous' are often found beside Celtic houses. They are also found in Scotland, where they are known as 'souterrains'.

This fogou at Boleigh in Cornwall is 12m long and 1.5m wide, with a small L-shaped side-passage. People went to a lot of trouble to build it, so it must have had an important use. Unfortunately, nobody knows what that use was. It is too dark and cramped to live in.

One idea is that the fogou was a place to hide if the settlement was attacked, but the entrance is very easy to find. Anyone hiding inside would have been trapped by their enemies.

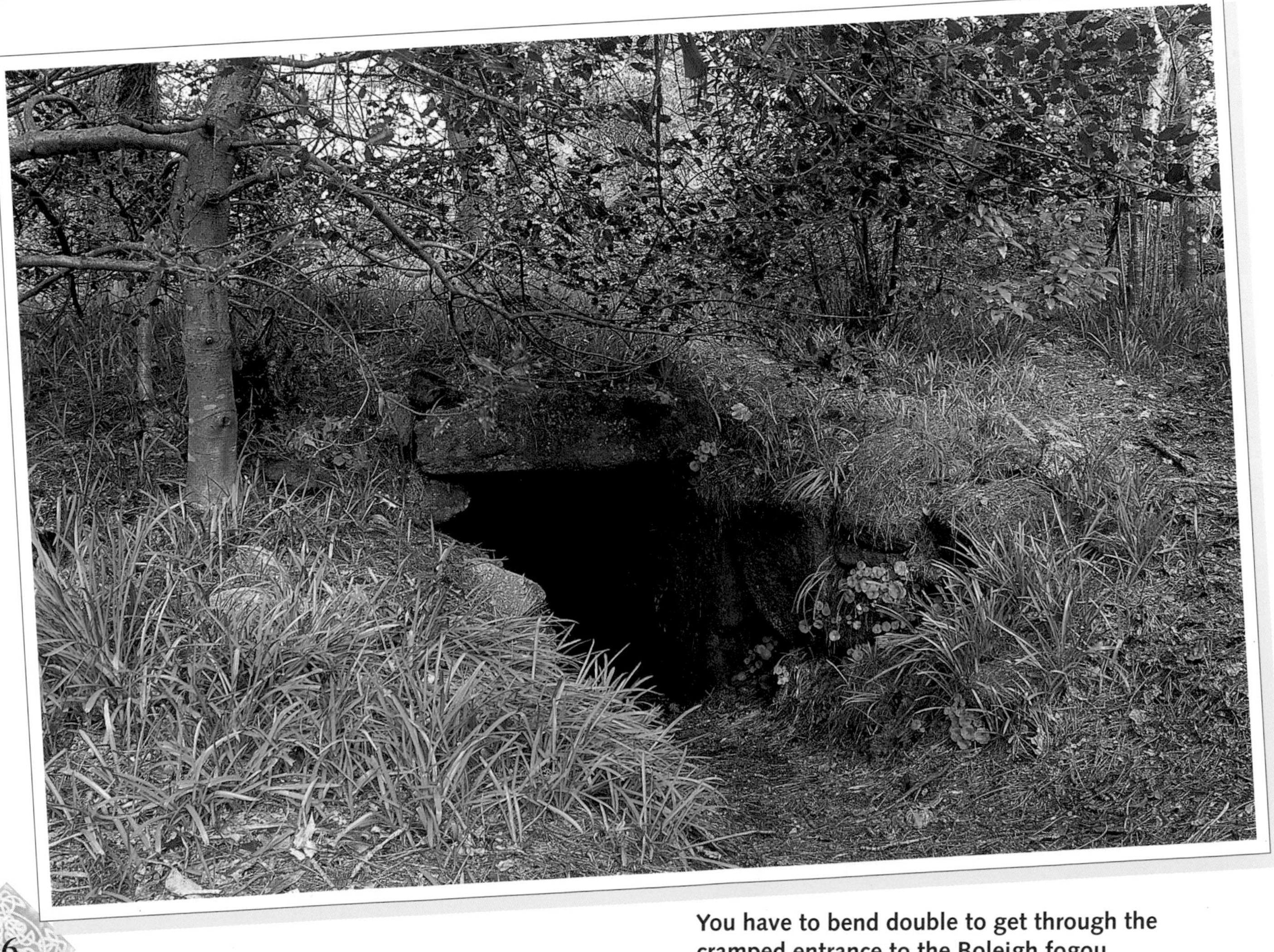

You have to bend double to get through the cramped entrance to the Boleigh fogou.

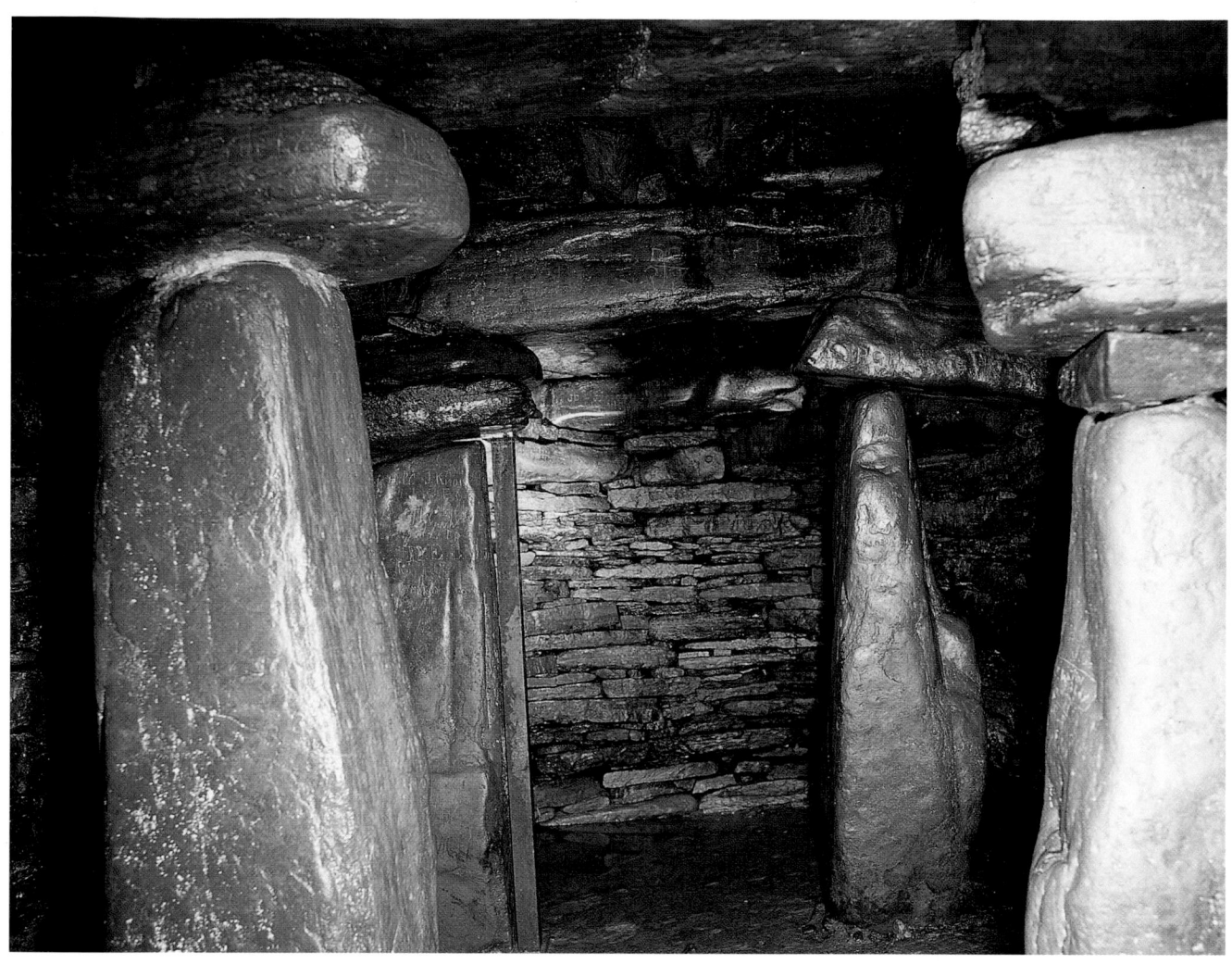

This is a Scottish stone tunnel, or souterrain, on Orkney.

Some people think that fogous were built for religious reasons. The Celts believed in gods who lived beneath the earth. Perhaps the fogou was a way of getting closer to the gods.

Many archaeologists believe that fogous were used for storage. A cool, dark tunnel would have been a good place to keep milk, cheese and grain.

TIN

The people who lived at Boleigh were farmers, like most Celts, but they had another way to make a living. They traded in tin, which they found lying in the local streams. Tin was valuable because it is only found in small areas of Britain. It was mixed with copper to make bronze, the metal used by the Celts for helmets, shields, mirrors and other decorative work.

A decorated bronze mirror. The other side was polished until it reflected the owner's face.

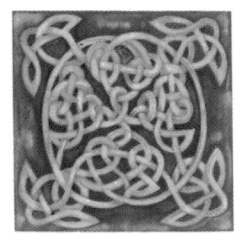

FARMING

Most Celtic people lived by farming. They grew their crops in small square fields, ploughing them using teams of oxen.

Like Celtic fields, the fields at Butser are small and square.

Butser Ancient Farm in Hampshire is a working farm, where crops are still being grown using Celtic methods. They grow wheat, barley, oats, peas and beans. We know that these were grown by the Celts because of finds of burnt grains and seeds in archaeological digs.

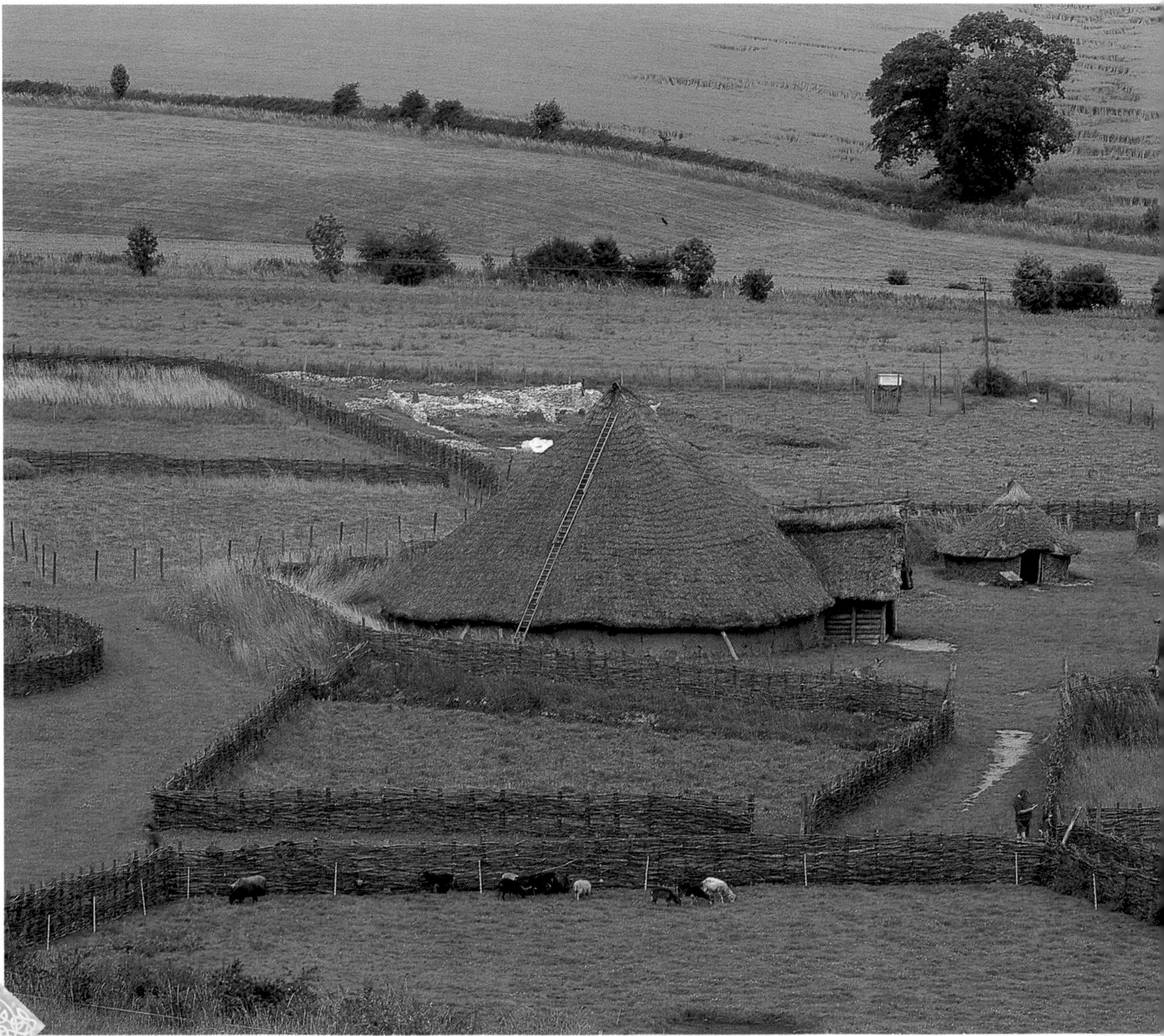

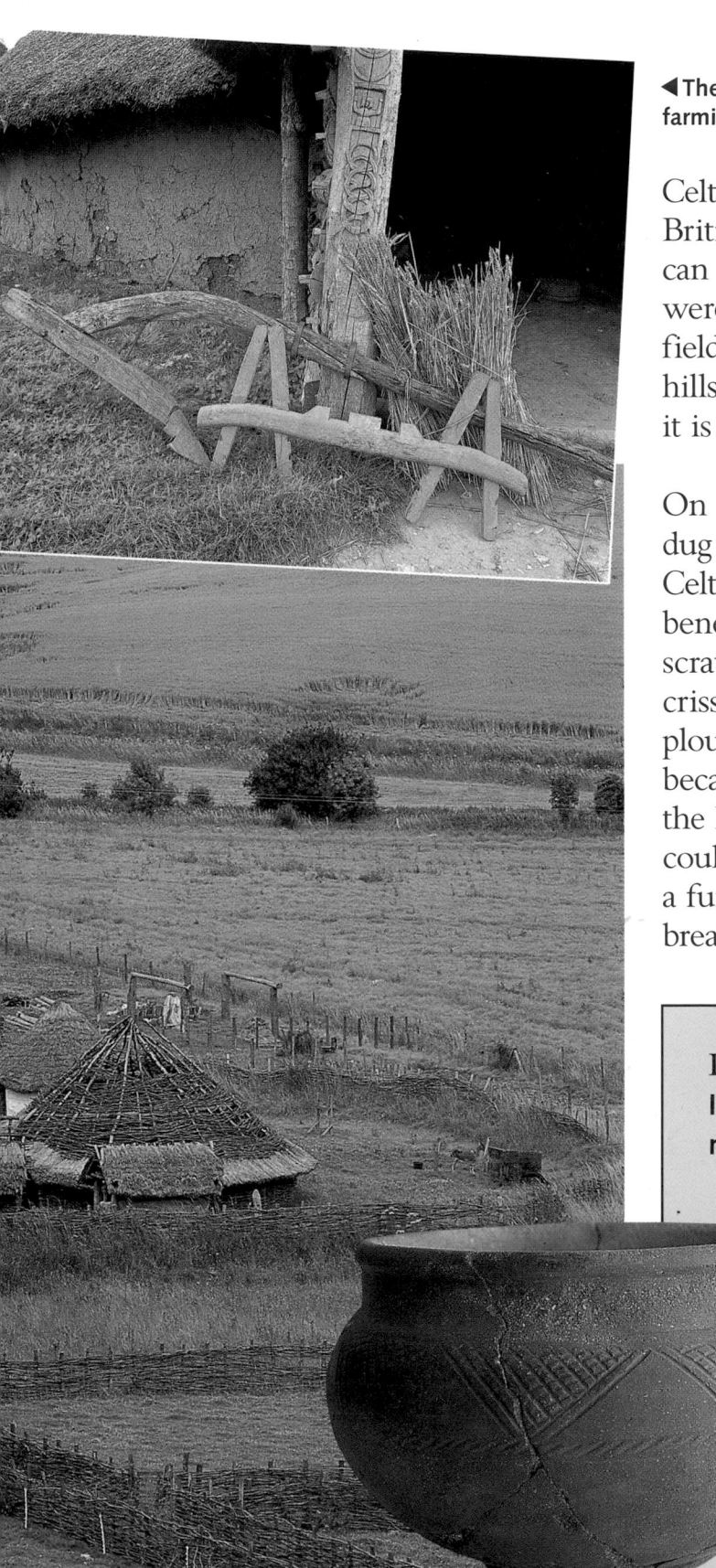

◄ The Butser farmers use reconstructions of Celtic farming tools, such as this wooden plough.

Celtic farming has left traces all over the British countryside. On many hillsides, you can see earth banks, called 'lynchets'. They were made by Celtic farmers, ploughing the fields. Gradually, soil slipped down the hillside to the lower edge of the field, where it is built up forming the bank.

On the chalk downlands, archaeologists have dug under Celtic fields and found signs of Celtic ploughing. The chalk surface, just beneath the soil, was scored with lines, scratched by ploughs. The lines were in a criss-cross pattern, showing that the farmers ploughed each field twice. They did this because they only had a light plough. Unlike the heavier plough used by later farmers, it could not turn over the soil, it just scratched a furrow. The Celts had to plough twice to break up the soil properly.

POTTERY

In the first century BC, the Celts learned to make pots by spinning them on a wheel – an idea brought across the sea from mainland Europe. We know this because they began to produce curved pots with a smooth finish. Previously, all pots had been shaped by hand. This did not produce as fine a finish.

This Celtic pot was made on a wheel. It was found in Somerset.

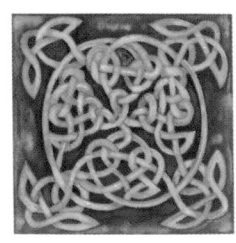

CHALK FIGURES

Chalk lies just beneath the green turf on many British hills. The Celts used the chalk to make huge white pictures on the hillsides.

One of the best chalk pictures lies just below a Celtic hill-fort, at Uffington in Oxfordshire. It shows a great white horse, 111m long. Seen from a distance, the horse looks as if it is galloping across the hills.

At Cerne Abbas in Dorset, you can see a chalk picture of a giant holding a club. At Wilmington in Sussex, there is a man holding two long poles. Nobody knows who made these pictures, or why they did it. Perhaps they were a warning to people from other tribes to stay away. Perhaps they were made to please the gods.

▼ This is how the Uffington White Horse looks from a distance.

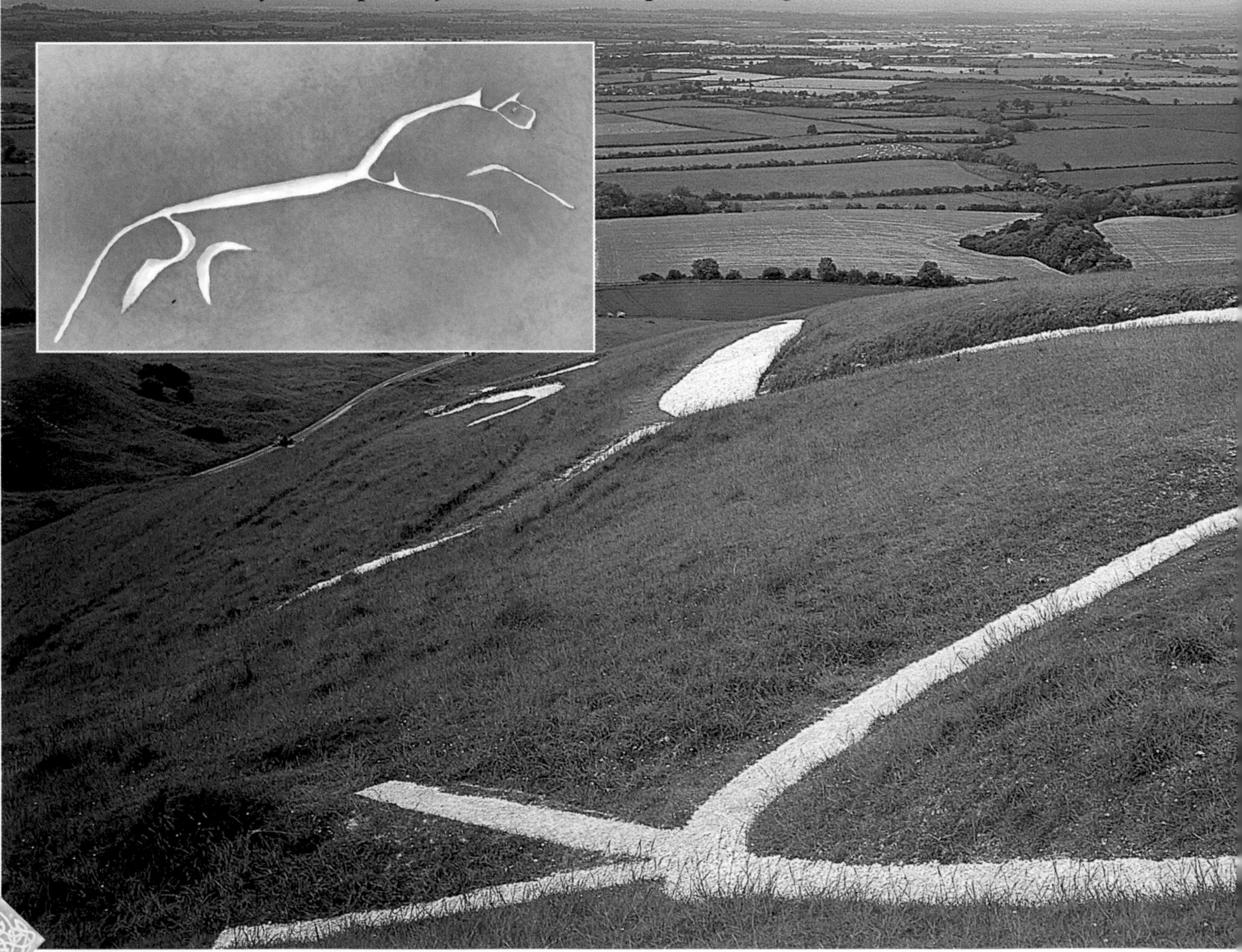

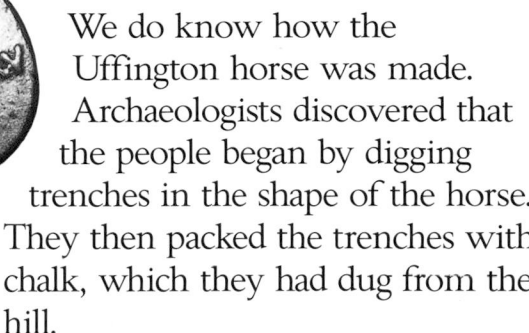

▼ This is the head of the White Horse, with its eye in the centre.

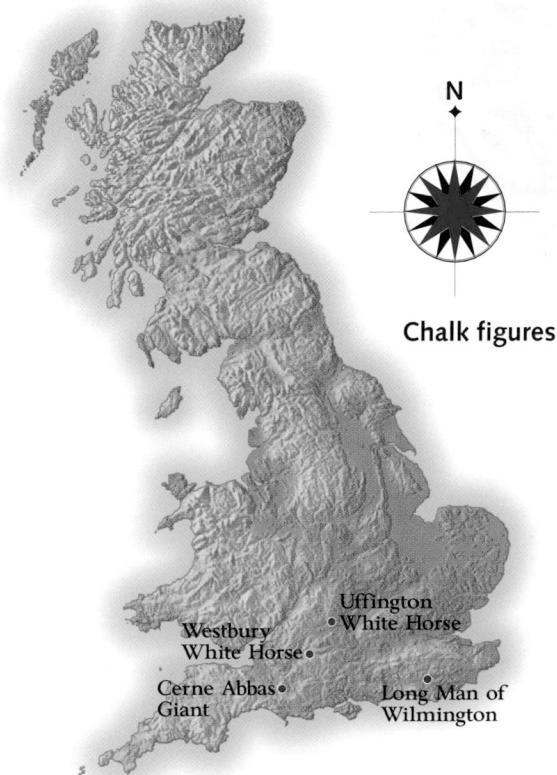

We do know how the Uffington horse was made. Archaeologists discovered that the people began by digging trenches in the shape of the horse. They then packed the trenches with chalk, which they had dug from the hill.

A new scientific method has been used to date the horse. It is called 'optical dating' and it tells us when sunlight last shone on buried soil. By testing soil from the trenches, the archaeologists discovered that the horse is at least 2,500 years old.

N

Chalk figures

Uffington
White Horse
Westbury
White Horse
Cerne Abbas
Giant
Long Man of
Wilmington

Not all of the chalk figures in Britain are Celtic. Some of them may be Roman. The White Horse at Westbury was made in the eighteenth century.

21

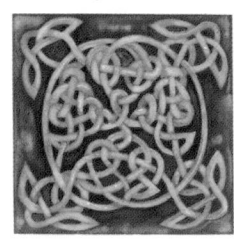

CELTIC RELIGION

The Celts seem to have believed that many of their Gods lived beneath the water.

Celtic people thought that rivers, lakes and springs were holy places. Treasures found beneath the water were probably offerings to Celtic gods, made to win their help.

These strips of cloth are called 'clouties'. They were left at Craigie Well in Inverness.

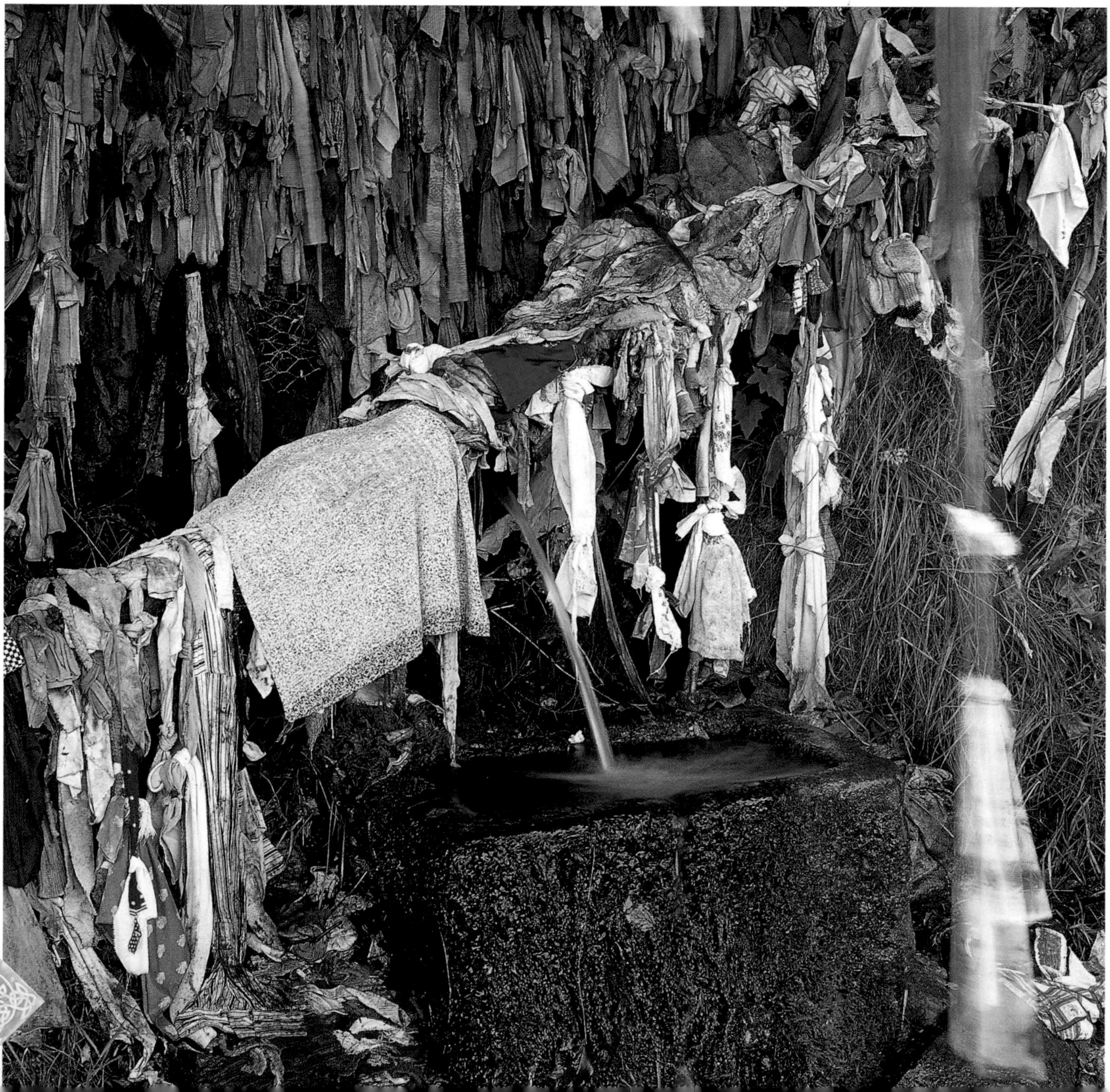

In some parts of the countryside, people still leave offerings at holy wells and springs. They may believe that this will cure them of an illness or bring them good luck.

All over Britain, valuable pieces of Celtic bronzework have been discovered by accident, in rivers, lakes, bogs and springs.

When the tide is low, you can sometimes find amazing things in the River Thames as it flows through London. People have picked up beautiful Celtic metalwork lying in the Thames mud. Finds include swords, spear-heads, shields, a cauldron and a helmet. Much more metalwork has been discovered in the river as it flows through the countryside on its way to the city.

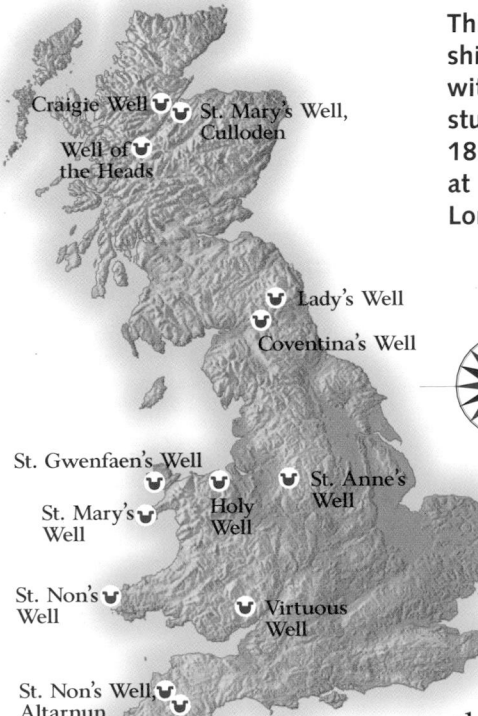

Ancient holy wells in Britain.

This bronze shield, decorated with red glass studs, was found in 1857 in the Thames at Battersea, London.

You can see several of the things that have been found on display in the British Museum and the Museum of London. There are so many of them that they cannot have been dropped into the river by accident. Celtic nobles may have wanted to show off their wealth by throwing some of it away.

BURYING THE DEAD

The Celts were often buried with their belongings. We can use these objects to build up a picture of their lives.

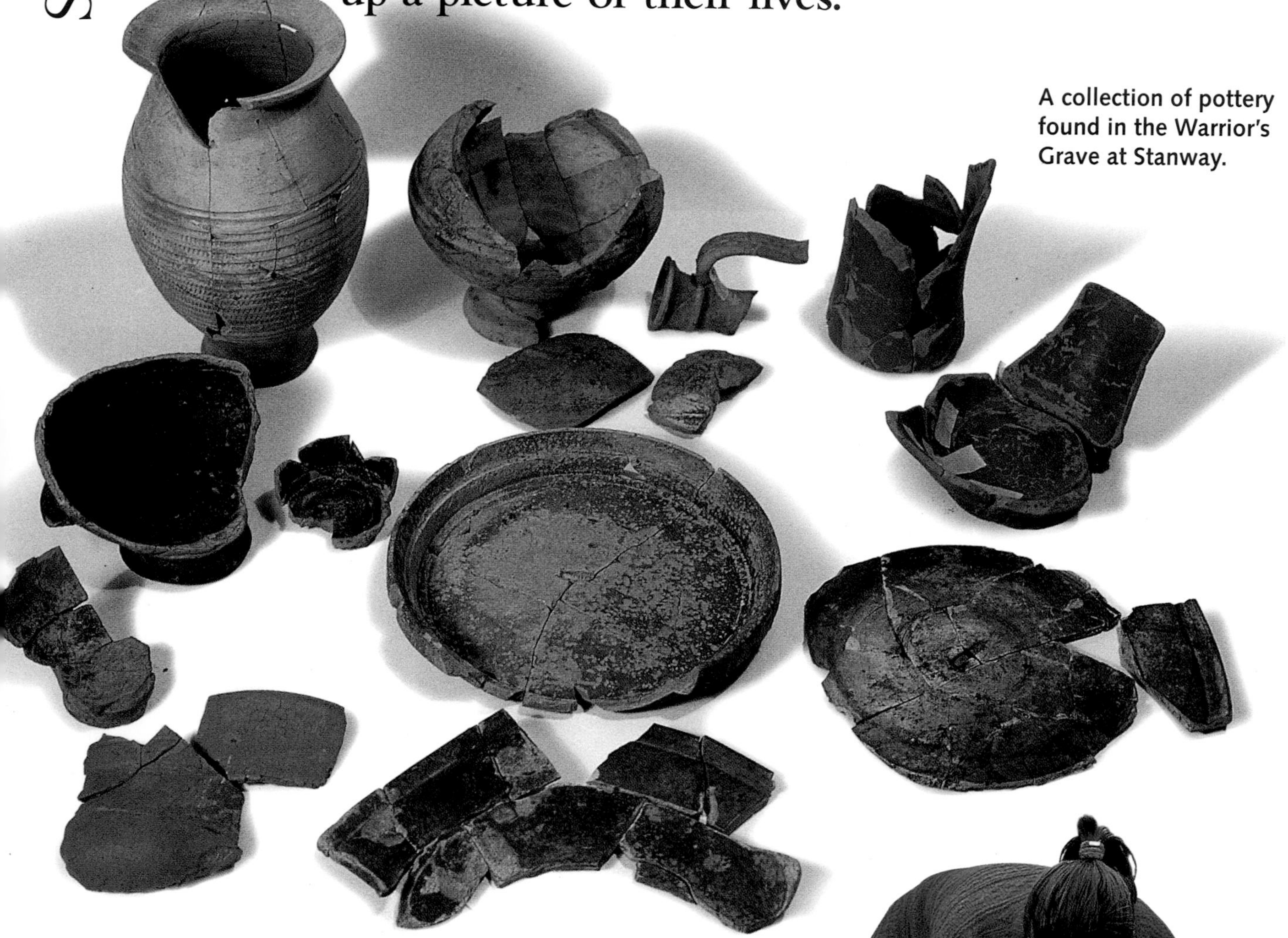

A collection of pottery found in the Warrior's Grave at Stanway.

At Stanway, in Essex, archaeologists have discovered a cemetery where wealthy Celts were buried. Their bodies were burned and the ashes placed in the earth with all sorts of goods, including pots, weapons, jewellery and gaming pieces.

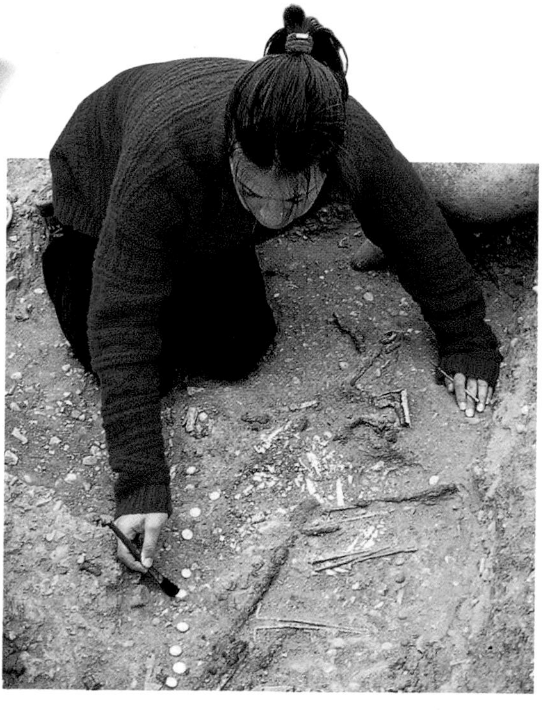

This archaeologists is excavating a game board and counters that were found in the Doctor's Grave at Stanway.

The wealth of the grave-goods shows that these Celts were important people. They must have been nobles from the local tribe, the Trinovantes.

The Stanway burials show that the Celts believed in an afterlife, another world where they could go on living the same sort of life that they had lived on earth. Many of the goods had been deliberately broken. This was a way of sending them into the next world.

▶A Roman glass bowl, which belonged to one of the Celts buried at Stanway.

At Wetwang Slack, in Yorkshire, archaeologists dug up the bodies of two Celtic men and women, each with their own war chariot. Perhaps this was done so that they could ride in style into the next world.

TRADE
Many of the goods buried at Stanway came across the sea from the Roman Empire. Roman writers tell us that their merchants sailed to Britain to buy wheat, slaves, tin and hunting dogs. In exchange, they supplied British nobles with wine, olive oil, precious glass like this bowl and metalwork.

▼ An iron spearhead found in the Warrior's Grave at Stanway. The wooden shaft had rotted away completely.

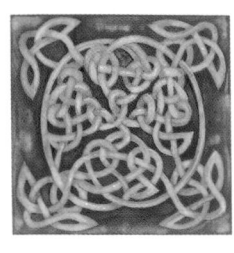

HUMAN SACRIFICE

According to Roman writers, the Celts killed people in special ways when they wanted to offer their bodies as gifts to the gods. Different kinds of death were chosen for different gods.

This is Lindow Moss, a peat bog near Manchester. In 1984, some peat diggers came across the body of a naked man in the bog. He was about 25 years old, 1.69m tall, with short hair and a beard, and neatly cut fingernails. The diggers called the police, thinking that they had found a recent murder victim.

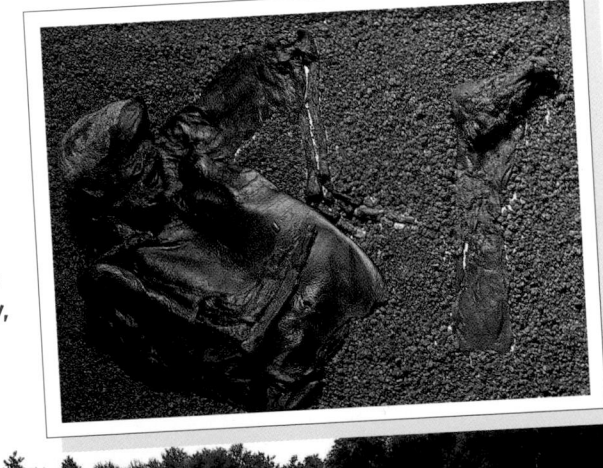

The brown peat of Lindow Moss, where the body (right) was found. If you look carefully, you can see the cord used to strangle the dead man, still tied around his neck.

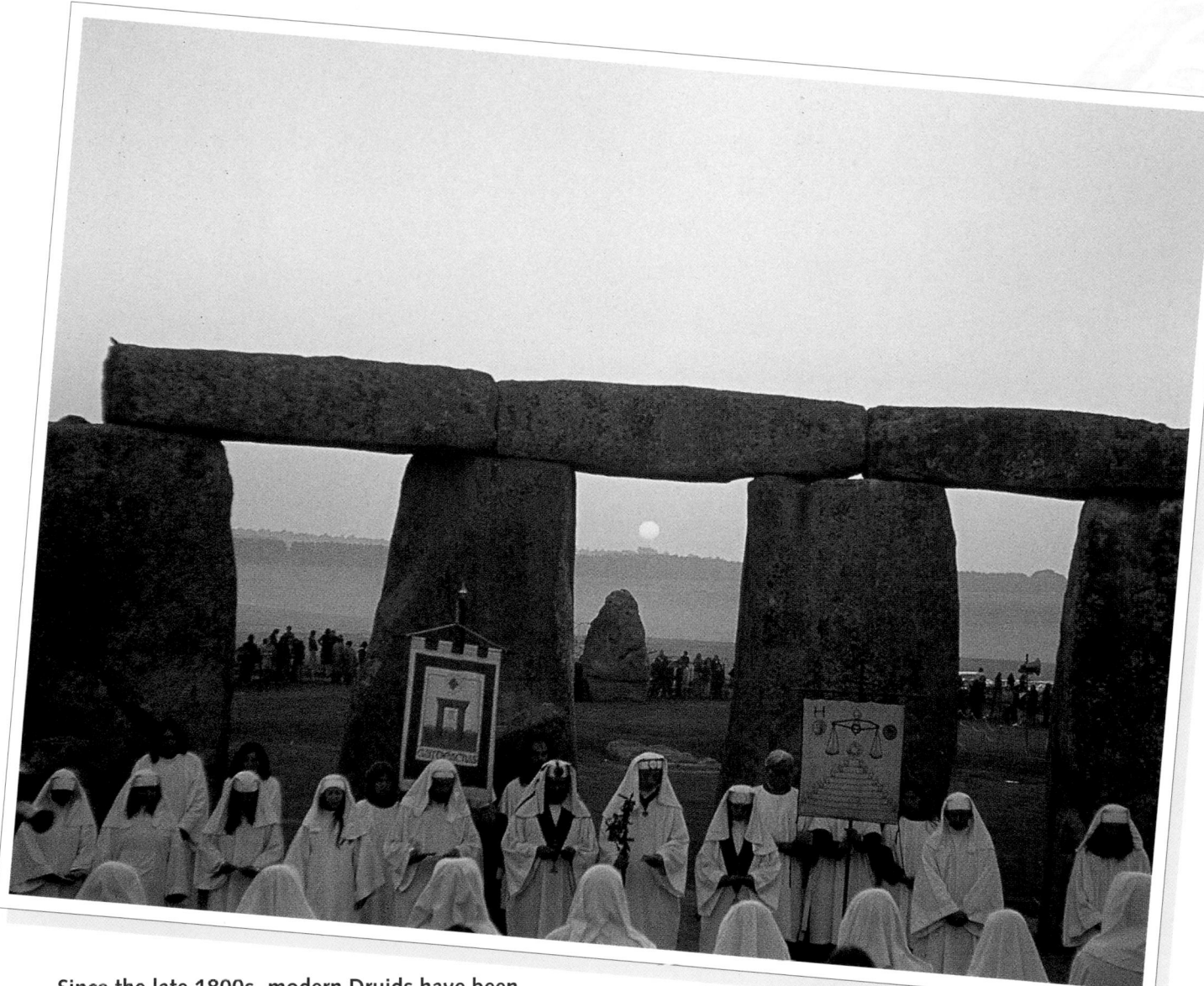

Since the late 1800s, modern Druids have been performing ceremonies at Stonehenge, which was wrongly believed to be a Druid temple. It is much older.

Peat, which is made from the partly rotted, squashed remains of plants, can preserve skin, hair and clothing for thousands of years. When tests were carried out on the man's body they showed that it was around 2,000 years old. He was a Celt.

This Celt died in a very strange way. First, he was hit on the head and knocked out and then he was strangled with a knotted cord and stabbed in the throat. Finally, he was thrown face down into a pool in the bog. This suggests that the man was a sacrifice. He had been thrown into water, just like the metalwork offered to the gods.

DRUIDS

The Celts' sacrifices were performed by priests called Druids. Pliny, a Roman writer, said that the Druids used mistletoe in their ceremonies. Mistletoe pollen was found in the stomach of the Lindow man. He had probably been given it mixed in a drink, shortly before he was killed.

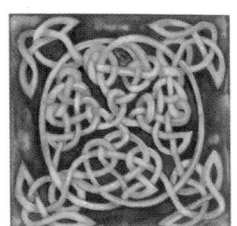

THE ROMAN INVASION

The Celtic way of life in southern Britain was shattered in AD 43. In that year, a Roman army crossed the English Channel.

Some of the southern tribes welcomed the invaders. Others fought fiercely, but they could not beat the Romans, who were much better organised. One by one, the Celtic hill-forts were captured and the tribes surrendered.

Roman rule brought big changes to Britain. The Romans built the first roads and proper towns in the country. They brought new styles of dress, a new language and a new religion, too. They stamped out the Druids and banned human sacrifice.

Key

Areas where Welsh spoken

Areas where Gaelic spoken

N

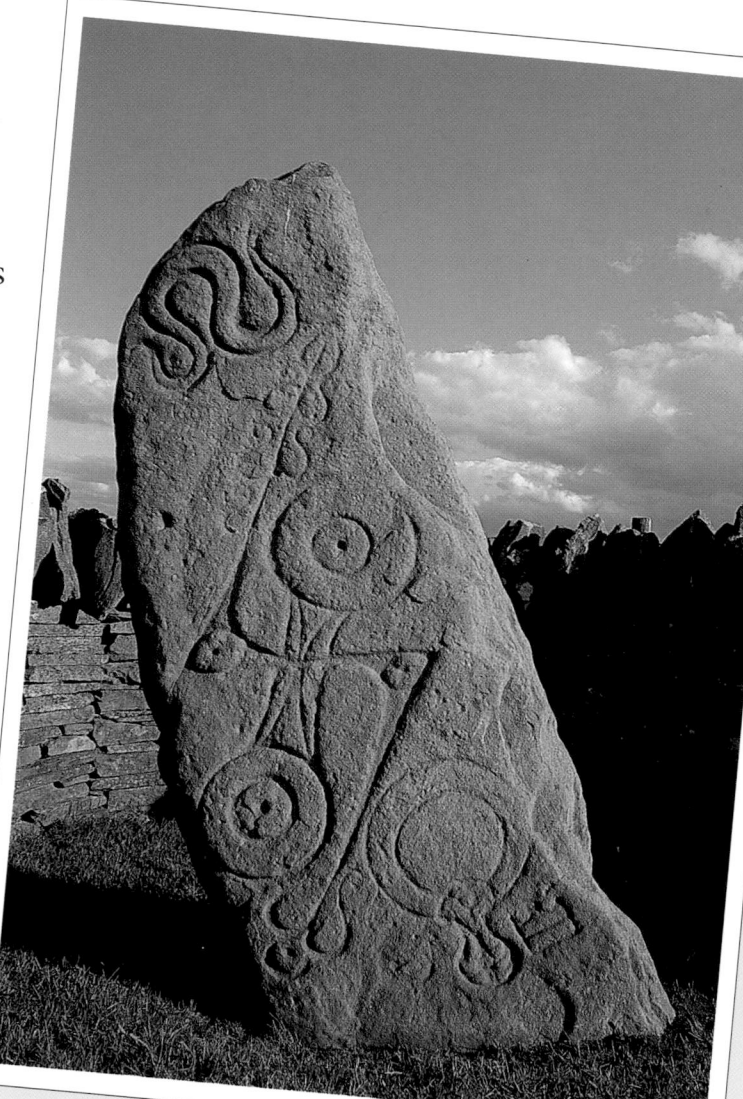

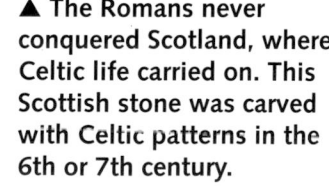
▲ The Romans never conquered Scotland, where Celtic life carried on. This Scottish stone was carved with Celtic patterns in the 6th or 7th century.

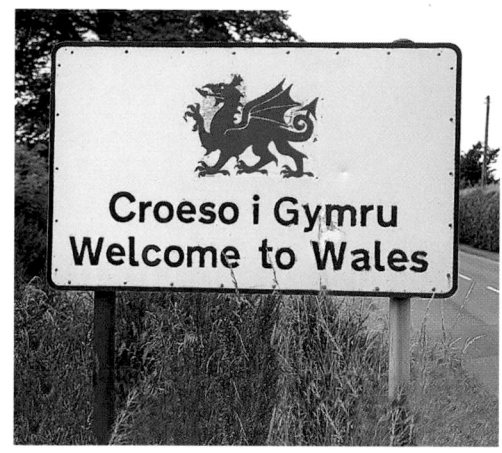

Welsh, a Celtic language, survives alongside English.

The Romans were the first of a series of foreign peoples who settled in Britain. They were followed by the Anglo-Saxons, the Vikings and the Normans. Over hundreds of years, people who spoke Celtic languages were pushed into the west and north. Despite everything, the old Celtic languages survived. Today, 650,000 people speak Welsh and 70,000 people speak Scottish Gaelic.

Until this century, many Scottish farmers lived in a type of house called a tigh dubh, or black house. It was built with the same methods used by the ancient Celts.

If you want to see the influence of the Celts, just look at a map of Britain. Place-names in Scotland, Wales and Cornwall are mostly Celtic. Almost all English rivers still have Celtic names. Avon and Tyne, for example, are both Celtic words, meaning 'river'.

GLOSSARY

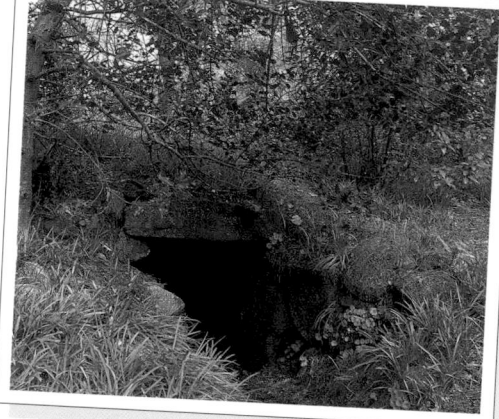

broch
a stone tower-house, found in the north of Scotland

bronze
a metal made from tin and copper, and harder than both. Prized by the Celts for mirrors, shields and other decorative metalwork

chariot
a horse-drawn vehicle with two wheels, usually used in battle

crannog
a small artificial island found in many Scottish lochs. It had a house on top and was usually joined to the shore by a wooden walkway

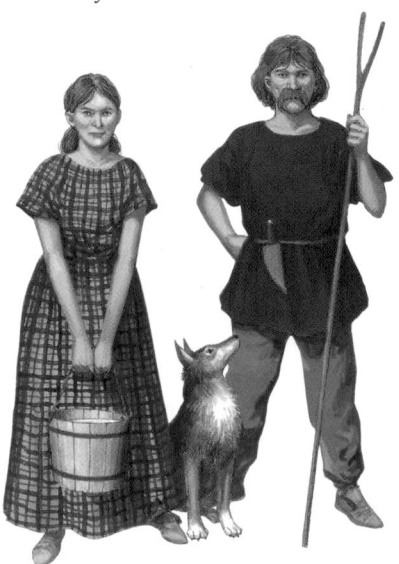

Druid
a Celtic priest. Druids performed religious ceremonies, and they were believed to be able to look into the future

fogou
a Cornish underground passage, lined and roofed with stone slabs

furrow
a narrow trench made by a plough

hill-fort
a settlement on a hilltop, defended by earth banks and ditches

iron
a metal, much harder than bronze, used for tools and weapons. The Celts were the first British people to use iron, and so the Celtic period is often called the 'Iron Age'

lynchet
an earth ridge or bank, formed by ploughing on hillsides

noble
a rich and powerful person

sacrifice
an offering made to a god. People, animals and precious objects could all be sacrifices

tribe
a group of families living together and being ruled by a chief

wattle
twigs or branches woven together to make a wall

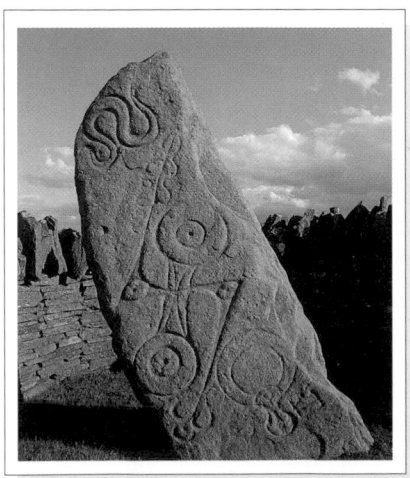

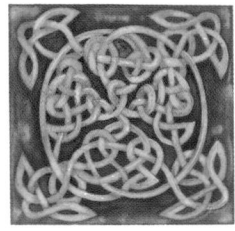

TIMELINE

c2000BC	British people begin to use bronze. The start of the 'Bronze Age'.
c1000BC	Bronze valuables, such as swords, begin to be placed in rivers, lakes and springs.
c800-700BC	British tribes begin to use iron. The start of the 'Iron Age'.
c700-500BC	Hill-forts built all over Britain.
c600BC	White Horse cut in the chalk at Uffington.
c100BC	Southern British tribes begin to use coins.
c80BC	Southern British tribes begin to make pottery using a wheel.
c100BC-AD50	'Lindow Man' killed.
55-54BC	Romans, led by Julius Caesar, make two expeditions to Britain.
AD43	Roman conquest of Britain begins.

PLACES TO VISIT

The British Museum, Great Russell St, London, WC1B 3DG: Includes the best collection of Celtic metalwork and the body found in the Lindow bog.

Butser Ancient Farm, near Chalton, Hampshire: A reconstruction of a Celtic farmstead which is also a working farm.

Chiltern Open Air Museum, Newlands Park, Gorelands Lane, Chalfont St Giles, Buckinghamshire, HP8 4AD: Includes a reconstruction of a Celtic round-house.

Colchester Museum, The Castle, Colchester, Essex, CO1 1TJ: Displays the treasures found in the Lexden grave-mound.

Iceni Village and Museum, Cockley Clay, Swaffham, Norfolk: A reconstructed settlement of the local tribe, the Iceni.

Maiden Castle, Winterborne St Martin, Dorset: One of the biggest hill-forts in the country.

Museum of the Iron Age, 6 Church Close, Andover, Hampshire, SP10 1DP: Includes finds from the nearby Danebury hill-fort, and reconstructions of life there. Visit the museum and then look at the hill-fort.

Museum of London, London Wall, London, EC2Y 5HN: Celtic metalwork found in the Thames.

Scottish Crannog Centre, Kenmore, Tayside, Scotland: A reconstruction of a crannog, with a visitors' centre displaying finds from the crannogs in the loch.

Welsh Folk Museum, St Fagans, Cardiff, CF5 6XB: Includes a Celtic village, with three round-houses.

INDEX

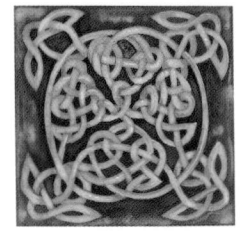